HARWICH LIFEBOATS

An Illustrated History

NICHOLAS LEACH

AMBERLEY

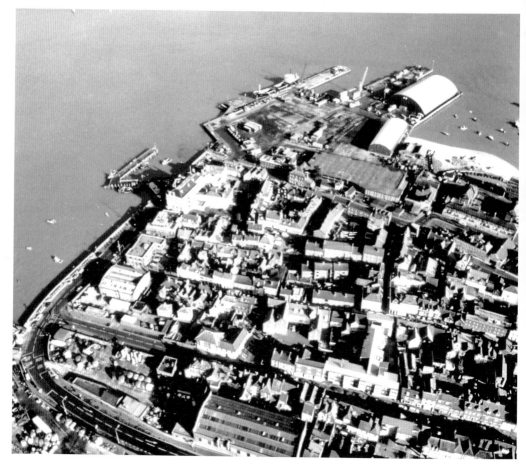

Aerial view of Harwich town, the Pound and Navyard Wharf. (By courtesy of the RNLI)

First published 2011

Amberley Publishing
The Hill, Stroud
Gloucestershire GL5 4EP

www.amberley-books.com

Copyright © Nicholas Leach 2011

The right of Nicholas Leach to be identified as
the Author of this work has been asserted in
accordance with the Copyrights, Designs and
Patents Act 1988.

ISBN 978 1 84868 876 6

British Library Cataloguing in Publication Data.
A catalogue record for this book is available
from the British Library.

Typesetting by Nicholas Leach.
Printed in Great Britain.

Contents

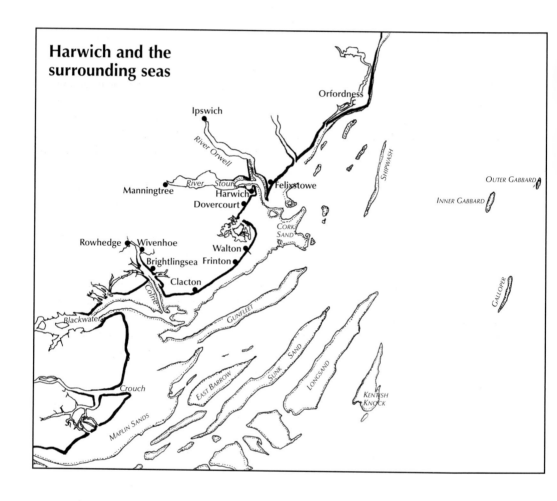

Harwich and the surrounding seas

Orfordness

Ipswich

River Orwell

SHIPWASH

Manningtree *River Stour* Felixstowe

OUTER GABBARD

Harwich

INNER GABBARD

Dovercourt

CORK SAND

Rowhedge Wivenhoe

Walton

Brightlingsea Frinton

Colne

Clacton

GUNFLEET

GALLOPER

Blackwater

EAST BARROW *SUNK SAND* *LONGSAND*

Crouch

KENTISH KNOCK

MAPLIN SANDS

This book has been partly funded by the estate of the late Clarice Ward (née Williams), a supporter of the RNLI and a lover of books and boats. It is dedicated to her and the brave lifeboat crews, past and present, who have served the Harwich lifeboat.

Introduction

Harwich lifeboat station operates two modern, fast, state-of-the-art lifeboats, manned by a twenty-eight-strong team of dedicated and enthusiastic volunteers, led by two full-timers who maintain the boats and equipment. The lifeboats work in the seas off the coast of Essex and Suffolk and have an unusual area of coverage in that they overlap with the neighbouring stations of Aldeburgh to the north and Walton & Frinton and Clacton-on-Sea to the south, without a clearly defined demarcation. They also cover the rivers Stour, Orwell and Deben, as well as the Walton Backwaters and well out into the Thames Estuary south of Harwich. The harbour and surrounding area is very popular, with leisure users coming in their hundreds, from bathers, yachts, power-boats, jet skis and popular tourist beaches.

The RNLI's declared area of coverage is up to fifty miles out, and while most services take place close to the coast, the 17m Severn goes out further when needed, and has even been as far as the Belgian port of Zeebrugge on service. The boat has also been on service to vessels at the Osterbank, sixty miles east of Harwich, a number of times, while the busy container port of Felixstowe and the Harwich International Ferry Port are also covered. Taking into account shipping coming from London and using the Sunk Traffic Separation Zone, which is twenty miles east of Harwich, this is one of the busiest areas of the North Sea for vessel movements. The most dangerous spots include the Cork Sand, the Shipwash Bank, the Gabbard Inner and Outer Sandbanks and the Galloper Bank, as well as several smaller sandbanks.

The history of the Harwich lifeboats is unusual in that for long periods the station was not operational and the town had no lifeboat, yet when a lifeboat was in service it was in great demand and performed many fine services. The three periods of operation – which opened in the 1820s, the 1870s and the 1960s – are characterised by new technology and design advances of their era. The station has therefore been in a position to operate lifeboats that were, of their era, at the cutting edge of technology. Harwich saw the first steam lifeboat built by the RNLI, one of the first motor lifeboats was sent there during trials, one of the first of the fast Waveney class steel self-righters was allocated to the station in the 1960s, and most recently the first 17m Severn to take up active station duty was the boat for Harwich. Many notable rescues have been performed by Harwich lifeboat crews, and sixteen silver and four bronze medals have been awarded since 1829.

Hundreds of sailing craft and steamers were wrecked on the dangerous sandbanks off the Essex coast during the nineteenth century, and the story of the sailing lifeboats at Harwich, and indeed of the other Essex lifeboats, is one of numerous launches to the outlying sands to help. Often the lifeboats were towed to a casualty by steam tugs, while at other times they were sailed, but in all instances the crew showed incredible endurance and bravery, and suffered hardships almost unimaginable by twenty-first century standards as they undertook their rescue duties. Harwich's sailing lifeboats, which served from 1876, were often at sea for more than twelve hours and undertook many fine services. It is hoped that the descriptions of these rescues do justice to the volunteer lifeboat crews of that era.

Today, Harwich lifeboat station is one of the 230 RNLI stations based about Britain's coast. The RNLI is a charity that provides a twenty-four-hour lifesaving service around the UK and Republic of Ireland . The RNLI operates solely from public donations and the crews and supporters are all volunteers. Because the lifeboat station is now so busy, and is in fact one of the RNLI's busiest, it has been possible to include descriptions of a handful of the services undertaken in the last two decades which it is intended will give a flavour of the kind of incidents to which the lifeboats are called. A full list of rescues by both all-weather and inshore lifeboats can be found in the appendixes.

ACKNOWLEDGEMENTS

Thanks to many people at Harwich lifeboat station, but in particular Coxswain Paul Smith and Andrew Moors, who have been extremely helpful in answering numerous questions and assisting with many requests for information. They were always welcoming and hospitable during my many visits to the station. Also at the lifeboat station, thanks to Graeme Ewens and Captain Rod Shaw, Lifeboat Operations Manager. At the RNLI, I am grateful to Brian Wead and his staff for supplying service listings, to Nathan Williams for providing images for possible inclusion, and to honorary librarian Barry Cox for facilitating my research at the RNLI Headquarters library in Poole. For assistance with other photographs, I am grateful to Peter Edey and V. H. Young. Finally, a special thanks to Ken Brand, crew member with various positions from June 1968 to December 2001, whose extensive research into the station's complex history has been invaluable. Suffolk Record Office accomodated him for the past ten years and his wife Ann kindly put up with him going there to undertake the research. Without his considerable input, it would have been impossible to compile such a comprehensive record of the Harwich station, and to him I owe the biggest debt. His knowledge of Harwich lifeboat history is second to none and he has guided me through the different eras in the station's history, producing additional and unusual material when needed and answering all my queries.

Nicholas Leach
Lichfield, April 2011

BIBLIOGRAPHY

Benham, Hervey (1980): *The Salvagers* (Essex County Newspapers).

Farr, Grahame (1981): *Papers on Life-boat History, No.5: The Steam Life-boats 1889-1928.* (Grahame Farr, Portishead).

Malster, Robert (1968): *Wreck and Rescue on the Essex Coast: The story of the Essex lifeboats* (D Bradford Barton Ltd, Truro).

ibid. (1969): Suffolk Lifeboats – The First Quarter Century, in *Mariners Mirror*, Vol.55, pp.263-280.

ibid. (1974): *Saved from the Sea: The story of life-saving services on the East Anglian coast* (Terence Dalton, Lavenham, Suffolk).

Moffat, H. W. (1963): The Landguard Life-boat of 1821, in *Sea Breezes*, Aug, pp.86-91.

Shaw, Willis (1990): *Launched on Service* (Harwich & Dovercourt RNLI Branch, Harwich).

Street, Sean (1992): *The Wreck of the Deutschland* (Souvenir, London).

Weaver, Leonard T. (1975): *The Harwich Story* (Harwich Printing Co).

The First Rescuers

The first lifeboats in Harwich, and indeed in Essex, were built at the start of the 1820s. By this time a number of lifeboat stations had already been established along England's east coast, with the nearest to Essex in Suffolk to the north. They dated from the early years of the nineteenth century, when the lifeboat design of the South Shields-based boatbuilder Henry Greathead was in widespread use, and the insurers Lloyds of London providing funding for many new lifeboats. Greathead-built boats were supplied to Cromer, Lowestoft, Hollesley Bay, Gorleston and Ramsgate, but their usefulness was varied and their fortunes mixed. The boat at Lowestoft was so disliked by the beachmen there that it was moved north to Gorleston, where she was liked no better so was sold for £10 in 1807 having never been used. Instead, a larger sailing lifeboat was built for Lowestoft, named *Frances Ann*, which proved to be considerably better suited to conditions off East Anglia and lasted for more than forty years.

That no lifeboat was provided to protect Harwich or the Essex during this early era of lifeboat building, from 1800 to 1805, is rather surprising given that it was the only natural safe haven of refuge of any size between the Thames and the Humber. When other factors are taken into account, however, the reasons for the lack of any rescue boat become evident: although the entrance to the harbour was full of shoals, few ships were wrecked within its confines, possibly because lights and beacons marked the area, or within the range of a oar-powered craft. A suitable place from which to launch a lifeboat, where sufficient crew was available, was also lacking, Offshore, matters were somewhat different as almost every winter gales caught out unwary vessels on the outlying sandbanks, which were both numerous and treacherous. A certain amount of rescue and salvage work was undertaken by the local smacks, although this was on an informal basis, and is described in the next chapter.

The impetus for having a lifeboat built for Harwich came as a result of several shipwrecks, with consequent loss of life, close to Harwich harbour. The *Suffolk Chronicle* for 28 October 1820 listed the vessels that had been lost off the Essex coast in the week prior to its publication:

> 'The Mary, on shore on the Gunfleet, full of water, crew arrived here safe; the
> Patriot, from Lynn to London, loss of two anchors and cables; the Curlew, coal, on
> shore on the Gunfleet; the Boyne, from Newcastle to London, coals and glass, on
> shore, likely to be lost; the Royal Oak, on shore on the West Rocks, since got off
> and brought in here; the Ann, of Whitby, Todd, coal, on shore and wrecked on the
> Main Back of Landguard Fort.'

As the crucial trade route from the north east to London passed the Essex coast, with much of the shipping approaching the capital using the narrow channels between the sandbanks off the county's shore, it is not surprising that many were caught out by bad weather, bad seamanship, bad luck, or a combination of the three, with usually tragic and disastrous consequences. The most reported of the wrecks from October 1820 was the last, which had occurred on 22 October, a Sunday, when a heavy gale from the south-west, increasing to almost hurricane force, whipped up heavy seas causing 'a most tremendous surf to break on the shore'. The casualty, *Ann*, was wrecked near Landguard Fort at the approaches to Harwich harbour, while making for the Essex port of Maldon from Newcastle. A detachment of the Sixth Royals, led by Captain Innes, assisted by men from the Revenue Service stationed at Landguard Fort, managed to save seven men from the wreck, with the *Suffolk Chronicle* concluding its report: 'When brought on shore, the poor sufferers were though the humanity of Captain Innes, taken to the Fort, and provided with comfortable food and lodging.'

Less than a month later, on 9 November, another vessel, the schooner *Constant Trader*, of Woodbridge, was wrecked, but this time offshore, on the Cork Sand. Several smacks were in the vicinity, but in the shoal water were unable to offer any help and the vessel broke up with the loss of its entire crew of nine. The *Suffolk Chronicle* for 18 November 1820 also reported the events:

> *'the sea being at that time so tremendous, that it was impossible to render them any assistance, although several vessels made the attempt. The poor men were observed to run up the rigging for safety; but such was the power of the waves, that they were alternately plunged into the sea, and then lifted into the air, till a heavy sea completely buried them and the vessel, and not a vestige was seen more! . . . It cannot be too deeply lamented, that . . . the establishment of Life-Boats, on the dangerous parts of our coast, has been so much neglected. Had there been a Life-Boat at Harwich, there is a strong reason to believe, that every man would have been rescued from destruction.'*

This incident seems to have been the catalyst for a campaign to have a lifeboat built for Harwich, with a letter, published in the same newspaper on 25 November 1820, from 'William', pushing the cause and arguing strongly in favour of a lifeboat for Harwich: 'Many reasons may be assigned why a Life Boat ought to be stationed at Harwich; there are many dangerous sands and shoals in the neighbourhood; there are always Smacks, Cutters, etc, to lead a Life Boat to the point where none but it can live; and there are always plenty of brave and dauntless hearts on the spot to man a Life Boat.' He stated that a lifeboat would have been able to save the lives of the schooner's crew on the Cork Sand, and concluded: 'a nation deriving a revenue of sixty millions of pounds per annum, could surely spare a few hundreds out of it, to station Life Boats round the coast, for the preservation of the brave men whose toils so materially contribute to that revenue.'

Another letter, this time in the *Colchester Gazette*, proposed that a county fund should be set up to establish lifeboats in Essex, and the same paper, on 2 December 1820, contained an advertisement calling for such a fund to be opened. The momentum for providing a lifeboat was gathering pace and George Graham, the Harwich shipbuilder, was next to contribute, writing from Harwich Navy Yard giving details of how a ship's boat could be fitted out as a lifeboat by the addition of air casks. Captain George Manby, who had in the preceding twenty years shown much interest in life-saving on the Norfolk coast, was contacted for his advice by the lifeboat advocates in Harwich, and on 7 December the town's mayor, Anthony Cox, called a meeting at the Moot Hall in Colchester to form an Essex Life Boat Association. The meeting agreed that lifeboats should be established at both Harwich and Brightlingsea, and the committee of Lloyd's voted £50 towards each, while Trinity House gave the association 100 guineas.

The Essex Life Boat Association was officially founded on the first day of 1821, and had sufficient funds to have a lifeboat constructed. A meeting of the Association in February 1821 held

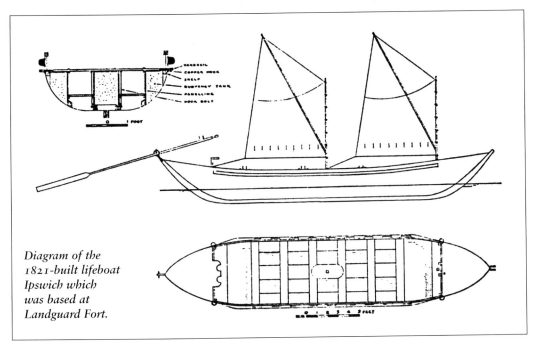

Diagram of the 1821-built lifeboat Ipswich which was based at Landguard Fort.

in Colchester was shown George Graham's model of a lifeboat, the design of which was approved by the committee, and which was of a boat was on the same lines as Lowestoft's *Frances Ann*. They immediately placed an order with Graham to begin constructing the boat for Harwich. However, the building of the Brightlingsea boat was 'unavoidably deferred until the benevolent object of the Association receives a more general support from the friends of humanity.'

Meanwhile, another subscription was being raised at Ipswich, completely independently of the efforts at Harwich, for a lifeboat to be stationed at Landguard Fort, at the entrance to the Suffolk side of Harwich harbour. The organisers had, like those at Harwich, been shocked into action by the *Constant Trader* disaster, and by the fact that the master of *Constant Trader* was the brother of the master of another Woodbridge vessel, *Sarah and Caroline*, which had been wrecked off Lowestoft three weeks earlier but whose entire crew had been saved by the Lowestoft lifeboat *Frances Ann*. The success demonstrated by *Frances Ann* was a spur to the organisers, who moved quickly as the *Ipswich Journal* of 3 February 1821 reported: 'The subscription for a Life-Boat, to be built and stationed at Landguard Fort, has been liberally contributed to by sixty-five of the Ladies and Gentlemen of this town and neighbourhood; and that on Sunday next, in the forenoon, a Sermon will be preached at the Tower Church, by the Rev Thomas Mills, of Stutton, Chaplain in Ordinary to his Majesty, in aid of that benevolent object.' The subscription, including the proceeds of the Sermon, amounted to an impressive £137 9s 0d.

At a meeting on 15 February 1821 the Ipswich subscribers accepted an offer by Jabez Bayley, a local boatbuilder, to construct a boat designed by Captain Richard Hall Gower (1767-1833), an ex-officer of the East India Company's service, who had original and usually successful ideas on naval architecture and been responsible for a number of unusual vessels. Bayley (c.1771-1834) was, at the time, the leading shipbuilder on the East Coast north of the Thames. At his larger Ipswich yard, in the hamlet of Halifax, he was building two 1,300-ton East Indiamen, and had already completed two vessels to Gower's designs. The boat destined for Landguard Fort, designed by Gower, was completed at his smaller Stoke Bridge yard.

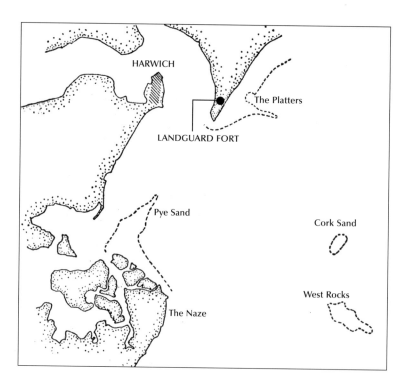

Map of Harwich, Landguard Fort and the sandbanks close to Harwich harbour entrance in the nineteenth century.

Gower wrote several pamphlets and books, one of which contained plans and a description of the lifeboat, which was, in contrast to the heavy lifeboat being built for Harwich, much lighter. It was similar to a whaleboat, and was capable of being transported over land or across the beach, if needed. Instead of the usual knees and fastenings, the thwarts were secured by a system of dovetailing, hooks and chocks. The boat was just over 31ft in length, only 6ft in beam, pulled by six oars, and the hull clinker built of half-inch oak plank with ash timbers three-quarter-inches square.

She was double-ended and rigged with two very short masts carrying spritsails, had two tubes for clearing water and her buoyancy came from eleven cubic feet of cork in her decked ends and fourteen copper tanks arranged in three rows along her sides. In the middle of the centre row was the step of the after mast, with a three-inch tube on either side for excess water from above the level of the thwarts to run off. The thwarts were held down amidships by iron hooks and ringbolts, with their ends dovetailed into a heavy shelf. A narrow canvas-covered cork fender ran along the sides of the boat and was fastened in place by copper bolts with nuts on the inside. There was a 220lb fixed iron keel. The helmsman steered with a long oar while standing on a raised platform, nearly as high as the thwarts, with his thighs in a crutch piece to help him stay on his feet. Gower's aim was that the boat should be fast enough to reach the scene of a wreck quickly, and her crew, just seven, be small in number so that assembling them could also be undertaken speedily while also meaning space was available for rescued persons. The boat was intended primarily for sailing, and the rig was chosen to avoid the work involved in rigging a dipping lugsail, much favoured by the longshoremen, when working to windward, as they would most likely have to do, if going to a wreck on the outlying sands.

The boat was launched from the yard of Jabez Bayley at Stoke Bridge, Ipswich, on 4 April 1821 watched by spectators in their hundreds lining the banks of the river and crowding onto ships at their moorings. She was officially named the 'Ipswich Life Boat' by Miss Daniel, daughter of the naval captain, although she has also been described as the 'Orwell lifeboat' in subsequent literature. After the launch, she was put through her paces in the river for the benefit of the crowds, with Benjamin Hamblin, master of the Ipswich smack Stevens, acting as coxswain. The rather rough launching , which involved the boat being pushed off the wharf and allowed to drop several feet into the water, was in itself a test of her sturdiness, after which six young seamen rowed her down river and back. Then further demonstrations of her capabilities were carried out: she was filled with water, but remained nearly as manageable as before; two men bailed water into her to test her self-relieving properties; and twenty-five men were taken aboard, in addition to her crew of seven, to show she was able to support this number.

After the demonstrations, the boat was taken to Landguard Fort, where her management committee had arranged with the military authorities for the Fort's garrison to fly flags by day or burn blue lights by night if a vessel in distress was sighted. Guns would be fired if the boat was to be launched. The soldiers would help launch the boat, but she would be manned by seamen and longshoremen and these could only be found in Harwich, over a mile away on the other side of the harbour, so their getting to Landguard would slow down any rescue efforts. Consequently, doubts were expressed as to whether such a scheme could work. However, the committee, undoubtedly aware of the rival boat nearing completion in Graham's yard at Harwich, adhered to their original plans and, to prove it was possible, organised a trial launch without notice. Seven 'waterfront idlers' from Harwich were ferried to Landguard, and launched the boat within an hour of the start of the operation. They rowed her across to Harwich, with the committee triumphant at the speed of launch, which was impressive considering the distances involved although probably not fast

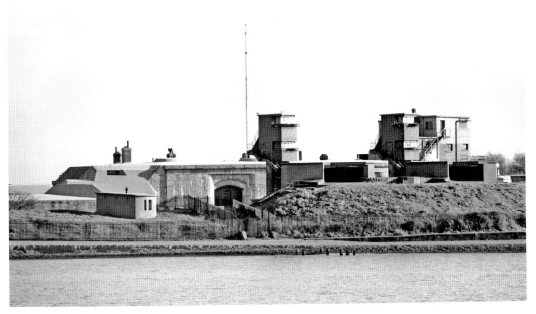

Landguard Fort, the location of one of the first lifeboats to cover Harwich harbour, dominated the navigable channel on the northern bank of the river Orwell, while the Redoubt at Harwich guarded the harbour entrance together with a battery at Shotley. The brick Fort of today dates from the eighteenth century but the first fortifications were built in 1543 by Henry VIII. No evidence exists today to show where the lifeboat of the 1820s was kept or to show how it was launched. (Nicholas Leach)

enough if lives were at stake. The committee stated, somewhat casually, that any seven or eight men could get the boat afloat when signals of distress had been seen, by 'going to the Fort, where every assistance will be given in launching her, and the men paid agreeable to the service they perform, by the Committee of Managers.'

The actual effectiveness of this lifeboat was questionable, and the boat launched at Harwich probably provided a better option. Whether the boats were rivals, however, seems unlikely for the *Orwell* lifeboat was brought across from Landguard Fort for the Harwich boat's official launching on 12 September 1821. *Orwell* also took part in a race against a lifeboat named *Melville*, at Harwich under the auspices of the Admiralty, and apparently beat her by several lengths. *Melville* was probably one of a number of boats, described as lifeboats, which the War Office kept at Harwich at least from 1821.

The events of 12 September 1821, which included 'a regatta worthy of the origin of the noble and generous undertaking', saw the new Harwich lifeboat named *Braybrooke* by the Mayoress of Harwich, Mrs Anthony Cox, in honour of the Lord Lieutenant of Essex. After the naming, she was launched from Graham's yard, formerly the naval dockyard, which the *Ipswich Journal* somewhat grandiosely reported: 'She swiftly glided into her natural element, amid the acclamations of the delighted spectators, who greeted her with re-iterated cheers. Various experiments were tried, in all of which she was found to answer admirably the intended purpose.' A public dinner and ball was held in the evening, at the Three Cups Inn, at which the Rev Archdeacon Jefferson presided, assisted by the stewards John Hopkins, R. W. Cox, Captain Dickens, RN and Captain Gore Brown. Between seventy and eighty attended the 'excellent dinner' and 110 at that ball at the tavern.

As the Essex Life Boat Association did not have sufficient funds to pay for a boathouse as well as a boat, *Braybrooke* had to lie at moorings in the harbour near the guard vessel. This was a far from ideal arrangement as in heavy weather the boat could not be reached from the shore, so it was not surprising that early in 1822 the Association asked for annual subscriptions to be paid promptly 'as funds are wanted to man the boat and enable her to act, should any case of peril call for her assistance'. Getting to *Braybrooke* was not straightforward, although the boatmen of Harwich no longer had to cross the harbour to the Fort to use a lifeboat. About a month after *Braybrooke* had been launched, experiments were undertaken under the direction of Rear Admiral Page to determine the best method for calling out the lifeboats when a ship was seen in distress. It was agreed that blue lights would be burned and guns fired at Landguard Fort at night, or the fort would fly two flags, one over the other, should help be required during the day.

So within the space of six months in 1821, the safety of those using Harwich harbour had been considerably enhanced, with two lifeboats available where before there had been none, although their careers proved to be short-lived. The boats performed relatively few services and on several occasions other boats were used for rescue work in the area, such as on 5 January 1822, when the brig *Ann* was wrecked on the Heap Sand. Its crews was saved by the smack *Providence*, whose master, John Matthews, was presented with a silver medal by the Essex Life Boat Association, which also gave twenty guineas to the crew.

Braybrooke did not perform her first service until May 1822, when a fishing vessel, bound for London, went grounded on the West Rocks in an easterly gale. Together with other boats, the lifeboat went out from Harwich after signals had been shown from Landguard Fort, and helped to refloat the vessel, which was little damaged and able to proceed on her way. She was involved in another salvage operation early in the following year, on 15 January 1823, when she assisted HM cutter *Surly* which had gone ashore. For the crew's 'meritorious exertions' on this occasion, the Commissioners of the Navy awarded them £10.

The only rescue performed by the Landguard lifeboat of which reports have been found took

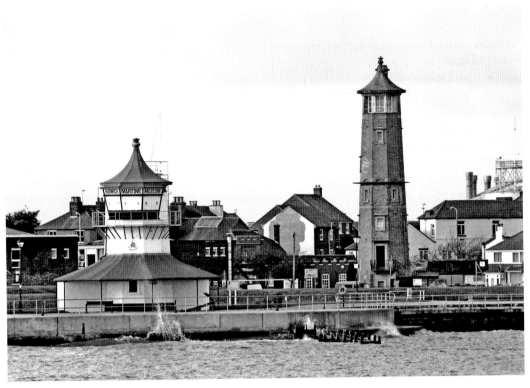

The two lighthouses at Harwich date from the early nineteenth century, and were used to guide ships through the entrance to the river Stour. The High Light was situated in the centre of the town, in what is now West Street, with the Low Light on what is now the promenade. (Nicholas Leach)

place on 19 February 1824, when the night-time signalling arrangements were also put into practice. The collier brig *Malvina*, of Newcastle bound for Southampton, went ashore on the Platters, off Felixstowe harbour mouth. The Landguard boat was launched, manned by seven Coast Blockade men, including a coxswain, all of whom had been summoned by the firing of guns and burning of blue lights at the fort and were close at hand. They reached the brig and, according to the *Ipswich Journal*, 'assistance being promptly rendered she was got off and brought into this harbour with loss of rudder add other damage'. A subscription for the men who crewed the lifeboat was raised in Ipswich, 'in reward of their alacrity and endeavours to be essentially useful'.

Braybrooke was in action on 8 November 1825, when she went out in a severe westerly gale to the brig *Northumberland*, of Sunderland, carrying coal, which had gone aground on the West Rocks. The brig's crew had abandoned their vessel and been picked up by another brig, *Caledonia*, of Sunderland, and from there were brought ashore by the lifeboat. The lifeboat had gone out a few days earlier to the brig, but found her abandoned and about to become a total wreck, so returned to Harwich. This incident appears to have been the last rescue work in which the lifeboat was involved and a few years later *Braybrooke* was in a state of disrepair, with the *Kent and Essex Mercury* of 22 December 1829 reporting on the 'disgracefully neglected state of the Essex lifeboat called the *Lady Braybrooke* (sic) . . . lying here rotting and breaking as fast as time and thieves can destroy it'. Lack of a sufficiently able and devoted local committee was the likely cause of her demise, although a local organisation with adequate annual income to ensure the crew practised and the lifeboat and its gear were maintained was missing despite the best intentions of those behind the Essex Life Boat Association.

The lifeboat at Landguard fared no better, despite coming under the auspices of Suffolk Association for Saving the Lives of Shipwrecked Seamen, which was founded at a meeting in the Shire Hall at Bury St Edmunds on 16 October 1824. The Suffolk Association brought a new focus to life-saving operations in the county and looked at providing new lifeboats and mortars along the coast. At a meeting in Stowmarket in November 1824, the organisation voted £35 to fund alterations and improvements to the Landguard Fort lifeboat. A further £20 was given to the stations at Landguard, Bawdsey and Lowestoft, while sub-committees were appointed for the three districts to meet at Lowestoft, Aldeburgh and Ipswich. The Landguard boat was altered by being broadened by 2ft 6in in the course of a refit by her builder, Jabez Bailey, to improve her stability. However, despite the alterations and financial support from the Suffolk Association, the Landguard lifeboat remained relatively ineffective, and when, in October 1825, the association appointed a committee to investigate the suitability of the station, and the committee soon reported that it was 'of no use whatever'. The Landguard boat was described by the committee as 'totally inefficient' and they recommended that she be sold. By March 1827 she had been converted to a yacht and was advertised for sale at the shipyard where she had been built.

Three launches in four years by two lifeboats based at a busy harbour could hardly justify having two such craft in Harwich, especially as many wrecks were given no assistance by either boat. For example, during the last week of December 1821, a few months after the boats had been built and approved of by the locals with such enthusiasm, numerous vessels were caught out by a week of severe gales, but none were helped by the lifeboats. *Methvin Castle*, bringing wheat to London, struck on the Platters on 22 December and was soon a complete wreck. Her crew escaped in the ship's boat, and with great difficulty reached the shore at Landguard Fort, with their the boat being swamped just as they reached land. On the same day *Friendship*, of and from Shields, struck on the Cutler Sand, and was holed with the crew escaping in the ship's boat just as their vessel sank. The lifeboats did not assist on this occasion, or on several subsequent occasions when ships were wrecked, and their ineffectiveness was probably one of the reasons for their short life-saving careers. As with many early lifeboats, lack of funds, poor organisation and difficulties with crewing all contributed to the Harwich boats' lack of success and ultimate demise, while their inability to get to the outlying sandbanks was also a factor.

The Admiralty lifeboats, stationed at Harwich in the first half of the nineteenth century, were occasionally mentioned in local newspapers, but never in connection with any rescue work. In 1821 when *Braybrooke* was launched at Harwich, a race was held between what was referred to as the Admiralty lifeboat *Melville* and the Landguard lifeboat. On another occasion not long afterwards a correspondent in the local press complained of the inactivity of 'The lifeboats in the storehouses at Harwich', apparently a reference to the Admiralty's craft. A return of 1848 gives details of a lifeboat, 28ft in length, built for the Admiralty in 1845 and stationed at Landguard Fort, on the north side of Harwich Harbour. However, no record has been found of her service, and she was 'condemned as useless' in 1864.

The Suffolk Association was eventually taken over by the national lifeboat organisation, the Royal National Institution for the Preservation of Life from Shipwreck (RNIPLS), which had been founded in March 1824. The new body was responsible for 'the preservation of lives and property from shipwreck'. This encompassed the funding, building, operation, maintenance and organisation of lifeboats and lifeboat stations. Initially quite successful, it added to the number of lifeboats in operation, but never got involved in any life-saving measures off Essex. As well as lifeboats, the new body presented medals to reward acts of outstanding bravery performed by lifeboat crews and meritorious actions by anyone saving lives at sea. The idea was first suggested by the Institution's founder, Sir William Hillary who believed that a medal or badge 'might have a very powerful effect (in inducing men) to render their utmost aid to the shipwrecked of every land, in the moment of their extreme distress.' The Gold and Silver Medals were introduced at the founding meeting of the Institution.

Although the two lifeboats' period of operation was short, when they were no longer available rescue work off the Essex coast was carried out by the salvaging smacks, whose masters and crews saved many lives despite a primary interest in salvage work. They were better suited to going to the outlying sandbanks the lifeboats, which were too small to cover the long distances. Indeed, even when the lifeboats were available the smacks undertook rescue work, such as on 23 October 1825 when the locally-based *Betty*, heading home to Harwich, went ashore yesterday on the East Barrows and the smacks helped her off. In February 1826 *Mentor*, of South Shields, was brought in by the salvage smacks having been driven past Harwich and found abandoned outside Deben Bar. Rewards, totalling 10s 6d to each of the sixteen smacksman who attempted to save the crew, were given by the Suffolk Association.

Another excellent life-saving rescue was undertaken just over three years later. At 7am on 30 April 1829 the Aberdeen brig *Superb* was seen by William Mudd, master of the smack *Samuel*, wrecked on the Shipwash Sand, with three men stranded in the rigging as the huge seas crashed over the wrecked hull. Since the boats of the smacks *Samuel*, of Ipswich, and *Lively*, which were on scene, were too small, Mudd sought help from the London smack *Paul Pry*, which was carrying a larger boat. Mudd and two of his crew, together with two men from *Paul Pry*, rowed the boat to the wreck, while *Lively* stood by. With great difficulty they managed to get two men on board, but the master of *Superb* was very tired and before he could get on board, the small boat was upset. Mudd and three men were thrown on to the wreck, where they clung to the rigging. The remaining men in the boat managed to reach *Lively*. Samuel Wordley, *Lively's* master, with two of his own crew, then launched his small boat and succeeded in getting everyone off. The master of *Superb*, almost unconscious, and the rescued men were finally landed ashore at 10pm after a rescue that had lasted fifteen hours. Three of the remaining crew of *Superb* had been in the rigging since 10pm on 28 April and two others had drowned. For their efforts during this rescue, Mudd and Wordley were awarded the Silver medal by the RNIPLS.

William Mudd was involved in a number of rescues during his time, but tragically he lost his life during one episode in January 1833 after the 230-ton collier brig *Eslington* went aground on the Gunfleet. She was boarded by men in two boats, but they left without any chance of salvage. In getting through the breakers to the casualty, however, one of the boats was upset and Mudd, two of his crew and three of the brig's crew lost their lives. The remainder were saved by the other boat. Mudd was master of one of many smacks operating off the Essex coast during the nineteenth century, and as well as salvage work many rescues were performed, with life-saving efforts rewarded on a number of occasions by the RNIPLS.

Another smacksmen to receive the Silver medal from the RNIPLS was Robert Cleave, master of *New Union*, for a rescue on 29 December 1829. The brig *Craig Elachie*, with a crew of six men and a boy, was driven on to the Gunfleet Sand during the night, in a heavy gale and snowstorm. Five died from cold and fatigue as the brig lay helpless in the face of the severe weather. The other two were saved by Cleave in his boat, who then brought ashore exhausted.

On 6-7 March 1832, in heavy rain and gale force winds, Captain William Jennings, master of the smack *Spy*, saw the brig *Faithful*, of Sunderland, on the Cork Sand, and set out to help. His smack reached the casualty at 6pm, and his boat, manned by himself and five others, was rowed towards the brig. But with the heavy seas on the sand, it was unable to get close enough to the casualty and was forced to return to the smack. Jennings then sailed the smack around the south of the Cork Sand and, at 10pm, manned his small boat for a second time, only to be forced back once more. After midnight, he made a third attempt, but found the wreck full of water, three men drowned in the longboat and the jolly boat gone. The master and four seamen survived, however, and they were taken aboard Jennings' smack and later landed safely at Harwich. For this fine rescue, Jennings was awarded the Silver medal by RNIPLS.

On 29 October 1838 the Guernsey vessel *Albion* went aground on Galloper Sand during a gale. Both of her boats were lost in the severe weather, and her hold was flooded. The master of the Boulogne fishing boat no.89, Captain John Antoine Delpierre, took off the casualty's crew of seven men in the face of the gale increasing to hurricane force, and landed them at Boulogne on 31 October. For this rescue, Delpierre was awarded the Silver medal by RNIPLS.

On 17 February 1843 the brig *Traveller* was wrecked on the Gunfleet Sand and was seen the next morning by the crews of two smacks, *Atalanta* and *New Gypsy*, both of Colchester. The brig was quickly breaking up and the crew had been forced to take to the rigging. The gale continued to rage all day, with heavy seas preventing the smacks from getting close enough to effect a rescue. At daybreak on 19 February the brig's crew could still be seen in the rigging, so the smacks attempted a rescue despite the fact that the seas were still running strongly through the area. A boat was

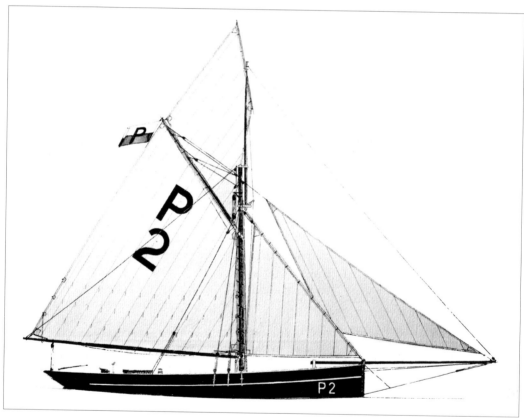

A line drawing of the Harwich bawleys which were employed under contract by Trinity House from 1866 to 1887 to land outward bound London District pilots in the vicinity of the Sunk lightvessel. Detail for the drawing was provided by H. A. Felgate, of Dovercourt. (Drawing by the late Captain Robert Sanders, former Superintendent of Pilots at Harwich, by courtesy of Andy Adams)

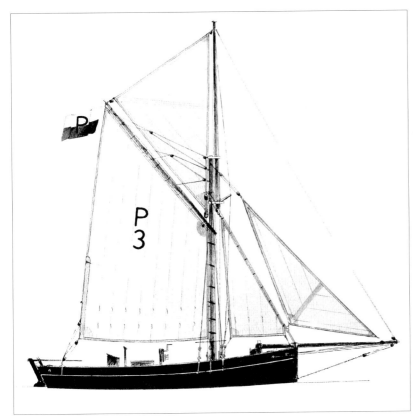

A line drawing of the Colne smacks employed under contract by Trinity House between 1885 and 1882 to land outward-bound London District pilots in the vicinity of the Sunk lightvessel. The smacks were cutter-rigged fishing vessels and were used for a variety of tasks, including sea rescue. Detail for the drawing was provided by John Leather, FRINA, of West Mersea. (Drawing by the late Captain Robert Sanders, former Superintendent of Pilots at Harwich, by courtesy of Andy Adams)

launched from each smack, manned by Captains John Glover and Stephen Hurry, as well as John Powell, master of the smack *Lord Howe*, and ten other men. After being buffeted for a considerable time, they succeeded in reaching the wreck and took on board all of those who were in the rigging, six into *New Gypsy*'s boat and four in *Atalanta*'s boat. After clearing the Sand, they ran alongside the steamer *Gazelle*, which was bound for London, and put the rescued men aboard her. For this outstanding rescue, the RNIPLS awarded Silver medals to all of the masters: Glover of *Atalanta*, Hurry of *New Gypsy* and Powell of *Lord Howe*.

On 20 February 1855 the Newcastle brig *Woodman* was driven ashore on the Shipwash Sand and wrecked in heavy seas. In two trips in his ship's boat, Captain William Newson, from the smack *Alfred*, rescued the brig's crew of eleven, for which he was awarded the Silver medal by the Royal National Lifeboat Institution (RNLI). By this time, the organisation responsible for lifeboats and sea rescue was known as the RNLI after the RNIPLS had been reformed and renamed in the 1850s. Indeed, the RNLI awarded another Silver medal for a rescue off Harwich in 1856 when the Goole ship *Maria* was wrecked on the Long Sand on 14 September. Captain William Lewis, of the smack *Tryall*, and four of his crew put off in their boat to rescue the sloop's three-man crew. The rescuers faced considerable danger in the face of a strong flood tide, and but for their actions the sloop's crew would have drowned.

One of the finest rescues undertaken by the smacks was effected on 3 November 1861 after the 329-ton barque *Darius*, of Shields, on her maiden voyage from Sunderland to Constantinople with coal, was wrecked on the Long Sand during a heavy gale. Five of the eleven crew were drowned, three when the long boat capsized and the other two after falling from the rigging having spent the night clinging to it. The remaining six were rescued by the smack *Volunteer*, of Harwich, which landed them at Harwich. *Volunteer's* crew had spent seven hours trying to reach the wreck during the night of 2-3 November, having several times been forced to put back because of the heavy sea on the sands. The survivors, when landed at Harwich, were 'in a very distressed state from exposure, having been in the rigging for more than eighteen hours', according to the *Suffolk Chronicle* of 9 November 1861.

When the RNLI's management committee heard about the efforts of the smacksmen, Silver medals were awarded to the master Thomas Adams and crew members Robert Scarlet, George Wyatt, John Lambert, Benjamin Lambeth and Henry Bacon, who manned the smack's boat and tried on several occasions to get to the wreck, 'in admiration of their daring and persevering services', with the thanks of the Institution inscribed on vellum to the remainder of the smack's six crew. The Board of Trade also recognised the efforts of the smack and gave £32 to be divided among the crew, of which £5 was given to Thomas Adams along with a telescope.

The other rescue off Harwich which gained formal recognition from the RNLI took place on 14 January 1893, by when the Institution had placed a lifeboat at Harwich. In a very heavy sea and strong northerly gale, the Glasgow ship *Enterkin* was wrecked on the Galloper Sands. The smack *Britain's Pride* went to help and, led by the master Captain Thomas Watson, the smack's crew managed to save an apprentice from the wreck. For their efforts, Captain Watson, and crew members William Burton, Edwin Hurle and Arthur Fisher were all awarded the Silver medal by the RNLI. This incident, and the other rescues by the smacks, show how active the smacksmen were in helping ships in difficulty, and how well suited their large vessels were to working on the outlying sands, particularly compared to the oar-powered lifeboats then in service with the RNLI.

NOTABLE RESCUES BY SMACKS OFF HARWICH 1822-1875

Date	Casualty	Smack(s) involved	Details of incident	Notes
6.1.1822	British brig Elegant of Sunderland.	Hero, of Woodbridge saved master, 8 drowned	Grounded on Rough off Harwich Harbour	
30.4.1829	British Brig Superb, of Aberdeen	Paul Pry, Samuel and Lively	Totally wrecked on Shipwash Sand	RNLI Silver medals awarded to William Mudd, master of Samuel and Samuel Wordley, master of Lively
24.12.1830	British brig Craig Elachie, of Leith	New Union, of Harwich; saved 3	Became total wreck on Gunfleet Sand	RNLI Silver medal awarded to Robert Cleave, master of New Union
27.10.1831	British brig Liberty, of Plymouth	Pearl, of Ipswich; saved all hands	Wrecked on Shipwash Sand	
6/7.3.1832	Brig Faithful, of Sunderland	Spy, of Ipswich; saved 5, 3 men drowned	Grounded on Cork Sand became total wreck	RNLI Silver medal awarded to William Jennings, master of Spy
18.12.1836	Dorothy Gray, of Hamburg	Pearl, of Ipswich saved all hands	Grounded and upset on Cork Sand	
21.11.1838	British schooner Ocean, of Sunderland	Beulah, of Colchester saved all hands	Totally wrecked on Middle Sunk	
30.11.1839	Endeavour, of Boston	Rumley, of Ipswich saved crew	Foundered on Ridge, off Harwich	
18/19.2.1843	Brig Traveller, of Hartlepool	New Gypsy, Atalanta and Lord Howe	Grounded and broke up on Gunfleet Sand	RNLI Silver medals to John Glover, master of Atalanta, Stephen Hurry, master of New Gypsy, and John Powell, master of Lord Howe
9.2.1846	Psyche, of Boston	Wonder, of Woodbridge saved 4 hands	Total loss on Shipwash Sand	
19.5.1846	Alert, of Whitby	William and Dorothy, of Dartmouth; saved 6, 9 drowned	Totally wrecked on Longsand	
13/14.11.1848	American emigrant schooner Burgundy, of Richmond, USA	Tryall, of Harwich, HM revenue cutter Desmond & other smacks	Grounded on Longsand, total wreck, all crew and 230 emigrants saved	

Date	Casualty	Smack(s) involved	Details of incident	Notes
24.11.1850	German emigrant barque Johan Frederick	Several Harwich & other smacks landed 140 emigrants and 16 hands	Totally wrecked on Gunfleet Sands	
30.10.1851	French brig Etoile de la Mer	Aurora's Increase, and Tryall, of Harwich	Grounded on Longsand, became total loss	Shipwrecked Mariners' Royal Benevolent Society Silver medals to masters and 3 crew of Aurora's Increase and Tryall, £5 between other crew; French Govt Gold medal to both masters of smacks, a Silver medal to both mates of smack
28.12.1851	Schooner Arrow, of Liverpool	Aurora's Increase, of Harwich	Grounded and upset on Longsand	RNLI awarded £5 to crew of Aurora's Increase
16.1.1855	British brig Stanton, of Shields	Aurora's Increase; and Tryall of Harwich	Wrecked on Gunfleet Sands	RNLI Silver medals to John Lewis, of Aurora's Increase and William Lewis, master of Tryall
20.2.1855	Brig Woodman, of Newcastle	Alfred, of Woodbridge; landed 11 men and boys	Grounded and upset on Shipwash Sand	RNLI Silver medal to William Newson, master of Alfred and £7 10s to be shared
20.5.1856	Brig Julia, of Whitby	Agenoria, of Ipswich; saved 2; 9 persons drowned	Totally lost on Shipwash Sand	RNLI awarded £12 to be shared between Adam Pinner, master of Agenoria, and crew
14.9.1856	Sloop Maria, of Goole	Tryall, of Harwich; landed crew of 3 hands	Total loss on Longsand	RNLI Silver medal to William Lewis, master of Tryall
27.3.1857	German barque Phoenix, of Hamburg	Running Rein and New Gypsy; saved 12 crew	Grounded and broke up on Longsand	
7.9.1859	Brig Fame, of South Shields	John and William of Harwich; saved all crew	Grounded and filled on Shipwash Sans	RNLI awarded £5 to be shared by master and crew of John and William
17.11.1860	British brigantine Charity, of Goole	Tryall of Harwich; landed 4; Master, his wife, daughter and 1 crew drowned	Grounded on Longsand and broke up	Board of Trade Bronze medal awarded to John Tye, master of Tryall, and 12s to be shared by 2 members of crew
3.11.1861	British barque Darius, of South Shields	Alfred, of Harwich; saved crew of 6	Aground on Longsand	RNLI Silver medals to Thomas Adams and 5 crew of Alfred, 3 other crew Thanks on Vellum
10/12.2.1869	Barque City of Carlisle, of Bristol	Aurora's Increase; Ranger of Harwich; 23 saved	Totally lost on Kentish Knock	
13.2.1869	Danish schooner Alvilda, of Holbeck	Alfred, of Harwich; George Wyatt, master, drowned in rescue attempt	Grounded and became total loss on Longsand	RNLI awarded £20 to widow of George Wyatt; Danish Govt £11 to widow and also £11 to be divided between crews of Agenoria, Celerity and Paragon
19.1.1870	Greek brig Tressithea	Ranger, of Harwich; saved all crew	Grounded on Longsand, total wreck	Greek Government awarded a Silver medal to Thomas Crane, master of Ranger
28.8.1870	British barque Alexander of Shields	Marco Polo, of Harwich; saved 10	Wrecked on Longsand	
18/19.12.1870	British brig Blyth, of Shields	Paragon; saved crew of 7	Grounded and total loss on Longsand	
29/30.1.1871	British steamer Battalion, of Leith	Battalion's crew saved by Unity, of Colchester	Wrecked on Longsand	Queen Victoria of Harwich lost 3 men in rescue attempt
7.6.1873	British barque Stornoway, of Newcastle	Ranger of Harwich landed crew at Harwich	Grounded on Kentish Knock, total wreck	
16.11.1874	British brigantine Grace Millie, of Lerwick	Crew saved by Violet, of Woodbridge; landed at Harwich	Grounded on Shipwash; became total loss	
22.5.1875	Brig Alacrity, of Whitby	Prince of Orange landed master and 5 at Harwich	Total loss on Gunfleet Sands.	
18.12.1875	Brig Aphrodite, of Newcastle	Violet, of Woodbridge landed crew of 8	Wrecked on Shipwash Sands	

Pulling and Sailing Lifeboats

Following the unsuccessful attempts to establish and operate a lifeboat at Harwich during the 1820s, a further half century passed before another lifeboat was supplied to the port. During that time the National Institution for the Preservation of Life from Shipwreck, established in 1824 but not involved in life-saving at Harwich hitherto, was reformed, reorganised and renamed, becoming the Royal National Lifeboat Institution (RNLI) in 1854. With a new secretary at its head and a new managing committee providing greater dynamism, the RNLI raised funds on a far greater scale than previously and considerably expanded its operations. The national economy, having recovered from the downturn of the 1830s and 1840s, prospered in the latter half of the century, and causes such as life-saving at sea gained a national prominence they had not before enjoyed. Many new lifeboat stations were established and a new design of lifeboat, the self-righter, was built in large numbers for stations nationwide.

On a local level, the modernisation of the RNLI meant that, at Harwich, operating and managing a lifeboat station would have been possible, and during this period of life-saving expansion the Institution offered a lifeboat to Harwich on several occasions. However, local support was not forthcoming, and no lifeboat was supplied despite ships getting into difficulty in the seas off the port, with the Suffolk and Ipswich-based newspapers often reporting shipwrecks off the Essex coast during the 1850s and 1860s. Among the worst incidents of shipwreck were those during the gales of November and December 1861, which claimed numerous victims along the entire length of England's east coast, particularly in the north-east, but vessels were not spared along the Thames Estuary and off the Essex coast.

In one of the more notable incidents, the barque *Darius*, of Shields, went aground and sank on the Long Sand during a severe storm on 3 November 1861. Only the vessel's mast remained standing, and five of the barque's crew of eleven lost their lives after clinging to the mast for more than twelve hours. However, in a particularly fine rescue the smack *Volunteer*, of Harwich, rescued the other six, although 'the poor men taken [off were] in a most helpless state'. The rescue was widely reported and the gallantry of the rescuers soon recognised. At the end of November 1861 the Board of Trade awarded them £32, to be divided between Thomas Adams, the master, the five men who went in the smack's boat to effect the rescue, and the rest of the smack's six crew. Adams was also presented with a telescope. Recognition was later forthcoming from the RNLI, which awarded its Silver medal and £5 to Thomas Adams, and the Thanks on Vellum to other men who had manned the small boat, in addition to a monetary award of £22 which was to be divided up, 'in admiration of their noble and persevering services in rescuing the barque'. At a public meeting at the Town Hall in Harwich the Mayor, Major Bowness, presented the awards to Adams, George

Wyatt, Benjamin Lambert, John Lambert, Robert Scarlett, Henry Bacon, William Harvey, John Mills, William Wyatt, Samuel Harris, William Redwood and James Owen. The meeting ended with 'cheers for the Royal National Lifeboat Institution and the Mayor' from the smacksmen.

In the days following the *Darius* incident, more vessels were caught out by terrible weather and the local salvage smacks had a busy few days. On 10 November 1861 the schooner *Friendship*, of London, lost both anchors and chains, but the smacks *Queen Victoria* and *Paragon*, of Harwich, got her clear of the Platters Sands and towed her to Harwich. The following day the sloop *Hannah*, of Rochester, also lost her anchors and chains, and was towed into Harwich by the smack *Paragon*. The brig *Thomas and Elizabeth*, bound from Sunderland to London with a cargo of coals, grounded on the Gunfleet Sand and was abandoned, but her crew were picked up by the schooner *Alert*. The brig was later got off by the crew of the smack *Orwell*, of Colchester, who brought her to Harwich the following morning. The Norwegian brig *Rata* also drove ashore on the Gunfleet Sand the same day, where she broke up despite the efforts of five smacks to try to save her. On 17 December 1861 the barque *Ganges*, of South Shields, bound to Havre with gas coals, was assisted into Harwich during the night by six smacks. The barque was leaking and part of her cargo had been thrown overboard after she had gone ashore on the Long Sand.

Despite the fact that ships continued to be wrecked and the shipping lanes off Essex were among the busiest in the country, no lifeboat was supplied for Harwich, and until well into the 1870s there were no lifeboat stations along the Essex's coast. The reasons put forward for not supplying a lifeboat to Harwich, and the same reasons could be applied to other Essex towns, were twofold. Firstly, it was believed that Harwich, as well as the adjacent coastline, was too far from the outlying sandbanks on which most wrecks occurred for a pulling lifeboat, with a limited range, to reach. Secondly, hovelling boats and salvaging smacks patrolled the coast looking for salvage work and these were also often used for life-saving. Some had made noteworthy rescues, as described above, and as they usually remained at sea in any weather, they were readily available for rescue and salvage work; with these vessels on hand the need for a lifeboat was apparently obviated. However, the wreck of the German emigrant steamship *Deutschland* on the Kentish Knock in December 1875, when fifty-seven lives were lost, convinced the RNLI that a lifeboat at Harwich was a necessity, despite some local opposition. And, after this tragedy, even if on some occasions a pulling and sailing lifeboat could not reach the sandbanks, it was realised that in many instances a lifeboat would be of use.

The wreck of the steamship *Deutschland*

While the wreck of the 3,000-ton steamer *Deutschland* was the main catalyst for the establishment of a lifeboat station at Harwich, the incident itself became particularly notorious at the time after accusations were made in the German press in the aftermath of the tragedy that the seafarers of Harwich made few attempts to save those on board the steamer. Strenuous denials were made by various local people in response to the accusations, and a Board of Trade inquiry was held to ascertain exactly what had happened. Not only that, but the RNLI acted with considerable speed in establishing a lifeboat station at Harwich within a little over a month after the event, suggesting that the Institution had realised their error in not providing the port with a lifeboat previously.

The events surrounding the *Deutschland* incident are these: the steamer, bound from Bremen for New York via Southampton, was wrecked on the morning of 6 December 1875 on the Kentish Knock sandbank, twenty-four miles from Harwich. She had 105 crew on board, and about 225 passengers, twenty-eight of whom were travelling first class. In the ensuing sinking, a total of fifty-seven of the passengers and crew lost their lives. The vessel had been caught out in heavy seas and gale force winds, which had driven her onto the sands at about 5.30am, while heavy snow showers greatly reduced visibility in the area. Signals of distress had been fired from the stranded ship, but these were not seen for well over twelve hours by any of the lightships in the area, the closest of which was the Kentish Knock, 'no doubt owing to the thickness of the weather, and almost continuous snowstorms', according to the RNLI's account. Crews on the Sunk and Cork lightships had seen rockets, but could not ascertain the exact position of the distressed ship, and the Sunk lightship's crew initially believed the vessel was on the Long Sand.

Once it was known that a vessel was in difficulty, however, the Harwich-based steam tug *Liverpool* was asked to help, and although her master did not immediately put to sea because of the gale force winds, he went at first light on 7 December as soon as the weather had moderated, and returned in the afternoon having rescued a large number of the passengers and crew from the steamer. Many of those on board the steamer who lost their lives had been washed off the decks by the heavy seas before the arrival of *Liverpool*. Two boats had been launched from the steamer, with three people in one and six in another, but these small craft were quickly swamped by heavy seas and their occupants drowned. When the tug first arrived at the sands and found the casualty, the steamer's decks were under water and the vessel was slowly breaking up. In its report on 8 December 1875, the *East Anglian Daily Times* stated that, 'the poor creatures who have been saved, about 150 all told, were for the most part found clinging to the rigging. A child died on board the tug during her return voyage.'

Once brought ashore, the survivors from the wrecked ship were attended to by people in Harwich, 'administering to their need in clothing and food, for which they received the hearty thanks of the poor people themselves; and by decently and reverentially interring in the town cemetery the bodies of the drowned which had been recovered and brought ashore', according to the *East Anglian Daily Times*. O. J. William, vice consul of Harwich, organised the task of looking after the survivors, and took 'measures to provide for the sufferers'. The steam tug *Liverpool* made many further trips to the vessel during the subsequent days, landing numerous bodies as well as bags of mail and other cargo.

But while the survivors were being given assistance and aid by various people and organisations in Harwich, the accusations were being made about the lack of help given to the steamer on the day she grounded. According to *The Lifeboat* journal, 'a portion of the German press' was advancing 'reckless charges against the town of Harwich and the boatmen of that port, accusing them of deliberately allowing the unfortunate emigrants to perish before their eyes and refusing them succour', mainly because the emigrants were German. The *Bourse Gazette*, of Berlin, claimed that *Deutschland* was wrecked close to the port of Harwich, where signals of distress could easily be seen, that she showed her German flag, and that the people of Harwich allowed many of her passengers and crew to perish, just because they were German. Quite why the newspaper made such accusations, trying to aggravate anti-British feeling in Germany, is not clear.

Whatever the motives of the German newspaper, several questions were raised following the tragedy. These were: (a) why was help so slow in reaching the wreck when it was relatively close to the mouth of the Thames, the country's busiest waterway, where signals of distress should have been seen and acted upon speedily?; (b) why was there no lifeboat at the nearest port, namely Harwich, ready to assist?; (c) where were the hovelling smacks that were supposedly patrolling the coast?; and (d) why was the steam tug so slow in putting out to help? To answer these points a Board of Trade enquiry was held into the wreck, and concluded that everything that could have been done by the people of Harwich was done.

Clearly the attack by the German newspapers on the people of Harwich, British seafarers and the British nation as a whole stung the British press into action. The accusations were reported in a letter which was published in *The Times* of 13 December 1875, which blamed the inadequacies of the local seafarers as well as the operators of the tug *Liverpool* for the loss of life. The Mayor of Harwich, Johnson Richmond, responded by writing a long and detailed letter, which appeared in the *East Anglian Daily Times* of 12 January 1876, stating, along with refutations of the accusations, 'that such allegations were unjustly made, and that when all allegations were brought to light, their [the seamen of Harwich] conduct would be found to be beyond reproach'.

The *Lifeboat* journal of 1 February 1876 also got involved, with the RNLI feeling compelled to furnish a complete explanation of events and devoted its first five pages to the incident and a defence of the actions of those involved. The journal began by stating:

> '*Perhaps no maritime disaster of modern times . . . has excited more general interest, arising partly from the circumstance of its having occurred so near the mouth of the Thames, and partly from the strange and reckless charges advanced by a portion of the German newspaper press against the town of Harwich and the boatmen of that port, maliciously accusing them of deliberately allowing the unfortunate emigrants to perish before their eyes and refusing them succour.*'

The accusations in the German press were countered by the RNLI's account. The German account seemed to be largely incorrect, as it stated the wreck was only four miles from Harwich, the steam tug put out too late to help, and, because the vessel's German flag could be seen, the people of Harwich deliberately refused to offer assistance. But, in fact, a combination of circumstances conspired against the passengers and crew on board *Deutschland*, and the people of Harwich were largely powerless to help. The ferocity of the gale had driven the hovelling smacks on this occasion into port, and the only available means of communication was by signals from the lightships. But none of the rockets fired by *Deutschland* had been seen by the lightships, even the closest one which was the Kentish Knock, owing to the very poor visibility caused by almost continuous snowstorms. Thus the *Deutschland*'s passengers and crew were left for fourteen hours in their perilous situation, aground and helpless on the sandbank, because 'no one knew of their danger'.

Accusations against the steam tug *Liverpool* and her master seem particularly unfair considering

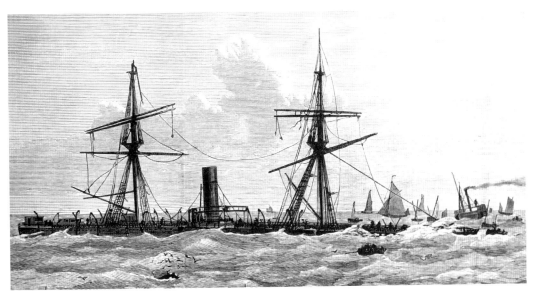

A contemporary illustration of the wreck of the steamship Deutschland.

the rescue work in which she had been involved during the months prior to the *Deutschland* tragedy. She had only arrived in Harwich on 1 September 1875 from Newcastle, where she had been built by James Rennoldson of South Shields. Her arrival was reported in the *East Anglian Daily Times*, in which she was described as 'powerful and commodious . . . and her power 60 horse nominal'. The 112ft vessel was purchased by W. J. Watts, of Harwich, and as soon as she arrived at her new home port was employed in towing the brig *Roska* from Harwich Harbour to the lock gates at Ipswich, and 'there can be little doubt that in the matter of saving lives she will be found of great service to vessels voyaging to Ipswich'. The newspaper summed up the description by saying, 'She is a stout, strongly built craft, a powerful and fast tug boat, and an advantageous vessel for pleasure excursions. She has two fore cabins, and a spacious well fitted saloon.'

In the time between her arrival and the wreck of the *Deutschland*, the steam tug was used to undertake a number of rescues. Among these rescues was that on 12 September 1875, when she towed the Swedish brig *Cleopatra* off the Kentish Knock and into Harwich Harbour. She went out to help another vessel on 29 October 1875, finding the schooner *Spectre*, of George Town, Prince Edwards Island, ashore in the Wallet. The casualty was a new vessel with a copper bottom and her crew had been landed at Clacton earlier in the day. When *Liverpool* reached the scene, both of the vessel's anchors had gone, so the tug attempted to tow her off, but without success, and the schooner sank the following day.

Of the *Deutschland* incident, the tug's master was criticised for not setting off to assist as soon as the rockets had been fired by the Cork Lightship. However, her master, Captain Carrington, 'an able and experienced seaman, who knew what he was about', realised that navigating

> 'in the intricate passages between the numerous shoals off the port in a dark night and gale of wind . . . could only [be done] at great risk of losing his owner's vessel and the lives of those entrusted to him'. Finding the vessel quickly in the night was also unlikely even if the tug had put out, and if the casualty was found, the small boats used to reach it by the tug would be unable 'to render any assistance to a vessel surrounded by broken water, in a dark night and heavy sea'.

Therefore, Carrington decided not to put to sea until shortly before daylight, leaving port at 6am by when the gale had moderated. He first went to the Cork Lightship, and then to the Sunk Lightship where he was informed that there was a steamer on the Long Sand. So he steamed to the Long Sand, but no vessel could be seen on it, so he headed for the Kentish Knock, and when halfway to it saw *Deutschland* aground. The tug was anchored about sixty fathoms away, and its boats went to the wreck, taking off three boat-loads of survivors.

The tug had proved to be a useful asset to help with incidents of shipwreck, but in the aftermath of the *Deutschland* disaster it was also asked what other means were available at Harwich for helping ships wrecked on the sands? No lifeboat was based at Harwich because, it was explained in *The Lifeboat* journal, 'the outlying sandbanks, on which vessels were liable to be wrecked, were all so distant that before a lifeboat from Harwich could reach them the shipwrecked persons would have been taken off by one of the numerous hovelling smacks which are almost always cruising about, or lying under shelter of the sands, on the look out for vessels in distress'. The smacks' work involved helping vessels in distress, assisting them to get afloat if they grounded on the sandbanks, recovering anchors and cables, and saving property which would otherwise be lost. They were also, as described above, often involved in saving lives. The smacksmen were not employed or paid to save lives, but put to sea at their own expense and risk in much the same way as the salvagers using luggers from Deal and Ramsgate and yawls from Yarmouth and Gorleston would go to the assistance of wrecked crews for a salvage reward. But in the case of the *Deutschland*, the smacks had been driven into port by the severity of the gale, although, even if they had been at sea, attempting to go alongside the wrecked ship in the teeth of the gale would have been almost impossible.

The lifeboat from Broadstairs did launch to help but was too late to be of service, and the Ramsgate lifeboat, notified by telegram from Harwich, was towed by the steam tug *Aid* forty-five miles north across the Thames Estuary to the scene, only to find on arrival there that the shipwrecked crew had already been saved by the tug. Another forty-five miles was covered on the return passage, with her fifteen crew suffering fourteen hours at sea, 'with the seas and spray breaking over them through their whole terrible voyage, in a freezing atmosphere and then landed in a benumbed, half frozen state, from the effects of which some of them may never entirely recover'.

The Board of Trade inquiry not only completely refuted the unfair German accusations, but explained that everything that could be done to help had been done, efforts to save lives from Harwich and elsewhere had been considerable, and that not only were the authorities and people of the port of Harwich free from blame, but they were entitled to much credit for their humane exertions on the occasion. However, the incident had clearly highlighted a lack of life-saving capability in the area and the RNLI wasted little time in getting a lifeboat stationed at the port, presumably wanting to avoid any negative questioning of their role in lifeboat provision should a future disaster occur.

The first RNLI lifeboat

The RNLI wasted no time in responding to the *Deutschland* incident. On 14 December 1875, just over a week after the tragedy, the Institution's Inspector, Rear Admiral John Ward, visited Harwich and met the Mayor, Johnson Richmond, to discuss establishing a lifeboat station. A public meeting was arranged, and Ward examined the foreshore between Harwich and Dovercourt, as well as the harbour, to find a site suitable for a lifeboat house. The best position was on ground that belonged to the Board of Ordnance. This site was sufficiently far from the sea to mean a carriage would be needed to transport the boat, so although the hovelling smacksmen had requested a large lifeboat, a boat light enough to be transported by a carriage would have to be provided. The Mayor took a great interest in the Inspector's work and supported establishing a lifeboat station.

The public meeting held at the Town Hall on 17 December was well attended, mostly by local seafarers, and those present supported the RNLI's plans, with the meeting resolving that a station should be established. It was also resolved to accept the offer to fund the lifeboat received via a letter sent to the Mayor from Miss E. Burmester, of Park Road Square, Regents Park, London, who was willing to pay for both the lifeboat and its equipment, with the boat to be named *Springwell*. A committee of management was formed, with several of those present at the meeting, including the Mayor, being enrolled onto it. The father of Mr Watts, the owner of the steam tug *Liverpool*, which had saved many lives from *Deutschland*, spoke on his son's behalf and said that the steamer would be available to tow the lifeboat to incidents free of charge.

The support of the local committee and community at Harwich was conveyed to the RNLI, and at a meeting of the Institution's Committee of Management on 6 January 1876, less than a month after the *Deutschland* tragedy, the establishment of the station at Harwich was formalised. Opening a new lifeboat station usually took several months, but when another ship was wrecked off Harwich, on the Shipwash Sands, the RNLI decided to send a lifeboat to the station immediately without waiting for the boathouse to be built, 'so as to be ready for any emergency which might arise'. No doubt stung by criticism following the *Deutschland* tragedy, the RNLI acted with considerable haste and the speed with which the Harwich station was opened suggests that a lifeboat should have been at such a major port as Harwich much earlier, and that those who failed to support it should have been ignored. Whether a lifeboat could have helped with *Deutschland* is a matter of conjecture, but undoubtedly had a lifeboat been on hand it would have removed the RNLI from criticism in the incident's aftermath.

The wreck which caused the RNLI to act so speedily took place on 8 January 1876 when the Norwegian barque *Hunter*, of Kragero, bound from Christiana for Rochester, was driven onto the Shipwash Sands in severe weather and filled with water. A smack reached the scene, but the seas were so bad that she could not get close to the casualty. For the rest of the day and throughout the night the captain and crew sheltered in the roundhouse. When news of the wreck reached Harwich, the steam tug *Liverpool* put out, with John Carrington in charge, and reached the Shipwash at about 1am the next day. The tug's crew could not see any vessel, but eventually spotted a French schooner, *Ville de Pontorson*, of Granville, which was on the point of sinking. The tug took her in tow, with some of the tug's crew assisting in pumping, and they reached Harwich at about 3am.

Liverpool then procured the boat from the smack *Ranger*, and left the harbour for a second time at 4.30am with the boat in tow. This time they found the stranded *Hunter*, with her crew standing on the top of the roundhouse signalling for assistance as the vessel was rapidly going to pieces. Several attempts were made to reach them, but pieces of wreckage initially made it too dangerous. The wreckage eventually dispersed, so a boat was launched from the tug, and, manned by Carrington, master of the tug, and several others, got close enough to the wreck to throw a line on board, which was used to haul eight of the men into the boat and to safety. They were then taken aboard the tug and landed at Harwich. For the rescue of the captain and crew of *Hunter*, Carrington was awarded the Silver medal by the RNLI.

Just three days after this rescue had been completed, moves were in hand to get the lifeboat to Harwich. The new boat, named *Springwell* in accordance with the donor's wishes, was a 35ft standard self-righter, had cost £433 to build and been completed by Woolfe at Shadwell, in London. She completed her harbour trial on 12 January 1876 and the following day was towed from London by the steamer *Secret*, of Hartlepool. However, bad weather forced the crew to abandon the short voyage and the lifeboat had to return to the Thames after being damaged, going to Blackwall for repairs on 15 January. Although the boat was delayed, the launching carriage, which was built by Frederick Chapman & Son, of Limehouse, and stores were forwarded to Harwich via the Great Eastern Railway, free of charge, and they arrived on 14 January.

The following afternoon the carriage was put together on the quay, under the supervision of the RNLI's Inspector Captain Ward. Once it was ready, it was taken through King's Quay Street to the Coastguard station, followed 'by a crowd of urchins who cheered lustily', according to the *East Anglian Daily Times* for 17 January 1876, which continued: 'In some places the street was scarcely wide enough, and as the vehicle proceeded its huge wheels ran on the edge of the pavement crushing off portions of the kerb stones as they slipped into the road again.' The carriage was taken to the site where the new boathouse was to be built and the gear was stored in the Coastguard house.

The business of getting the station up and running continued over the next few days and on 17 January the local committee met to organise a crew with harbour boatmen, who were described as 'good rowers', being enrolled. John Tye, a local mariner, was appointed Coxswain in 1876 and he served in the post until 1881, although he missed the service on 18 January 1881 in which *Springwell* capsized, as described below, as he was at home with his wife who was very ill; he resigned the position shortly afterwards. Thomas Thompson was appointed as the first second coxswain and Matthew Scarlett became bowman.

On 20 January 1876 *Springwell*, having had the minor damage repaired, again left the Thames and was towed to Harwich, this time by the steamer *Lord Alfred Paget*, and again free of charge.

26

This time, she reached her new station safely, arriving at 6pm, and was placed on moorings. The following day she was taken to sea by the Assistant Inspector for a short trial before being recovered and placed on her carriage, had her equipment loaded on board, and cleaned ready for service. The Assistant Inspector met the local committee, and, although it was usual practice at the time for an inauguration to take place within a few days of a new lifeboat's arrival, the formal ceremony was deferred until the boathouse was completed.

The boathouse was built on the sea bank east of the town. Various sites had been considered but the most suitable, in the shipbuilder's yard, was not available, so an alternative was found on War Office land for which a nominal rent had to be paid to the War Department of one shilling per annum. During the first few months of 1876, while the building was under construction, the gear was kept in the Coastguard boathouse and the lifeboat under a tarpaulin cover. A tender for the building work of £247 10s 0d from I. J. Newton was accepted by the RNLI on 2 March 1876, and construction took place during the first few months of the year. On 4 May 1876 the Corporate Seal of the Institution was affixed on the counterpart of the lifeboat house lease, and three months later the building was ready for the lifeboat.

With the boathouse complete, plans were made for the station's inauguration ceremony on 7 September 1876, which was declared a holiday with the shops closed 'and bunting profusely decorating every street', as the whole town turning out to watch the lifeboat procession. The event was overseen by Rear-Admiral D. Robertson-MacDonald, the RNLI's Assistant Inspector, with the Mayor, Johnson Richmond, and the local committee keen to formally recognise Miss Ellen Burmester's generous gift by giving her the honour of christening the new boat. However, the donor could not be present, but she wrote to the Mayor expressing

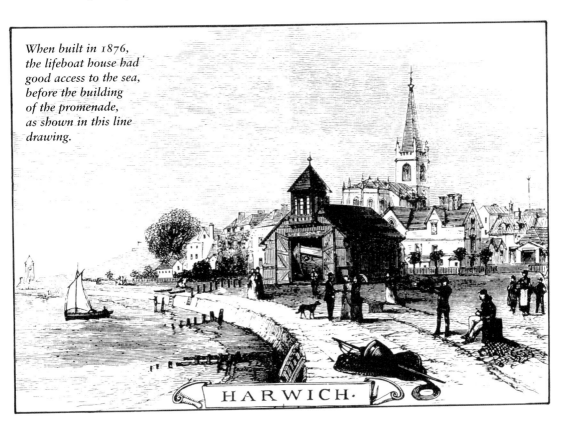

When built in 1876, the lifeboat house had good access to the sea, before the building of the promenade, as shown in this line drawing.

HARWICH.

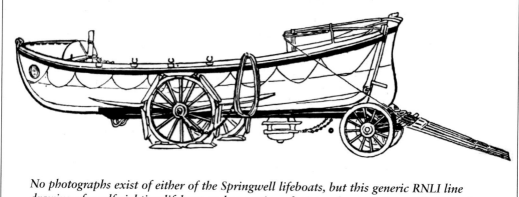

No photographs exist of either of the Springwell lifeboats, but this generic RNLI line drawing of a self-righting lifeboat on her carriage depicts a boat similar to the first of the Springwell lifeboats at Harwich.

'my hope that all may go off well on Thursday, and that the events of the day may give pleasure to a large number. It will interest me greatly to hear all details of the inauguration of the lifeboat station; and I shall be at Harwich in thought, though not in presence.'

The *East Anglian Daily Times* for 8 September 1876 gave a full account of the day's events, with people from all the local towns and villages attending helped by 'The Great Eastern Company . . . [which] ran a special boat from Ipswich, while a late train to Manningtree and Colchester gave the inhabitants of those towns an opportunity of witnessing the whole of the proceedings. Notwithstanding the cloudy weather everything passed off admirably, a successful result for which the energetic and hospitable Mayor, Johnson Richmond, Esq, cannot be too highly thanked.' The procession started at midday, and was composed of the band of the 1st Essex Volunteers, the lifeboat on her carriage drawn by horses, local clergy, the Mayor and Corporation, the Lifeboat Committee, and friendly societies. Despite the rain, the procession went through the town and was watched by hundreds of local people.

The boat was formally presented to the Mayor by Admiral Robertson, on behalf of the donor. After a service of dedication read by the Rev J. Farman, the boat was launched by the Angel Gate Battery, and rowed by her crew to the barge of the Regatta Committee. She was then deliberately capsized to show her self-righting powers, and she 'quickly and satisfactorily righted herself'. Admiral Robertson afterwards said he had 'never before seen a more enthusiastic reception and as there was a first-rate crew he felt that if they continued as they had begun no chance of doing their duty would be lost', according to the report given to the RNLI's Committee of Management. With the lifeboat naming concluded, a regatta was held along the esplanade consisting of races between cutters and gigs from HMS *Challenger*, as well as a swimming match and duck hunt. At the end of proceedings, the Mayor entertained the Town Council and friends to a lunch at the Great Eastern Hotel, and Mr J. H. Vaux, local shipbuilder, gave a supper to the Committee and lifeboat crew at the Three Cups Hotel in the evening. This grand ceremony concluded when Admiral Robertson 'expressed the pride he felt in having the honour of handing the lifeboat to the committee'.

Springwell served at Harwich for just over five years, but in that short time she gained an impressive record, performing twenty-six services and saving sixty-one lives. The following accounts detail her effective services, the first of which was not undertaken until 29 December 1876, almost a year after she arrived. After fires had been seen in the direction of the Platters Sand,

Springwell was launched, and was rowed out of the harbour some way until taken in tow by the steam tug *Liverpool*. The brigantine *Willie*, of Llanelli, was flying the distress signals, and the vessel was found in a dangerous position near Landguard Point. The lifeboat was taken alongside the casualty and the lifeboat men went aboard. With the assistance of a pilot cutter, they got a rope to the tug, after which the vessel's anchors and chains were slipped and she was towed into Harwich.

Springwell's next service was almost exactly a year later, on 2 December 1877. She put out 10.30pm after flares from the Sunk lightship had been seen and, on reaching the lightship, the lifeboat crew were told that the signals had actually been made from the Kentish Knock. So the lifeboat proceeded to the Long Sand, where the wreck of the Swedish barque *Jacob Lanstrum* was found. The eight men on the barque were rescued by the lifeboat, albeit with some difficulty in heavy seas and strong north-easterly wind. The lifeboat remained with the ship until daylight, when the steam tug *Harwich* arrived. The rescued crew were then transferred onto the tug, which towed the lifeboat back to her Harwich.

Fourteen months later *Springwell* was in action again, launching on 16 February 1879 after the barque *Pasithea*, of Liverpool, bound from Hamburg to Cardiff, went ashore on the Long Sand. The lifeboat immediately launched but, once on scene, because it was low tide, could not get alongside the wreck. At high tide the steam tug Harwich arrived, and, with the lifeboat's help, managed to got a rope to the stranded ship, but was unable to get the schooner off. With the weather worsening and heavy seas crashing over the casualty, the lifeboat went alongside and succeeded in taking off thirteen of the crew as well as ten smacksmen, who had gone on board to assist. Two of the men fell between the vessel and the lifeboat as they were trying to get across, but they were rescued. The lifeboat remained by the wreck until daylight, when it was found that the steward was missing, but he was seen in the rigging. So the shipwrecked sailors were put aboard a smack, and the lifeboat returned to the ship to save the steward, who lowered himself by a rope to safety. The lifeboat was then towed back to Harwich by the steam tug.

Further launches by *Springwell* during 1879 failed to result in any effective services being performed, but the routine inspections of the station, undertaken by Captain St Vincent Nepean, RN, the RNLI's Inspector, took place. On 30 August 1879 he found the station 'in good order' apart from a few minor defects. He did not take the lifeboat out for her quarterly exercise because she had been launched for a visit of the donor earlier in the month. The way that the lifeboat was hauled up the slipway was considered unsatisfactory as there was insufficient room to place the boat on her carriage until she had been hauled up on skids to the top of the narrow slipway. On 25 November 1879 Nepean visited again and during the evening some of Captain Very's patent rockets, used for signalling by the lifeboat crew, were tried and 'found to answer satisfactorily', according to the *East Anglian Daily Times*. The following day *Springwell* was taken out on exercise to the Rolling Grounds in a strong wind with moderate sea and snow falling, and the crew were 'exercised in the use of the heaving lines, and after two hours of anything but agreeable work, the lifeboat returned to harbour, and was safely housed'. The station was found to be in good order, apart from three defective lifebelts, which were replaced.

During the Inspector's visits in 1880 various problems had to be addressed, although on the whole the station's operation was deemed satisfactory. A visit by the District Inspector in March found the station in good order, but the lifeboat was not launched as the Coxswain had taken the boat out for exercise a few days earlier without authority from the Honorary Secretary. The boat was 'beginning to show a battered appearance', as the slope down a passage to the launching site was only just wide enough for the carriage and when getting through the passage the boat had been damaged. The Honorary Secretary was asked to get the wooden roadway leading to the beach levelled. Another inspection visit was made to the station on 29 April 1880, this time by

Chief Inspector Admiral Ward. He inspected the boat and station and found them in good order, although repairs to the boat were required as it had been damaged when being taken through a narrow gapway leading to the beach and when alongside a casualty. One of the main issues that was addressed was the unauthorised exercise launch, which was explained by the Coxswains saying that some of the crew wanted to take the lifeboat out as they were 'much impoverished at the time' and they needed the small payment made for an exercise. However, after further discussions, the Coxswains promised not to launch again without the sanction of the Honorary Secretary and the matter was closed.

The final year *Springwell* was at Harwich, 1881, proved to be an eventful one, beginning on 5 January when the barque *Indian Chief*, of Liverpool, went aground on the Long Sands, at the mouth of the Thames, off Clacton-on-Sea. Springwell launched to assist, as did the Clacton lifeboat, but neither could reach the casualty because of the severity of the easterly gale. Although *Springwell* put out again at 9.30pm, she was still unable to reach the barque. However, the Ramsgate lifeboat *Bradford* was towed to the scene by the steam tug *Vulcan* and, under Coxswain Charles Fish, was able to effect a rescue. Fish was awarded the RNLI's Gold Medal for his courage and bravery, with Silver medals going to the rest of the Ramsgate crew and those who manned the steam tug, and the rescue became one of the most famous in the history of the RNLI.

The following day, 6 January 1881, *Springwell* was out on service again, launching after reports had been received that the Spanish brigantine *Rosita*, bound from Hamburg to Porto Rico with a general cargo, had gone ashore on the Halliday Sands. The vessel soon drifted onto Pye Sand, where the masts were cut away. After the brigantine's signals of distress had been seen, *Springwell* was launched at about 7.30am and, arriving on scene, the lifeboatmen found the brigantine was sinking. Seven of the crew and a woman were taken into the lifeboat, but the master, mate, and boatswain, refused to leave. So the eight rescued persons were landed at midday, and, as the weather had not improved, the lifeboat returned to the scene to get the remaining crew. By the time *Springwell* reached the casualty again, the seas were sweeping over the vessel, and the three men had no choice but to abandon ship and so they were brought ashore by the lifeboat.

The dangers of nineteenth century lifeboat work were evident less than two weeks later when *Springwell* was again launched on service, putting out during the late morning on 18 January 1881 to a vessel in distress on the sands. The weather was so bad that she could not be launched from her carriage and instead had to be lowered into the water by crane from the Continental Pier. But she was got away and her sails were set as she headed out to sea. However, when she was about half a mile from the shore, the full force of the gale struck her and she was capsized, with all but two of her crew thrown into the water. Righting took about half a minute, during which time lifeboat man William Wink was washed away although the rest of the crew clung on to the hull. Some onlookers saw what had happened and immediately went to help, going out in a cutter from HMS *Penelope* having seen Wink drift away. Although he was picked up about a quarter of an hour later and every was made to revive him, he died shortly afterwards from exhaustion and exposure. The remaining eleven men were taken on board the smack *Ranger* and the lifeboat had to be towed ashore as most of her gear had been lost. The lifeboat was landed at Ray Island and the crew walked to Harwich, arriving just as William Wink's body was being brought ashore.

An inquest into Wink's death was held on 21 January at which Coxswain William Britton explained the events as he saw them, stating that, when the lifeboat capsized, 'none of the men were lashed in, I had to set sail because it would have been impossible to get to the distressed vessel without. We could get no steamer to tow us. The foresail was close reefed, and the mizen double reefed. As soon as the boat righted, I ordered the sheets to be let go to ease the strain, and this was done. I did not see Wink after I got into the boat.' The jury returned a verdict of accidental death, and added that no blame was attached to any of the lifeboat crew, but that 'the highest commendation was due to them for the way in which they attempted to carry out their heroic work of saving life'. The RNLI's Committee of Management expressed their sympathy with the widow of Wink and voted £100 for her benefit as well as paying the funeral expenses of £13 8s 6d.

The day before the inquest, despite the tragedy, *Springwell* had been out on service again and this time completed a fine service in very difficult conditions. She put to sea just before 7pm after signals from the Cork lightship indicated a vessel was on the sands. She was manned by a crew of twelve under the command of the Coxswain William Britton, with Captain Nepean, RN, the district inspector, also on board. Just getting out of the harbour was difficult because a severe frost had frozen the sea, so a passage had to be cut through the ice before the lifeboat could reach the harbour entrance. Once out at sea, the lifeboat initially headed for the Cork lightvessel, but

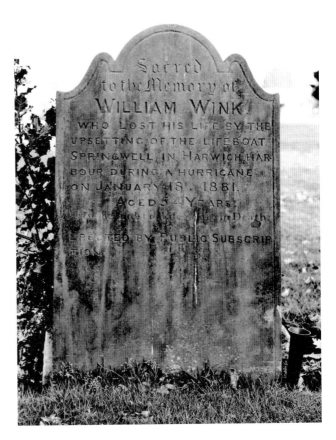

The gravestone for William Wink in Dovercourt Cemetery, with the inscription reading 'who lost his life by the upsetting of the lifeboat'. (Nicholas Leach)

put about after learning that the vessel was on the Sunk Sand with her crew lashed to the rigging. *Springwell* was towed some of the way by the smack *Albatross*, whose master gave them directions to the wreck. After leaving the smack, the lifeboat crew set sail and, between 4am and 5am, spotted the wreck. The vessel turned out to be the 438-ton screw steamship *Ingerid*, of Rotterdam, which was carrying fish from Norway for Naples.

The steamer had gone aground on Monday 17 January, and her condition had gradually worsened thereafter. Of the sixteen crew, seven left in a boat and were drowned, while two others were drowned helping to get another boat away. The captain and six men who were left on board were forced to take to the foremast, 'lashing themselves to it for fear of falling into the boiling sea beneath them', and remained there until the lifeboat arrived on scene in the early hours of Friday 21 January. The newspaper account succinctly summed up their subsequent plight: 'What their sufferings were none can tell during the four nights and three days they were on the sands in the searching wind and biting frost, without any possibility of getting either food or drink.'

The lifeboat crew found the seven men lashed to the foremast and the vessel almost completely under water. After it had been established that the men on board were alive, a line was made fast to the wreck, but it broke as the lifeboat was being hauled towards the survivors. At this point, according to the *East Anglian Daily Times*' account, 'The poor fellows in the rigging, seeing the

The Sunk lightvessel has been operational from 1802. The vessel illustrated is one of the early wooden or composite boats, possible LV 64 which was stationed at the Sunk for some time. (By courtesy of Ken Brand)

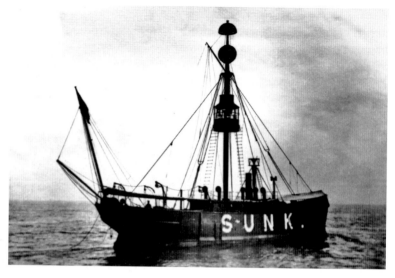

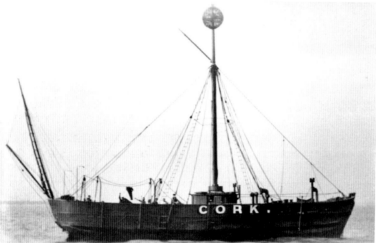

The Cork lightvessel was first established in 1844. This wooden-hulled vessel was typical of those stationed off the east coast during the nineteenth and twentieth centuries. It was often the signal guns fired by these lightships that gave the first news of a ship wrecked on the sandbanks. (By courtesy of Ken Brand)

The Cork lightvessel LV 86, built by J. S. White, Cowes in 1931 was 86ft overall and 185grt. This vessel also served as the Edinburgh lightvessel in the Thames Estuary and at Calshot Spit. Her main station was the Nore from 1931. (By courtesy of Ken Brand)

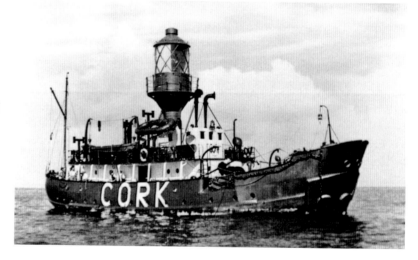

lifeboat receding from them, cried out in their fear, 'Don't leave us, or we shall fall into the sea directly. Come this moment, or we shall drop off. We can't hold out any longer'.' A second line was immediately secured, and this time it held, enabling the lifeboat to get close enough to the stranded vessel for her crew to board the wreck, help the survivors down, and get them into the lifeboat.

During the passage back to station, *Springwell* came across the Lowestoft tug *Despatch*, which was leaving Harwich with the Lowestoft lifeboat in tow. The tug and lifeboat had come over on Thursday 20 January after a telegram had been sent asking for assistance because *Springwell* had been damaged during the capsize three days before. Finding that the lifeboat had the seven survivors on board and in fact no assistance was required to help the casualty, the tug towed *Springwell* into harbour, reaching the pier at 9.45am. *Springwell* had been out for more than fifteen hours, and her appearance in the port was 'greeted with a loud cheer from the crowd assembled awaiting her return.' The survivors had suffered greatly during their ordeal, and their faces were 'so blackened with frost that they looked as if they had all been in a horrible fighting affray, whilst their limbs were stiff and useless', having been severely frost-bitten. The rescued men were taken care of at the Great Eastern Hotel, where the lifeboat crew were also given a hot breakfast.

For this outstanding rescue, the RNLI awarded Silver medals to Coxswain William Britton and Captain St Vincent Nepean, together with £4 to each of the crew, 'in acknowledgement of their brave and determined services in saving seven of the crew of the Dutch steamer *Ingerid*. . . This service was the more creditable on account of the fact that the lifeboat had capsized two or three days previously, and the meeting much applauded the noble example of Captain Nepean and the lifeboat crew in thus unhesitatingly proceeding in her on a long and dangerous service.' The Netherlands lifeboat society, the South Holland Society for the Preservation of Life from Shipwreck, also recognised the lifeboat crew's effort and awarded each a silver medal. The presentations were formally made at a public meeting held on 9 April 1881 at the Town Hall presided over by Sir Henry W. Tyler, MP, with the Dutch Consul O. J. Williams also in attendance.

Despite the outstanding success of *Springwell* and her crew in saving the men from the Dutch steamer within days of the capsize, calls for a larger boat for Harwich became more vociferous as a result of the accident that had overtaken *Springwell*. At the inquest into the death of Wink, several witnesses stated that she was too small and 'not fit for use at Harwich . . . if she had been a boat like those at Aldeburgh and Yarmouth, the accident would not have occurred.' The jury was almost unanimous in its opinion that the boat was not large enough for the station, with the distances to the outlying sands making a larger and more powerful boat an 'absolutely necessary'. These statements were passed to RNLI and on 15 February 1881 the Chief Inspector of Lifeboats, Admiral John Ross Ward, visited the station to assess the situation.

For some time the Coxswain and crew had been dissatisfied with the boat, not only considering her too small but also complaining that she could not work to windward in rough weather and was 'comparatively useless at a place where outlying sands were so distant and assistance of a steam tug cannot be depended on'. Since the capsize, which occurred when she was under close-reefed sail, the crew had even less confidence in the boat and so providing a larger one was essential, all of which was explained to Ward during his visit. A safe mooring for a larger boat was available near the pier in the Inner Pound, and keeping the lifeboat afloat would greatly reduce the time taken to get to sea; the current launching arrangements meant that a launch could take up to half an hour to an hour, depending on the tide. No site suitable for a boathouse and launching slipway was available. This was the RNLI's preferred option, so keeping the boat on moorings was the only option if a larger boat were to be provided.

Following his visit, Ward recommended that a new boat, the same size as the Ramsgate boat, 45ft long by 11ft in beam, be built for the station and these recommendations were agreed by the

RNLI's Committee of Management at a meeting held on 3 March, with a new boat being ordered a week later. Meanwhile, the *East Anglian Daily Times* for 18 February 1881 reported that:

'The necessary arrangements having been made for stationing a larger lifeboat at this important station, it is expected that one will shortly be sent. The difficulty hitherto has been with regard to a suitable spot for mooring the boat, but this has been overcome by the selection of a site in the Lower Pound, where the boat will be kept afloat. This will render her available for service at much shorter notice than when lodged in the boathouse, the launching generally occupying valuable time. The question of procuring steam power to assist remains in abeyance for the present, although every effort has been made to secure the aid of a Government steamer.'

While the new lifeboat was under construction for the station, *Springwell* continued on station throughout the summer of 1881, and was mostly kept at the moorings her successor would occupy. However, she only completed one more effective service, on 23 October 1881, when she launched to the Swedish barque *Iris*, of Gefle, putting out at 5am in response to signals from the Cork Lightship and proceeding under sail to the Cork Sands, where the timber-laden barque was found ashore full of water. The lifeboat stood by the casualty throughout the day and, when it was realised that the vessel could not be saved, brought the twelve crew to Harwich, reaching port at 9pm having been out for the whole day.

Although the service to the barque *Iris* was *Springwell's* last effective service, during her six years on station she had undertaken numerous launches when no lives or vessels were saved, and of the twenty-six launches with which she is credited not all were 'effective' services. The statistics behind her service are therefore somewhat misleading, as the *East Anglian Daily Times* for 19 June 1878, reporting the RNLI's *Annual Report* for 1878, explained by stating that the figures

'do not represent fairly the stupendous exertions which have from time to time been put forth in the humane work by the Coxswain and crew of the Harwich lifeboat. Frequently has it been their lot to turn out on dark stormy nights, and put off in answer to signals of distress, only to find, after going a journey of from twenty to thirty miles, that their services were not required. Such things are very discouraging to the stoutest hearts, but then, on the other hand, this should only act as an incentive to further efforts, because, even though they be unsuccessful in the majority of cases, there is every cause for feeling gratified when they prove to be of service. . . As in former years, the launches of the lifeboats unattended with positive results have been very frequent, and accompanied by a large expense to the Institution. Nevertheless, it is no time for hesitation when a ship's signal of distress is either seen or heard; but, on the contrary, it is a period when judgement and promptitude are absolutely needed. Besides, lifeboat men can never tell, till they actually reach an apparently distressed vessel, that their help is not required; while, in many doubtful cases, failure to act may mean disastrous results.'

The newspaper pointed out a number of other factors that should be taken into consideration when assessing the work of the Harwich lifeboat men, explaining:

'Harwich stands at a disadvantage, so far as comparison in the actual number of lives saved is concerned, but there are few ports where a lifeboat is called upon to undertake such long journeys. At many places along the coast, such as Yarmouth, people can stand at their doors and see ships go ashore, and the work of saving life is a much shorter process there than it is here. We are not trying to throw *cold water upon or to disparage the work done by the crews of lifeboats on these stations – it is quite as much deserving praise as if their task was more arduous; but, what we desire to point out is that the Harwich lifeboat crew should be credited with that amount of eulogy which they so well merit for their gallantry.'*

Springwell (second) Lifeboat

Following the decision, taken in February 1881, to station a larger lifeboat at Harwich, an order was placed on 10 March 1881 with Woolfe & Son, the Shadwell-based boatbuilders, for a new boat measuring 45ft by 11ft, with a depth of 5ft 5in. These dimensions made her one of the largest self-righters ever built. The boat was ready by the autumn and successfully completed her harbour trials on the Thames on 27 October 1881. Sent to Harwich on 7 November 1881, she was towed to the port by the steamship *John Bowes*. The *Woodbridge Reporter* newspaper of 17 November 1881 described the arrival:

'The new boat arrived under sail, and looked in every way fit for the service of this port. The Sands are far away, and no crew can row to them in time for saving life, and in too many cases a tug is out of the question. The new boat is large and handy and will be less dependent on steam tugs. The old Springwell has been returned to London. She was sent up in tow of the tug Pacific.'

The new lifeboat, which was un-named during the first few months of her career at Harwich, was taken out on exercise for the first time on 25 November 1881, with the *East Anglian Daily Times* reporting, 'The wind was from a strong breeze to a moderate gale, and the sea was consequently rough. Starting at 11 o'clock, the boat was taken off to the Cork Sand and tried in the broken water. She behaved in a very successful manner, and the crew place great confidence in her.' Afterwards Coxswain William Britton and the crew stated that they 'were quite satisfied with her behaviour and expressed confidence in her capacity and stability'. Because she was too large to be carriage launched, the new lifeboat had to lie afloat at moorings in the Inner Pound, near the Pier, and the lifeboat house was then used as a gear store.

The new lifeboat remained unnamed until April 1882 when, 'on the strong recommendation of the local committee', the RNLI decided to name the new lifeboat *Springwell*, like her predecessor, in consideration of Miss Burmester's gift of £550 on 22 December 1875. She had also given £52 10s 0d to the RNLI towards cost of the new boat. Although a legacy of £500, bequeathed by late Mrs Fawcett of Paddington, had also been received to fund for a lifeboat for Harwich, it was arranged with Mrs Fawcett's executors that this bequest should be appropriated accordingly when the present boat was replaced or that a lifeboat bearing that name should be placed elsewhere if suitable station could be found first.

The first effective service by the second *Springwell* took place on 25 April 1882 after reports were received that a schooner was aground on the Cork Sand. *Springwell* was immediately launched and arrived on scene at about 8pm to find the schooner *Henrietta*, of London, bound from that port to Newcastle with a cargo of gunpowder. As the stranded vessel was not leaking, her crew wanted to stay on board, so the lifeboat stood by throughout the night. The schooner had been holed and so, as she was gradually sinking, her crew signalled to the lifeboat crew that they needed assistance. The lifeboat went alongside as soon as there was enough water on the Sand, took off the four crew, and landed them at Harwich at about 6.30am on 26 April. This was the first time the new lifeboat has undertaken service on the sandbanks, and afterwards the crew 'expressed themselves fully satisfied with her'.

The next service was undertaken in early 1883. At noon on 7 February 1883 *Springwell* was launched to a vessel ashore on the Shipwash Sand in strong south-easterly winds and heavy seas. The tug *Harwich* towed the lifeboat from just outside the harbour to the Sands, where the coxswain communicated with the master of a large screw steamer, *Sea*, of Aberdeen, which had been standing by the wreck and which had made several unsuccessful attempts to rescue the exhausted crew, who been in the rigging for several hours. The vessel was a total wreck, her foremast and mainmast had been carried away and she had lost her boats. The tug towed the lifeboat to windward so that she could sail down to the wreck. On arriving alongside the vessel, the barque *Lorely*, of Memel, bound from Memel to London, with a cargo of timber. The lifeboat anchored, the crew threw a grappling rope across, and, with much difficulty and danger caused by the floating wreckage, rescued her eleven-man crew, by means of the rope. The tug then towed the lifeboat back to harbour, arriving at about 6pm.

In August 1883 discussions were held with Mr Vaux, owner of the steam tug *Harwich*, who agreed to allow his steam tug to always be used to tow the lifeboat, when he considered it safe for the tug to go to sea. Enquiries were made about obtaining the services of local tugs or other steamers for helping the lifeboat get to the outlying sands when required, but the tug *Harwich* was the only viable option. Vaux was prepared to guarantee his vessel if the RNLI would agree to pay the insurance premium for the six winter months to her value of £5,000 as well as his outlay in coal, which would be £5 if the tug went to the Cork, Shipwash, Sunk or Gunfleet Sands, and £10 to the Kentish Knock. If the tug were on any such occasion to receive salvage money, Vaux agreed not to make any claim on the RNLI for towage and would donate a percentage of any salvage money to the Institution towards defraying the cost of the insurance. Enquiries had been made of Messrs Dunn, Dumas and Vylie, Insurance Brokers, Birchin Lane, and the lowest quotation obtained for insuring the tug from 1 October to 31 March was five guineas per cent, which meant an outlay each year of £262 10s 0d. The RNLI committee therefore decided that payment should be made to Vaux for each occasion when his tug was employed to tow the lifeboat, and this arrangement continued until the RNLI's own steam lifeboat was sent to Harwich.

Springwell's next service took place on 24 January 1884 when she was launched at 5.30pm into rough seas to the barge *Jessie*, of Rochester, which was carrying a cargo of stone and had gone aground on the Gunfleet Sand. Signals had been fired from the Gunfleet lightship indicating that a vessel was in difficulty, and information given to the lifeboat crew by the lightship stated that the vessel was on the 'Heaps', another part of the Sands. With a strong head wind and the tide against them, the lifeboat crew laid to until 3am the next morning, and at about 7am were able to board the vessel, which was labouring heavily in the rough seas about a mile from the Heaps Buoy. The barge was found to have lost all her sails and steering gear, and had been abandoned by her crew. The lifeboat men rigged a temporary steering gear, and then towed the vessel into Harwich harbour, arriving at about 1pm having been out on service for twenty hours. While the lifeboat was alongside the barge, two of the lifeboat men were washed overboard, but clung to the sail and were pulled on board again. As this was a salvage case, the lifeboat crew were subsequently paid £90 for their services by the owner of the barge.

Later in the same year *Springwell* completed another service, launching at about 6.30pm on 11 October 1884, in a strong wind and a heavy sea after signals had been fired from the Cork lightvessel. The three-mast schooner *Moreford and Trubey*, of Aberdeen, bound from Grangemouth to Devonport with a cargo of coal, had gone aground on the Sunk Sand and her crew had taken to the rigging. The lifeboat reached the wreck at about 3am the following morning, but it was only with difficulty that the shipwrecked men could be made to understand that help had arrived, as they were wrapped up in canvas and did not see the boat approach. Two of the men were eventually got safely into the lifeboat, but saving a third from the mizen mast proved to be extremely dangerous as a heavy sea caught the lifeboat and lifted her keel onto the wreck. Four oars were broken, the anchor was lost, and several fathoms of cable had to be cut away to prevent the boat being completely wrecked. The captain was lashed to the casualty's maintop, but the mate informed the coxswain that he had been dead some hours. So the lifeboat, with the three survivors on board, set sail for home, and near the Sunk lightvessel fell came upon the screw collier *Nereid*, of Newcastle, which towed her as far as the Cork, after which she sailed back to Harwich, arriving there at 11am after another long and difficult service.

Just over a month later *Springwell* was called out again but her crew were unable to effect any service. She put out at about 10pm on 21 November 1884 in response to signals from the sands, and was towed out by the Great Eastern Railway Company's passenger steamer *Avalon*, which was on her way to Rotterdam. However, no distressed vessel could be seen and the lifeboat returned to Harwich, arriving at 12 noon on 22 November. The Coxswain and crew subsequently reported that, throughout this service, they had to endure severe discomfort because, not only had they faced a very heavy easterly gale, but the steamer had also towed the boat too fast, meaning that:

> 'a continuous sea was flowing over them [the crew] and they were compelled to keep their heads under the thwarts, the Coxswain and another man being lashed to the bollard heads with the lifelines to enable them to steer the boat. Had they seen a wreck, they were so exhausted they feared they would have been unable to render any assistance.'

The crew were clearly upset by what had happened, understandably so, and also stated that they would not volunteer for the lifeboat again in such circumstance unless they were provided with 'proper steam towage'. Edward Birkbeck, the RNLI's Chairman, became involved and wrote to the Chairman of the Great Eastern Railway Company about the provision of better steam towage for the lifeboat. However, the Railway Company were unable to assist as they had no steam tug at Harwich and their requirements were insufficient to justify them in placing one there. So the situation persisted

The next service performed by *Springwell*, on 4 December 1886, saw her arrive at the casualty after the Walton & Frinton lifeboat *Honourable Artillery Company*, a standard 37ft self-righter that had been built in 1884. The Walton lifeboat put off at about 9.15pm and headed for the Gunfleet, then for the Long Sand, but as no signals had been seen she headed towards the Long Sand Head. Eventually the crew spotted rockets being fired, and the lifeboat found the full-rigged ship *Constanze*, of Hamburg, bound for Cardiff in ballast, carrying a crew of nineteen. The lifeboat reached the casualty, which was stranded on the Kentish Knock, at 2am and stood by for two hours. But when the weather worsened, the ship's crew were taken off and landed at 4pm the following afternoon. Meanwhile, *Springwell* had also launched, and was towed to the ship by the tug *Harwich*, but her crew found 'nothing alive . . . excepting a dog, a pig and canary'. Showing considerable skill and hard work, the Harwich crew got the vessel off so that it could be towed into Harwich by the tug.

The year 1888 proved to be a busy one for *Springwell*, with the first request for her services coming on 17 January when she went to a three-masted schooner on the Kentish Knock, but her services were not required. In the early hours of 14 March she was launched at 1.15am into a strong south-easterly gale and heavy seas to the brig *William and Anthony*, of Folkestone, which was in difficulty below Platters Buoy. The lifeboat went alongside the vessel and discovered that she had been in collision with a steamer and was leaking. So her anchor was slipped, and the lifeboat assisted her, together with her crew of eight, into harbour. On 4 June *Springwell* went to the Genoan barque *Raffaele Ligure*, which was on the Long Sand in heavy seas, but the lifeboat's service were declined.

The final service of the year came on 9 November 1888, when *Springwell* was called out after news was received that a vessel was in distress on the Gunfleet Sands. She put out at 9.30am into a gale and heavy seas, and proceeded towards the sands. However, she was unable to reach the stranded vessel, the brig *Carl Gustaf*, of Christianstad, which laden with deals from the Baltic for the Mediterranean, because of the strong tide. However, the Trinity steamer *Satellite* arrived on scene soon afterwards and towed the lifeboat into a position to effect a rescue. When the tide rose, the lifeboat was able to get close enough to the vessel to rescue her crew of nine, although the rescue proved to be extremely difficult because of the large amount of wreckage drifting around the brig. The lifeboat returned to station at 6pm, she immediately put out again after signals of distress were seen. She was recalled soon after launching, however, as the Walton lifeboat had put off instead.

The next effective service was undertaken on 2 March 1890, when *Springwell* was launched at 4.30pm and was towed by the steam tug *Harwich* to help the schooner *Mary and Maria*, of Hull, bound for London, laden with oil-cake, which had shown signals of distress while lying at anchor in Mill Bay, off Dovercourt, during stormy weather and heavy seas. On reaching the casualty, the lifeboat crew found that she was bumping heavily on the sands, so six of the lifeboat men boarded her, and helped her crew of three attach the tug's hawser, slip both anchors and chains, and enable her to be towed to Harwich, where she was safely moored alongside the pier.

Just over six months after this service, on 19 September 1890, *Springwell* was returned to London for alterations and improvements to be undertaken by Woolfe & Sons and a temporary lifeboat was sent to the station. The temporary boat was a brand new 38ft self-righting lifeboat which had been completed earlier in 1890 by Livie & Sons. Designated *Reserve No.3* during her time at Harwich, she was later stationed at Grimsby and named *Manchester Unity*. While at Harwich, she undertook several services, all in conjunction with the steam lifeboat, which are described in the following chapter.

The alterations and improvements by Woolfe were completed by June 1891 and on 5 June the boat successfully completed her harbour trial. At the end of July 1891 she was returned to station, arriving by sea and manned by the Harwich crew, after which *Reserve No.3* was withdrawn and subsequently reallocated to Grimsby. *Springwell* was out on service on 31 August 1891 in a strong south-westerly gale, but found nothing despite being at sea for fifteen hours. Upon returning to station, the crew stated that they were 'delighted with behaviour of the large sailing lifeboat' in the heavy weather after the alterations made to her.

No more effective services were performed in 1891, although the lifeboat put out on a number of occasions, including on 5 October when she was almost twelve hours searching for the reported casualty. Her next effective rescue was undertaken on 5 June 1892, when she launched, together with the Aldeburgh lifeboat *Aldeburgh*, to the barque *Ephrussi*, of Brevig, bound from Dram for London with a cargo of ice, which was stranded on the Shipwash Sands. A smack was already on scene by the time the lifeboats arrived, and the crew had been helping to throw some of the cargo overboard in order to lighten the vessel. The lifeboats stood by until the tide flowed, by when their services were not required and the ship was eventually towed off by the steam tug Harwich, which had brought *Springwell* on her outward passage from Harwich.

On the morning of 17 January 1893 *Springwell* was launched in snowy conditions after rockets fired by the Cork and Sunk lightvessel had been seen. In moderate seas the lifeboat made for the Cork lightship, being taken in tow on her way by the Ipswich steam tug *Merrimac*, which, according to the local newspaper account, 'in the absence of the much-needed steam lifeboat [described below], is able to render invaluable service in these emergencies'. Once at the Cork

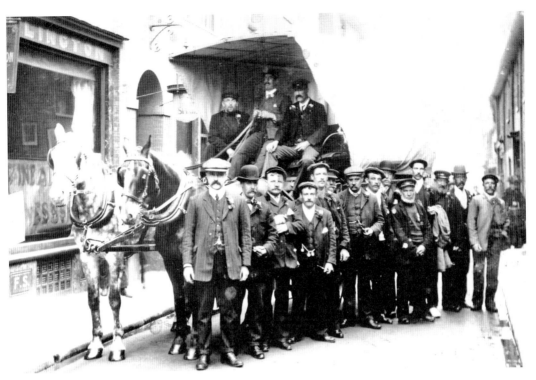

The lifeboat crew from the late nineteenth century outside the Wellington Public House in King's Head Street. (By courtesy of the late Tony Eaton)

lightvessel, the lifeboat crew found that the signals had been made in response to signals from the Sunk, and on proceeding there it was ascertained that they were in turn answering the Long Sand lightship. So the lifeboat was towed to the Long Sand vessel and found that she had a shipwrecked crew of eighteen. The wrecked ship was the steamship *Helsingor*, of Elsinore, which had stranded and sunk. The survivors were taken on board the lifeboat, which was towed back to Harwich, reaching her station at about 2.30pm.

During November 1893 *Springwell* was called out twice in the space of a week. On 4 November she was towed by the steam tug *Harwich* to help the 1,400-ton steamship *Rockcliff*, of West Hartlepool, which was stranded on the Long Sand while in ballast, bound from Rotterdam to Constantinople. The master of the tug went aboard the steamer while the lifeboat stood by for about four hours. Five lifeboat men then boarded the tug, a hawser to *Rockcliff* was rigged, and at high water the steamer was towed off the sands and proceeded under her own steam to Falmouth. The lifeboat was towed back to station by the tug, arriving at 2am the following morning.

Less than a week after the *Rockcliff* service, *Springwell* was launched again, under the command of Coxswain William Tyrrell, putting out at 2.45am on 10 November 1893 to a vessel reportedly ashore on the Long Sand, and performing a fine service. As she left harbour, she was taken in tow by the steam tug *Merrimac*, of Ipswich, and on arrival at the Longsand the lifeboat men found a large vessel aground, the 500-ton barque *St Olof*, of Mariehamn. However, the lifeboat crew could not get their boat close to the wrecked vessel until the tide rose. The fore and mizen masts of the barque were standing, but the rest of the rigging had been washed away. After waiting for sufficient water to get the boat across the sands, she was taken alongside and quickly took off nine of the

39

barque's crew, with the master and one man following, but having to be dragged through the surf to the lifeboat. As the lifeboat lay alongside, the barque began to break up, with the masts threatening to fall on *Springwell*. To avoid the risk of damaging the lifeboat, the cable had to be cut to free the boat from the wreck, and the lifeboat was then towed back to Harwich by the tug *Merrimac*.

This service was undertaken in difficult and dangerous conditions with a heavy easterly gale and high seas make the work of the rescuers particularly difficult. The lifeboat was out for more than fourteen hours and did not return to its station until 5pm. The following letter appeared in the *Shipping and Mercantile Gazette* of 13 November 1893:

> Sir, I shall be glad if you will allow me, through your valuable paper, to tender
> my own and my crew's heartfelt thanks to the coxswain and crew of the Harwich
> lifeboat, and also to Captain Tovee, of the tug Merrimac, for the brave and gallant
> manner in which they rescued us from the barque St Olof, of Mariehamn, wrecked
> on the Long Sand during a heavy gale of wind from the E. N. E., on the 10th
> November, 1893. — I am, dear Sir, your obedient servant,
> (Signed) E. J. Kahlsson. Master of barque St Olof, of Mariehamn.

At the end of November 1893, Captain E. W. Tovee, master of the tug *Merrimac*, was sent a letter by Charles Dibdin, Secretary of the RNLI, in recognition of his efforts during this service:

> I have very great pleasure in conveying to you the best thanks of the Committee
> of the Royal National Lifeboat Institution for the exceedingly kind assistance
> which you rendered to the Harwich lifeboat on the occasion of the wreck of the
> barque St Olof, of Mariehamn, on the Longsand, on the 10th inst., in a heavy
> easterly gale and a heavy sea. You and your crew of the steam tug Merrimac, under
> your command, have the satisfaction of knowing that on the occasion in question
> your kind help materially contributed to the saving of twelve fellow-sailors lives,
> and I assure you that the kind co-operation of yourself and your crew are most
> appreciated by my Committee and the crew of the Springwell.

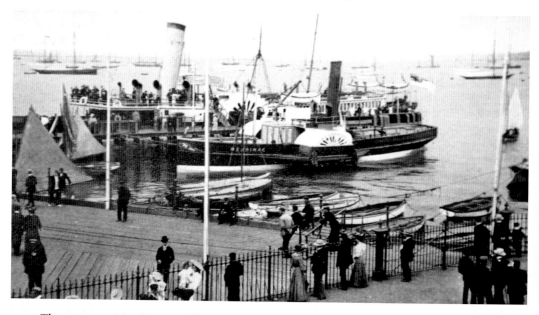

The steam tug Merrimac, used in conjunction with the pulling lifeboats for many rescues, in the Pound. (By courtesy of Ken Brand)

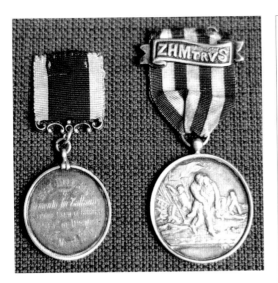

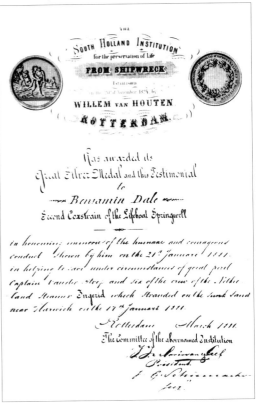

The Silver medal (above) and testimonial certificate (right) presented to Benjamin Dale by the South Holland Lifeboat Service for the service to the steamer Ingerid. (By courtesy of Ken Brand and Harwich RNLI)

On 19 February 1894 another vessel was helped off the sands by *Springwell*, which put out at 8.45am in response to a telephone message received from the Gunfleet lightvessel and signals shown by the Sunk lightvessel. The lifeboat was towed by the steam tug *Harwich* to the Sunk, and then on to the Long Sand where they found the barque *Eboe*, of Liverpool, bound from Rotterdam for the West Coast of Africa with a general cargo, stranded. To help get her afloat, eleven lifeboat men went aboard, stowed the sails, got up the anchors, and attached tow ropes from the steam tugs *Harwich* and *Merrimac*, which were both on scene. The barque was successfully towed off the sand and taken into Harwich harbour.

By the time of this service, the steam lifeboats had become established at Harwich, and after the station's second such boat, *City of Glasgow*, had arrived in November 1894, as described in the following chapter, she was used for the majority of services during the 1890s. However, the sailing lifeboat was still called out, but it was almost three years after the *Eboe* service that *Springwell* and her crew completed another effective service. During the intervening years, the lifeboat had been out to a number of vessels, mostly unknown, which had stranded on the sands, but none of the launches resulted in the casualty being found.

Her next effective service took place on 23 January 1897 after the schooner *Sancho Panza*, of Faversham, carrying coal from Sunderland for Ramsgate, broke adrift from her anchors in a north-easterly gale and very heavy seas, and stranded on the Pye Sands. She hoisted a signal of distress, and at 9.30am *Springwell* launched to her assistance and rescued her six crew. The lifeboat also picked up a smack's boat, with five men on board, who had attempted to rescue the schooner's crew but their small boat been overwhelmed by the wind and sea, putting them in considerable danger. The lifeboat returned to station at 1pm with the survivors, with her own crew having

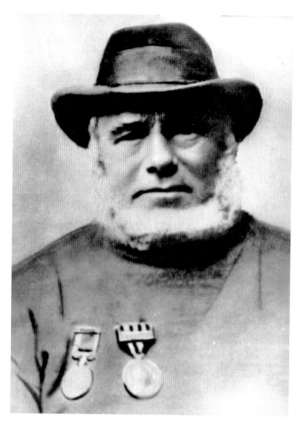

William Britton, Coxswain from 1880 to 1883, was voted £10 on his retirement. During his three years in the post, the lifeboat had assisted to save seventy lives from shipwreck. During the service to Lorely in February 1883 he had been injured causing a rupture which would necessitate his constantly wearing a truss. (By courtesy of Harwich RNLI)

endured a very difficult time in intensely cold weather accompanied by blinding snow squalls. The schooner subsequently became a total wreck.

In December 1898 an unusual matter was brought to the attention of the RNLI when the local committee expressed concern about 'the large amount of spirits consumed by the crew of the lifeboat whenever they were out in the boat'. The amount spent on spirits was recorded as being £4 8s 9d in 1895, £3 7s 7d in 1896 and £4 1s 3d in 1897, and it was not stated where this money came from. The practice had been going on for a number of years, but in 1898 the crew were informed that it must be discontinued for exercises. Towards the end of December 1898 the Honorary Secretary reported to the RNLI that 'he had been unable to obtain a satisfactory explanation from the Coxswains on this subject, but he was taking such steps as he thought would prevent an improper consumption of spirits in future'. After this, the matter seems to have been closed and the money spent on alcohol is not recorded.

The last two services undertaken by the 1881-built *Springwell* came in the last two years of the nineteenth century. On 17 October 1898 she launched at 6.45am to the barque *Inga*, of Laurvig, and stood by the vessel until 4pm. The barque had gone aground on the Gunfleet in moderate seas. The last service was undertaken on 2 November 1899, when *Springwell* saved five crew from the barquentine *Pactolus*, of London, which had grounded on the West Rocks. The following day, HM gunboat *Onyx* landed the captain and three other men, who had remained with the vessel but been forced to abandon her after she filled with water, making it impossible to get her off the rocks.

Although this was the last effective service rendered by *Springwell*, she undertook several more service launches, none of which resulted in any assistance being rendered. On 8 December 1899 *Springwell* was called out in a severe storm, undertaking a fruitless search at the Shingle Street, close to Bawdsey. During the search undertaken in pitch darkness, as the lifeboat was towed by the tug *Merrimac*, the Coxswain's son William Dale was washed overboard, while attending the ropes, near the Shipwash sands. The severe gale force winds and darkness made it very difficult for the lifeboat crew to find their fellow crewman, but the tow rope to the tug was immediately cut and the man was rescued after spending twenty minutes in the water. He could not swim, but fortuitously was kept afloat by his lifebelt.

At the beginning of the twentieth century, the usefulness of the sailing lifeboat, when a steam lifeboat was also on station, was being called into question but not before the lifeboat was badly damaged by a barge, which broke adrift in the Pound on the night of 28 January 1901. The boat was taken to McLearon's yard in Harwich to be repaired, after being examined by the RNLI's Assistant Surveyor. The owners of the barge paid the cost of the repairs, which amounted to £46. While the boat was being repaired, it was decided she should undergo her triennial overhaul under the supervision of an Assistant Surveyor, and this was completed by September 1901, after which she was returned to service.

Once *Springwell* was back on station after being repaired, consideration was given as to her replacement. She was almost twenty years old and was more or less at the end of her service life. However, when the question of a replacement was raised in January 1902, the District Inspector stated that he considered the No.1 Station was no longer necessary as 'the new steam lifeboat was most efficient and could render all the assistance required, and while she was being repaired, the Aldeburgh, Walton and Clacton boats could do the work'. A decision was deferred by the Chief Inspector, who believed that the sailing lifeboat should be replaced by a new boat.

Meanwhile, *Springwell* remained in service but in something of a poor condition, and in June 1902, after the Surveyor of Lifeboats had found she was need of various repairs but as she was twenty-one years old she was not worth spending more money on, she was withdrawn from service. In August 1902 the local committee expressed their wish for a new boat, and in October the crew of the sailing lifeboat agree to man the *Reserve No.3* lifeboat, a 39ft by 9ft self-righting type, until a new sailing lifeboat had been built and while the steam lifeboat was away being repaired. As the steam lifeboat could not always be relied upon to be operational, providing a new sailing lifeboat for the station was essential, and towards the end of 1902 the Coxswain and crew were asked to decide on the type most suitable for service at Harwich. Meanwhile, the question of closing the No.1 station was not raised again.

Ann Fawcett Lifeboat

Once the decision had been made to provide a new lifeboat for Harwich, a deputation from the crew visited various neighbouring stations in November 1902 to look at other lifeboats. Having assessed the various boats, they asked for one similar to that at Clacton-on-Sea but 3ft longer and 1ft wider with two water ballast tanks, and for it to be decked like the Walton-on-the-Naze lifeboat. The District Inspector did not concur with this request, and as the crew disliked the 39ft x 9ft self-righting lifeboat on temporary duty at Harwich, they were agreed to have a boat designed by and named after the RNLI's Consulting Naval Architect, George L. Watson. The Watson type boat measured 43ft by 12ft 6in, carried ten oars double-banked and was fitted with two sliding or drop keels to 'increase her weatherly qualities whilst in deep water', according to the *East Anglian Daily Times*. The newspaper explained, 'she belongs to the class of powerful sailing life-boats' making her ideally suited for service to the outlying sands.

Funding for the new boat had been agreed in July 1902, when it was appropriated to the legacy of £450 bequeathed by the late Mrs Fawcett of Norfolk Terrace, West London, to provide a lifeboat named *Ann Fawcett* for the Harwich station. A further donation was received towards the end of 1902, this one from John S. C. Chadwick of Rochdale, who presented £543 to the RNLI towards the cost of a new lifeboat, stating that he did not want his name to be disclosed or have anything to do with the naming of the boat, so he remained anonymous at the time. The Committee therefore decided to appropriate this contribution towards the cost of the new lifeboat by adding it to the late Mrs Fawcett's bequest, with the boat expected to cost more than £1,000.

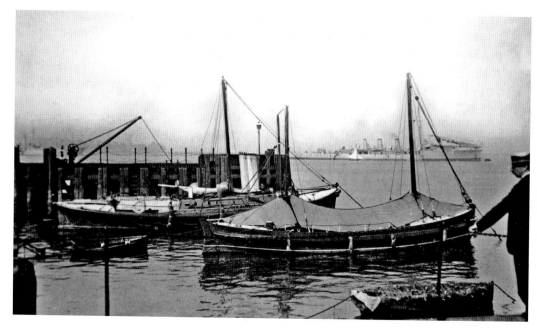

Ann Fawcett, covered with a tarpaulin, and City of Glasgow at moorings in the Pound, which provided a sheltered mooring for both boats. During the early years of the twentieth century it as unusual for lifeboats to be kept afloat at moorings.

The new Watson lifeboat was built by Thames Ironworks at Blackwall, London, and completed her harbour trials satisfactorily on 3 March 1904. She was one of a number of new boats completed in 1904 by Thames Ironworks, with the others going to Polkerris, Bull Bay, Troon and Port Erroll. *Ann Fawcett* successfully completed her harbour trial on 3 March 1904 and two weeks later left for Harwich, being sailed to her new station by Coxswain Ben Dale and some of the Harwich crew. On 6 April 1904 she was taken out on exercise by the District Inspector for the first time, putting out in a south-westerly wind force seven with little sea. The Coxswain and crew stated afterwards that they were 'satisfied on the whole' with the new boat, but thought the sails were small.

With the steam lifeboat being used for the majority of services, *Ann Fawcett's* first effective rescue was not undertaken until 1911, more than seven years after she had arrived at Harwich. Although she had been called out a few times before, her services had never been required with the casualty either not found or getting to safety unaided. In an easterly gale, accompanied by snow and sleet showers, creating very rough seas off Harwich, the brigantine *Lenore*, of Faversham, got into difficulty at the mouth of the harbour on 5 April 1911. *Ann Fawcett* put out at 5pm and rescued the brigantine's six crew, returning to station at 7.30pm to land the survivors.

The lifeboat completed another service shortly afterwards, on 25 June 1911, after the Coastguard telephoned to say that a vessel was burning flares and in need of assistance off East Lane Point during a heavy south-westerly gale. *Ann Fawcett* proceeded to Shingle Street and found the schooner *L'Espoir de L'Avenir*, of Rotterdam, with six men aboard, aground and her rudder gone. The captain of the schooner gave charge of the vessel to the Coxswain so that he could try to save her. The lifeboat stood by for two hours while efforts were made, and the Coxswain then sent to Harwich for the help of a tug. The tug *Garnet* succeeded in getting the schooner afloat, and the lifeboat then took up station astern to act as a rudder for the damaged craft, so tug and lifeboat worked together to bring the vessel safely into Harwich. This service, undertaken in very heavy seas, tested the endurance of the lifeboat crew, who were at sea for twelve hours.

The next service launch by *Ann Fawcett* was an even longer one for the lifeboat men, even though the outcome saw no service being effected. The lifeboat launched at 6.30pm on 26 September 1911 to the steamship *James Bennett*, of Goole, and was towed by the tug *W. D. Satellite* as far as the Cork End Buoy. Then, because of very light winds, the crew had to row the next part of the journey. Good progress was made and the lifeboat reached the West Rocks about 8pm, but the crew found no sign of a vessel needing assistance. They went on to the Sunk Light, where they were told that a light steam trader had been ashore on the West Rocks, but had floated off unaided. A torpedo boat was also seen at the West Rocks, and so the lifeboat men signalled to it, requesting a tow back to the harbour, but the lifeboat's signals were not understood and ignored. As the boat remained becalmed, the lifeboat men had to use the oars, and they rowed throughout the night, covering an estimated thirty miles until a breeze started again enabling them to set the sails. *Ann Fawcett* returned to harbour at 10am on 27 September, taking up her moorings in the Pound having been out for fifteen hours on a fruitless search.

The final service performed by *Ann Fawcett* took place on 6 January 1912, when the spritsail barge *Monarch*, of London, got into difficulties off Harwich while bound from London to Yarmouth. Her steering gear failed and, when three miles south east of the port, she fired distress signals which were seen by the Coastguard who passed the information to Coxswain Dale. *Ann Fawcett* was launched at 12.50pm and soon reached the vessel, which the lifeboat men were engaged to salvage. They went aboard and successfully brought her into the harbour at 3.45pm, having had to contend with rough seas and a moderate gale throughout a difficult service.

Just over a month after this service, on 8 February 1912, the District Inspector again considered the necessity of retaining the sailing lifeboat at Harwich and believed that closing either the Harwich No.1 or Walton-on-the-Naze stations should be considered. The decision was made on 9 May 1912 at an RNLI Committee of Management meeting, when it was decided to close the No.1 station and withdraw *Ann Fawcett*. The Deputy Chief Inspector had recommended this course of action, while also suggesting that the Reserve boat at Clacton be stored at Harwich in the care of

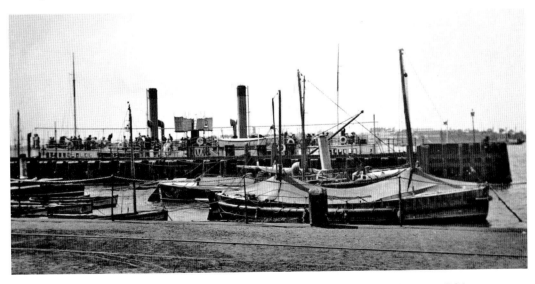

Another view of the Pound with Ann Fawcett at moorings alongside the steam lifeboat City of Glasgow and a steamer at the other side of the pier.

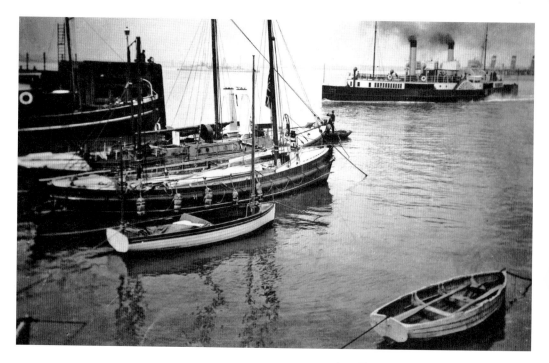

Ann Fawcett at moorings alongside the steam lifeboat City of Glasgow in the Pound, with a steamer about to pass the pier. (Supplied by Ken Brand)

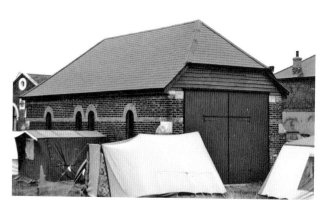

(Left) Very few photos were taken of the 1871 boathouse as the whole area of Harwich promenade, from Naval Yard to Dovercourt, was managed by the government's War Department. The boathouse, pictured in 1989, was later bought by Essex County Council and passed to the Harwich Society in 1993. (Nicholas Leach)

the permanent crew of the steam lifeboat so that, during extensive overhauls or repairs of either the steam boat or the Clacton motor boat, the Reserve boat could be placed at either station as necessary. However, the committee did not think that a Reserve boat was required at Harwich and so none was supplied.

The station was officially closed in October 1912 and *Ann Fawcett* was sailed to London, where she was taken to the RNLI's Depot, having gained a record in her eight years at Harwich of fifteen lives saved in sixteen service launches. She was later allocated to Dun Laoghaire, a station covering Dublin Bay, where she served for a further six years before being sold out of service in 1920. The moorings were left at Harwich so that they could be used by motor lifeboats calling at the port while on trials. Meanwhile, in August 1912 the retiring Coxswain, Benjamin Dale, was given a gratuity of £11 5s 0d and the Second Coxswain, James Dale, a pension of £5 17s 6d per annum.

Steam Lifeboats

Harwich was one of only a handful of lifeboat stations that were served by steam lifeboats, which were designed and built towards the end of the nineteenth century to become the RNLI's first powered lifeboats. A steam lifeboat seemed the obvious way forward considering the number of times the pulling and sailing lifeboats were towed to a rescue by steam-powered tugs. At a number of the major ports on the east coast this arrangement existed, with pulling and sailing lifeboats working in conjunction with a local steam tug at Ramsgate, Gorleston and Harwich. Many coxswains and crews regarded this as an ideal arrangement, as the close-quarters manoeuvrability of a pulling lifeboat when attending a wreck was better than that

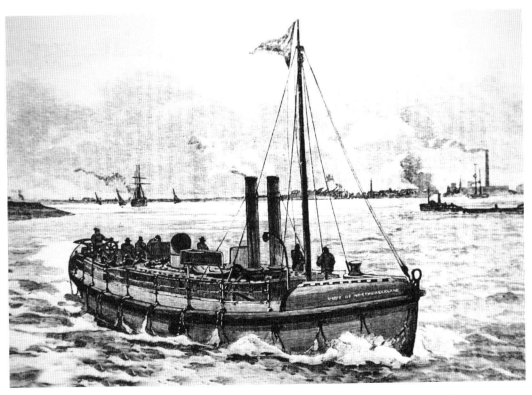

The RNLI's first steam lifeboat Duke of Northumberland from a contemporary drawing.

of a larger and more cumbersome steam tug, which itself was ideal in getting to a distant casualty. However, a steam lifeboat, operated by the RNLI and thus ready specifically for life-saving duties, would offer many advantages over a lifeboat relying on sails, oars or a combination of the two.

By the 1880s steam had been used for many years to power ships of all sizes, but doubts existed about the efficiency of steam-powered craft when used for life-saving and designing and building a steam powered lifeboat presented lifeboat naval architects with a difficult set of challenges to those of pulling lifeboat design. However, the advantages it offered convinced the RNLI to go ahead with construction and a special sub-committee was set up to examine designs for a mechanically-drive lifeboat. Although none of the plans was deemed practicable, a design by the London-based boatbuilder R. and H. Green, of Blackwall, in June 1888 was found to be more suitable. Green's plans were then modified by the RNLI, which then ordered Green to build a steam lifeboat.

This prototype steam lifeboat was completed in 1889 and, after being launched from her builder's yard on the Thames in the spring, made her first trial trip on 31 May 1889. She was named *Duke of Northumberland* in honour of the sixth Duke, who was president of the Institution at the time, and the fourth Duke, who had been heavily involved in improving the fortunes of the RNLI in the 1850s. The Thornycroft engine with which she was fitted, with its 'patent tubulous pattern' boiler, produced 170hp and drove hydraulic pumps, which were in effect water jets. She was built of mild steel and was very strongly riveted, having a third more rivets than a torpedo boat of comparable size. She measured 50ft in length, had a moulded breadth of 12ft and an extreme breadth, over the wales, of 14ft 3¾in. Her extreme draught with thirty passengers, all her crew and full bunkers was 3ft 6in, in which condition her displacement was twenty-three tons. On 4 August 1890 she was taken to the Maplin measured mile for speed trials, averaging more than nine knots. With a full bunker of three tons of coal, her radius of action was 254 miles at eight and a half knots.

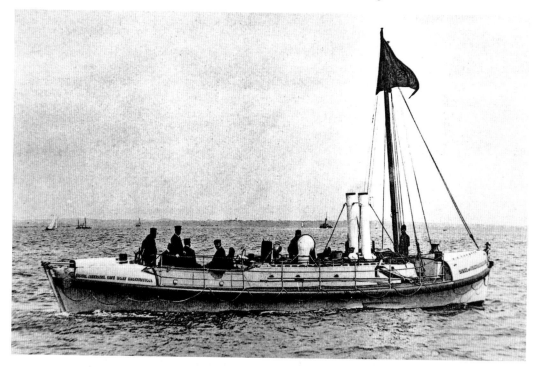

The RNLI's first steam lifeboat Duke of Northumberland on trials in the early 1890s after being built by R. & H. Green. (By courtesy of the RNLI)

Duke of Northumberland soon proved that steam had many advantages over pulling and sailing. Not only were steam lifeboats able to head into the wind, they could also tow a sailing or pulling lifeboat if necessary. But their drawbacks included their size, 50ft in length and more than 30 tons in weight, which restricted the number of places where they could be stationed. They had to be kept moored afloat at a time when lifeboats were kept afloat only as a last resort as anti-fouling paints were not as effective as now. Getting up the steam necessary before setting out could take twenty minutes and even then the boats were comparatively slow, making no more than seven knots in practice despite better speeds reached during trials. Manning was also problematic as they required specialist engineers to service the boiler whilst their relatively large draught meant they were not ideal for shallow water operation. But despite the difficulties, steam lifeboats remained in RNLI service for almost three decades and are credited with saving more than 600 lives.

During a summer running trials in and around the Thames estuary, the prototype steam lifeboat *Duke of Northumberland* called at Sheerness, Southend and Harwich a number of times. One of her visits to Harwich was described in the *East Anglian Daily Times* for 26 July 1890:

> The Royal National Lifeboat Institution has produced the latest novelty in shipbuilding in the shape of a steam lifeboat, and on Thursday (24th) afternoon this wonderful little craft was on view. She lay in the Thames at Blackwall Pier, and attracted a considerable amount of attention. Visitors were received on board by Charles Dibdin, RNLI Secretary, and Captain The Right Hon H. W. Chetwynd, RN, chief Inspector of Lifeboats. At three o'clock precisely the order was given to get under way, and the lifeboat at once steamed easily down the river, returning to Blackwall after a very successful run of rather more than a couple of hours. Those who had the good fortune to be on board were charmed with the handiness of the boat and the ingenuity of its construction and machinery.

As steam lifeboats had to be kept afloat, Harwich, with its sailing lifeboat already at moorings, was in an ideal position to receive one. In fact, three of the RNLI's six steam lifeboats went on to serve the station, over almost three decades, and undertook numerous rescues, with *Duke of Northumberland* being placed on station in September 1890. When she was first placed at Harwich, the RNLI imposed the condition that, whenever she went out on service, she would take the sailing lifeboat with her. As a result, all her services involved the station's self-righting lifeboat *Reserve No.3*, which was temporarily on station while Harwich's own boat was undergoing alterations, being fitted with the latest improvements. *Duke of Northumberland* undertook her first service on 8 October, within a month of arriving at Harwich, when she went to the Cork Sand and stood by the brigantine *Ada*, of Faversham, which was aground. The lifeboats went to the Cork lightship, and from there found the brigantine, which was bound from Hartlepool for London, with a crew of six. At the master's request the lifeboats stood by the ship until high water, when the brigantine was towed off by a steam tug and taken to Harwich.

Less than two weeks later, *Duke of Northumberland* was in action again, taking *Reserve No.3* in tow after signals had been fired by the Cork lightvessel. The lifeboats put out at 4am on 20 October 1890 and found the 913-ton steamship *Achilles*, of Sunderland, aground on the middle of the Shipwash Sand in a moderate north-westerly gale and heavy seas. The vessel was bound from *Riga* for London carrying railway sleepers, with a crew of twenty-one. On nearing the sand, the lifeboat men saw a tar-barrel burning on the vessel, and *Reserve No.3* was towed alongside. The master asked the lifeboat crews to lighten the ship, so some of the cargo of railway sleepers was thrown overboard, which enabled the vessel to float off at high tide. The steam lifeboat, working with the steam tug Harwich, then towed the steamer clear of the sands, so the vessel could resume

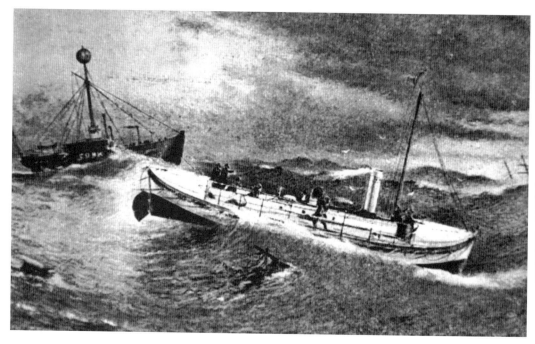

Print of Duke of Northumberland on service in rough seas by the Cork lightvessel. (By courtesy of Ken Brand)

her voyage to London. The lifeboat men went back to their respective boats and returned to their station, arriving at 6pm. The weekly publication *Vanity Fair* summed up the benefits of the steam lifeboat after this rescue, saying 'Apart from doing her own work, the *Duke* towed one of the Institution's lifeboats to the rescue of the wreck, arriving there three hours sooner than a boat rowing and sailing could possibly have done'.

Duke of Northumberland was called out again soon afterwards, launching at 10am on 13 November 1890 and taking *Reserve No.3* in tow. They went to the upper part of the Long Sand, where the three-masted schooner *Christine Elisabeth*, of Haugesund, bound from Rotterdam for Moluccas, East Indies, with a general cargo, had stranded. A pilot cutter and a steam tug were lying alongside the casualty, with the ship's crew on one of these two vessels. The four men who were in the tug's boat were taken on board the steam lifeboat, after which the lifeboat men got on board the vessel, worked the pumps, and prepared her for towing off at the next tide. At midnight the schooner was towed clear, but when a heavy fog descended she was anchored until daybreak, when the fog cleared off. The vessel was then got underway, and she reached Harwich at 8.30am.

In early 1891 *Duke of Northumberland* completed two effective services, both with Reserve No.3 lifeboat. The first was on the morning of 6 January, in a fresh gale from the north east, snow squalls and a very heavy sea. The ketch *Day's*, of Barrow, carrying scrap iron from London for Newcastle, was wrecked on the Cork Sands. As the lifeboats neared the casualty, the lifeboat men saw three men in the rigging, two of whom waved for help. *Reserve No.3* was towed close to the sunken wreck, and her crew threw grappling irons and life lines to the two men, who tied them round themselves, jumped into the water, and were pulled into the lifeboat, exhausted and numb. The third man in the rigging was dead. The boats then promptly returned to their station, where the men were landed and looked after. The coxswain of the steam lifeboat then decided to return to the wreck to bring ashore the dead body, which had been left in the rigging. The boat therefore returned to the wreck, and one of the crew of *Reserve No.3* jumped onto the rigging, untied the man's body which was then dragged on board the lifeboat using a line.

What proved to be the final service by *Duke of Northumberland* while she was at Harwich came on 3 March 1891, when she went to the three-masted schooner *Mercury*, of Aberdeen, taking the *Reserve No.3* lifeboat with her. The schooner had stranded on the Long Sand in a moderate north-westerly gale, heavy seas and steady rain. The lifeboats reached the Sunk lightvessel, which confirmed the casualty's position. The boats reached the casualty quickly and the schooner's twelve crew were taken into the steam lifeboat and landed at Harwich at 1.30am.

On 17 April 1891 the RNLI's Chief Inspector came to Harwich with representatives of the KZHMRS, the South Holland Lifeboat Society, and were taken out by the steam lifeboat. The Dutch visitors requested not to go out to sea but instead to go upriver to Parkeston as they were later going to be travelling back to their home country and wanted to stay dry. During their short trip in calm waters they were reported to be 'much pleased with the boat', while the station's Chief Engineer and Coxswain 'spoke in very high terms of her'. Subsequently the Dutch Lifeboat Society had two steam lifeboats built, the first by Thornycroft at Chiswick, named *President van Heel*. Both boats were operated from the important Hook of Holland station.

Although *Duke of Northumberland* remained on service at Harwich for a further sixteen months after this service, for much of that time she was undergoing repairs and was also sent to Lowestoft to participate in the lifeboat trials held there in March 1892. The first problem with the boat was found at the same time as the Dutch visitors came to Harwich, with the dial plates for directing the discharge of water found to be unsatisfactory. Further problems were found in August 1891 when *Duke of Northumberland* was hauled up for painting. The heads of bolts securing the intake near the pump were worn away, probably by galvanic action caused by copper grating at the intake's mouth. The intake was replaced by a cast steel one of a different pattern by Thornycroft, who undertook the necessary repairs at their Chiswick yard on the Thames in September 1891 at a cost of £199 19s 0d. They also gave the boat a thorough examination before she was sent back to station. Soon after these repairs had been completed, the District Inspector discussed with the RNLI's Committee of Management a request from the local committee and Coxswain that the

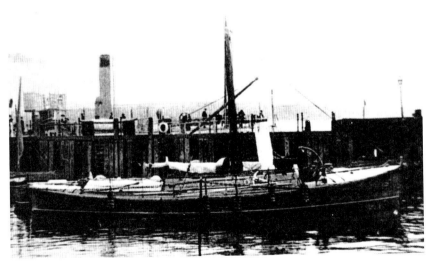

Duke of Northumberland at moorings in the Pound while on duty at Harwich. She was on station for less than two years but saved thirty-three lives in that time. (By courtesy of Ken Brand)

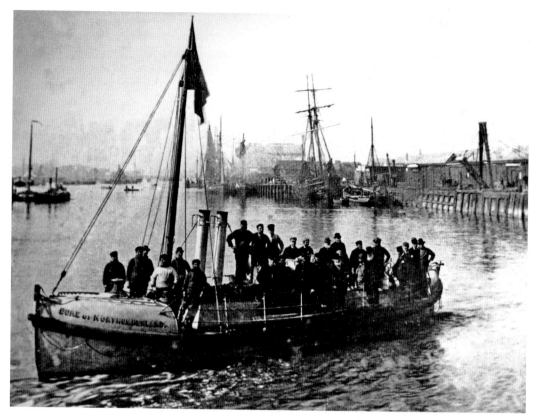

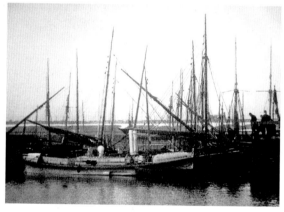

Duke of Northumberland at Lowestoft during the lifeboat trials in 1892. She did not participate in the trials to be compared with the other lifeboat types, but was mainly used for towing the heavy tubular lifeboat. (By courtesy of Ken Brand)

steam lifeboat be allowed to go out on service independently of the sailing lifeboat. The Committee consented to this request in February 1892 with the condition that, when the boat was out on service alone, an additional crew member must be taken.

Before *Duke of Northumberland* could undertake any services alone, however, she was sent to Lowestoft for a fortnight to take part in the competitive trials of lifeboats. She arrived at Lowestoft on 19 February 1892 after a passage from Harwich, during which her feed pump broke down, and remained there throughout the trials, which lasted from 12 February until 19 April, being used mainly for towing the heavy tubular lifeboat. The trials involved assessing four different types pulling and sailing lifeboats – a Norfolk & Suffolk sailing lifeboat, a Watson sailing lifeboat,

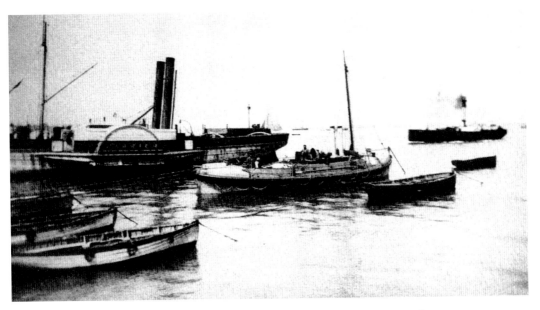

Duke of Northumberland in the harbour, 1891. (By courtesy of Ken Brand)

a self-righter and the Tubular – to ascertain which best coped with the variety of sea conditions encountered. The tests did not involve assessing the steam lifeboat, other than in her capacity to tow the lifeboats. *Duke of Northumberland* was used to tow the lifeboats through heavy break seas as well as steaming against a tug towing a lifeboat in bad weather and a heavy sea, with the steam lifeboat's performance considered 'most satisfactory'. The tug reached a top speed of seven and a half knots an hour and the steam lifeboat was able to kept up with her, 'the tug being then pressed as hard against the sea as prudent'.

After the trials, *Duke of Northumberland* returned to Harwich, but on 25 May 1892 she was taken out of the water to be examined on the slip by a Lloyd's surveyor, who recommended various repairs be carried out. After a further month at Harwich, during which she was not used on service, the RNLI decided that the boat should be taken elsewhere to be assessed at other stations. So she left Harwich on 22 July 1892, with a record of thirty-three lives saved in less than two years, and was initially sent to Cowes Regatta, where she was opened up for visitors to look over. After some repairs had been completed at Cowes, she was reallocated to the Holyhead station on Anglesey, where she served from October 1892 to May 1893. She then had a brief stint at New Brighton, at the entrance to the river Mersey, before returning to Holyhead in December 1897 and staying at the Anglesey station until November 1922.

City of Glasgow

Meanwhile, at Harwich, where a steam lifeboat was regarded as important, a new craft was placed on station on 7 November 1894. The new boat, named *City of Glasgow*, was the RNLI's second steam lifeboat and had been funded through the Glasgow Lifeboat Saturday Fund. Designed by the RNLI's Naval Architect, George Lennox Watson, she was built by R. & H. Green at Blackwall, builders of *Duke of Northumberland*, at a cost of £2,639 10s 0d. She had different machinery to *Duke of Northumberland*, although she was still jet-propelled, but was slightly larger than the prototype at 53ft long with a 16ft beam. Her machinery installation consisted of a Penn patent water-tube boiler, which drove two vertical turbines via a 200hp compound engine. The danger of having the intakes fouled was obviated by making the intakes flush with the full plating, in place of the Thornycroft patent scope which was used on the first steam boat. The engines operated at 358-420rpm and produced 220-230 indicated horse power, giving a maximum speed of 9.3 knots and an economical speed of 7.34 knots. Her bunkers carried four tons of coal and half a ton of fresh water, and she could accommodate up to forty survivors.

City of Glasgow visited her namesake city on 16 June 1894 for a Lifeboat Saturday demonstration and publicity visit, during which she was officially named by Mrs Bell, the wife of the city's Lord Provost. She then had to return to her builder's for a few finishing touches before being sent to Harwich, arriving at the port on 7 November 1894. Her construction was reported by the *East Anglian Daily Times* in April 1894, which was describing general developments within the RNLI, and concluded that: 'The [RNLI's] Committee are sanguine that the new steam lifeboat will quite fulfil their favourable anticipations, as they believe she will possess many material improvements on the old boat, suggested by experience.'

However, their confidence in the new boat was somewhat misplaced, and throughout her time at Harwich many problems with the boat were experienced. In March 1895, while she was returning to station from service, the tubes of the condensers started leaking, a defect which the Chief Engineer repaired. In June 1895 the crew expressed their dissatisfaction with the boat's trim, which was down by the stern, while the Chief Engineer stated that the after tank could not be used as a reserve for fresh water, which was needed because of the amount of water wasted by the inefficiency of the boiler. Alterations were made as a result of these comments, and these, according to the deckhands and engine room staff, 'greatly improved the boat'. However, the problems persisted and on 31 October 1895, again while returning from service, the lifeboat's exhaust pipe cracked round the flange and further repairs were needed. A year later the joint of the low pressure valve casing cover of the boat burst, and more repairs had to be carried out.

Perhaps the most serious incident occurred in January 1897 after the port inlet joint started leaking two hours after *City of Glasgow* had returned from exercise. This was so serious that the lifeboat had to be taken to London for the repairs to be effected. Although the Chief Engineer effected temporary repairs for the passage, when the lifeboat reached Sheerness during her journey south, so much water was coming into the engine room that the Deputy Chief Inspector, who was in charge, had to ground her on a mudbank in Sheerness. The Chief Engineer improvised a further repair, with help from dockyard storekeepers at Sheerness, using Portland cement to stop the leak, but as mud had leaked in as well as water, it was impossible to use the engines. So the following day, 6 January, she had to be towed to R. & H. Green's yard at Blackwall. The repairs took three months and *City of Glasgow* did not return to station until 14 April 1897, the work having cost £235, with the return journey from Blackwall to Harwich undertaken at seven knots per hour. Following the near sinking of the boat off Sheerness, the engine room staff were formally thanked by the RNLI's Committee of Management 'for their arduous duties in bringing the boat up', and Captain Brunell RN, Captain Superintendent of Sheerness Dockyard, and the dockyard storekeeper were also thanked 'for their courtesy and assistance'.

But only three months later, on 10 July 1897, a severe leak developed in *City of Glasgow's* steel starboard pipe, flooding the engine room when the lifeboat was undertaking a Lifeboat Saturday demonstration at Ipswich. Although the leak was plugged, the boat had to be taken to London on 13 July for repairs. However, before arriving at Blackwall the other pipe developed a serious leak. The repairs by Green took two months to complete, and *City of Glasgow* returned to station on 8 September 1897 under the command of the District Inspector. The journey took thirteen hours during which time the engines worked satisfactorily.

From 24 November 1897 to 1 February 1898 *City of Glasgow* went to Gorleston for trials to ascertain whether that station could operate a steam lifeboat. However, on one occasion, she suffered the ignominy of being swept backwards while trying to negotiate a strong tide rip, and the Gorleston crew soon returned her to Harwich. The persistent mechanical and technical problems from which she suffered eventually led to her replacement and withdrawal in May 1901, and then her sale from service five months later for £100.

Despite *City of Glasgow* needing so many repairs, she undertook a number of services while at Harwich, saving four lives during her first stint, from 1894 to November 1897, and a further twenty-eight between February 1898 and October 1901. The following descriptions cover the majority of her effective services, the first of which was completed on 6 June 1895, although she had been out a number of times before this without completing any service, including spending almost ten hours at sea on 13 March 1895 attending to the steamer *Roumania*, of West Hartlepool, which was aground on the Kentish Knock. But her service in June proved more successful, when she went out in the morning through rough seas to the schooner *Hans*, of Rendsburg, bound for Colchester, laden with oil cake and manned by four crew. The vessel had lost her steering gear and, leaking badly, was aground on the West Rocks. Some of the lifeboat men boarded her, and she was taken in tow, with the vessels reaching Harwich at 5.35am on 7 June.

More than two years passed until another effective service was completed. On 25 October 1897 *City of Glasgow* went to the barque *Triton*, of Rostock, bound from Raumo in Finland for Port Natal. The barque had grounded on the Shipwash Sands but had managed to get off unaided only to go aground again, this time on the Cork Sands, while making for Harwich. *City of Glasgow*

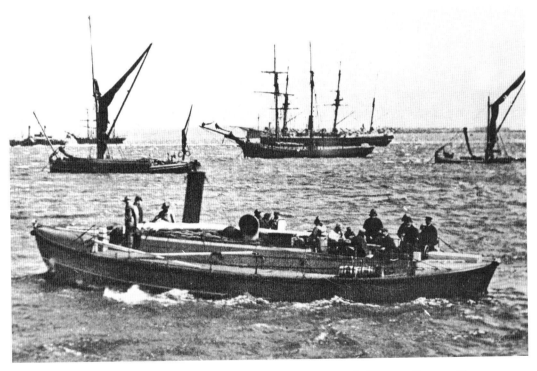

The first City of Glasgow on trials, probably somewhere in the Thames Estuary. She proved to be less than satisfactory and her career at Harwich was blighted by technical problems (By courtesy of the RNLI)

launched at 2.45am to go to her aid and, assisted by the volunteer lifeboat *True to the Core* from Walton, a 40ft Norfolk & Suffolk sailing lifeboat, stood by the casualty until 8.30am. The lifeboat crews then helped to refloat the barque before bringing her into Harwich harbour at 10am.

On 30 January 1899 *City of Glasgow* performed a messenger service after the Long Sand lightvessel was seen flying a distress signal. The lifeboat put out and the Harwich crew found two mechanics were on the lightship and they needed to get ashore. Although the lightship's crew had tried to communicate with a passing steamer, the steamer reported to the Kentish Knock lightvessel that the Long Sand was signalling but misunderstanding the message resulting in the signals misinterpreted as distress signals. However, the two men were taken into the lifeboat and landed at Harwich by the steam lifeboat.

The final service undertaken by *City of Glasgow* during her stop-start career at Harwich came on the morning of 30 March 1901 and saw her crew complete a fine rescue. With a southerly gale raging, whipping up heavy seas off the harbour entrance, a telephone message was received from Felixstowe stating that a schooner was aground on the St Andrew's Shoal, off Felixstowe, flying signals of distress. *City of Glasgow* left her moorings at 9.10am and found the ninety-seven-ton schooner *Rose*, of and for Ipswich, laden with granite from Guernsey. Hundreds of people had gathered on the beach to watch as men from the Coastguard, under Chief Officer King, launched their galley. After several attempts, they managed to get their craft afloat, but it was driven back by the gale. Further attempts also proved fruitless and the boat was eventually capsized in the breakers, leaving it useless.

By this time *City of Glasgow* had arrived on scene, but the strong winds and heavy seas made approaching the wreck difficult and dangerous. After several attempts, and with the crowd cheering them on, the lifeboat crew succeeded in getting a line aboard the wreck. With the lifeboat then able to approach the wreck, she got close enough for the sailors, one by one, to jump to safety. Three men were rescued, but the fourth slipped between the lifeboat and the casualty as he stepped across. Fortunately, one of the lifeboat men caught hold of his arm, and with the help of another lifeboat man got him on board the lifeboat, although he had been seriously injured in the incident. The lifeboat then headed back to station, escorted by the tug *Merrimac*, landing the four survivors at Harwich at about 11.45am.

Following this service, which had been witnessed from the shore by many local people, reports of the lifeboat men's gallantry were received by a Mr J. Flory, missionary of the Missions to Seamen, who determined that the crew should receive formal recognition for their work. And so, at the Grand Nautical Fair at Ipswich on 30 Aril 1901, with the Mayor overseeing proceedings, the Mayoress presented silver medals to the twelve lifeboat men involved. The name of each man was inscribed in capital letters on the medal, together with the words, 'Memento for gallantry in saving the crew of the schooner *Rose*, of Ipswich, 30th March 1901. Let not the deep swallow me up'. The recipients were Coxswains Benjamin Dale and William Tyrrell, James Dale, Matt Scarlett, Ben Dale, jnr, A. Garnett, John Garnett, George Fenner, R. B. Scott, P. Harley, James Melville, and Charles Knights. The medals were supplied by Messrs R. D. and J. B. Fraser. These medals were nothing to do with the RNLI, but were funded and presented through the efforts of local people.

The second City of Glasgow

As the first *City of Glasgow* had suffered from so many reliability and mechanical problems, a new steam lifeboat was completed in 1901 for Harwich, which was considered such an important station that a steam lifeboat was seen as essential in order for the outlying sandbanks to be adequately covered. A boat identical to the RNLI's two steam lifeboats built in 1898 and 1899, and named *James Stevens No.3* and *James Stevens No.4* respectively, was ordered from J. Samuel White at Cowes in 1900. The new boat was 56ft 6in in length, with a breadth of 14ft and depth of 5ft 8in. She had a 12ft gunwale, ten relieving tubes, iron side keels 34ft long and 25ft bilge keels. She was powered by a compound vertical type engine of 180hp running at 410rpm, while she also carried sails, and had a displacement of 32.6 tons.

Unlike the two previous steam lifeboats to served the station, the third one was powered by screws, not waterjets, with the screws recessed in tunnels so she could 'proceed in shallow water or rocks in perfect safety'. Like the boat being replaced, she was named *City of Glasgow* in recognition of the gift of the first boat by the citizens of Glasgow, following the Lifeboat Saturday demonstrations of 1893 and 1894. The new lifeboat and her machinery were put through a series of trials off the Isle of Wight in May 1901, which went very well, after which she left for Harwich. The trials showed that, compared to the other steam lifeboats built by the RNLI, *City of Glasgow* was the fastest. She achieved an average maximum full speed on the measured mile of 9.66 knots per hour, with an ordinary working full speed of 9.143 knots.

Following the trials off Cowes, *City of Glasgow* left her builders yard and headed east and then north across the Thames estuary for her station. She was placed on station at Harwich on 9 May 1901, and on the morning of 13 May, as taken on a trial trip to Walton in a stiff breeze and choppy seas. The nine miles was covered in fifty minutes on an ebb tide, and, according to the local newspaper report, 'the manner in which the boat behaved was extremely gratifying to the crew'. She was showed to the lifeboat crew at Walton before returning to Harwich to be ready for service.

City of Glasgow was soon called into action. A few days after her trip to Walton, on 17 May 1901, she performed her first service, which proved to be a routine call. At 7.05pm she slipped her moorings, watched by a 'large crowd of interested spectators . . . and as she slipped away lusty cheers were raised', according to the *East Anglian Daily Times*' report and left the harbour. She proceeded the sands and stood by the schooner *Harriet*, of Goole, bound from London for Great Yarmouth, which floated off unaided. The steam lifeboat returned to station, and afterwards it was reported that 'her behaviour and speed gave great satisfaction'.

She did not complete another effective service until 1904, when she went out throughout the night of 23-24 November to assist the chalk-laden steamer *Tyne*, of Newcastle, which was on

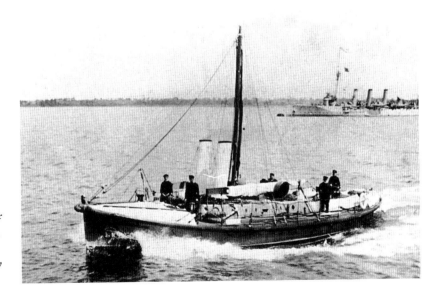

The second City of Glasgow shows an impressive turn of speed. (By courtesy of Harwich RNLI)

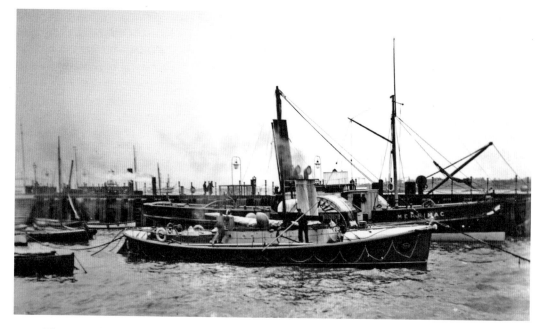

The steam lifeboat City of Glasgow in the Pound, with her engineers aboard, and the steam tug Merrimac moored behind. (Supplied by Ken Brand)

passage from Grays to Middlesbrough, and had grounded on the Shipwash Sands at noon on 23 November. The crew of the steam lifeboat helped to refloat her at about 11pm on 24 November, after which the vessel was able to continue on her voyage having sustained no damage. A similar service was carried out on 21 January 1905, when the lifeboat assisted to get the schooner *Dashing Wave*, of Fowey, bound from Dunkirk to Ipswich, off the Cork Sands.

Exactly a year later *City of Glasgow* completed her next service, launching to the brigantine *Thirza*, of Faversham, which stranded in rough weather south-east of Platters Buoy while bound from the Tyne to Whitstable with a cargo of coal. The steam tug *Spray* went out with the lifeboat in case the casualty needed to be towed. Once on scene, the lifeboat took off six of the crew, while the captain remained on board hoping to be able to save the vessel. The tug's crew managed to get a rope aboard the casualty, albeit with some difficulty, thus enabling the brigantine to be towed into harbour. As the vessel was leaking and in danger of sinking, with her decks almost under water, the lifeboat assisted with the tow. As she was in danger of sinking, she was taken up the river Stour and brought ashore close by the Old Continental Pier at Harwich. But as the brigantine was being moored safely by the tug, the tow rope fouled the tug's propeller, so the lifeboat crew had to assist in clearing the rope.

The steam lifeboats at Harwich, and other stations, were generally regarded as a success and clearly demonstrated the advantages that a powered lifeboat offered. However, steam power also brought with it a number of problems and by the early years of the twentieth century the use of the internal combustion engine in lifeboats was being explored by RNLI designers. Motor lifeboat development began in 1904 when an existing lifeboat, the 1893-built *J. McConnell Hussey* from Folkestone, was fitted with a two-stroke Fay & Bowen petrol engine, which gave her a speed of approximately six knots. This first motor lifeboat then went to the coast for evaluation at a number of stations and proved quite a success. Numerous technical problems had to be overcome to successfully operate an engine on board a lifeboat, however, including keeping the engine dry, even in the event of a capsize; ensuring it was totally reliable both when starting and running; and ensuring the propellers were protected from damage. As the problems were gradually surmounted, lifeboats powered by the internal combustion engine began to be built. Several pulling and Sailing lifeboats were converted to motor during the 1900s and a number of these pioneering craft were based at Harwich for trials.

Among the first lifeboats converted to power were those from Newhaven, Walton and Clacton, the latter two stations being Harwich's neighbours. The Walton boat, *James Stevens No.14*, had been fitted with a single 40hp Blake four-cylinder in 1906 while the Clacton boat, *Albert Edward*, had a single 40hp Tylor engine installed, also with four cylinders. They were joined by the Newhaven boat, *Michael Henry*, during trials out of Harwich. The boats left Blackwall on 26 October 1906 and reached Harwich the following day, after an overnight stop at Sheerness. The trials saw the boats running together, sometimes on long passages, as a result of which problems with the engines could be found and rectified, with modifications and improvements subsequently made to the engines. The *East Essex Advertiser* for 10 November 1906 reported on the trials:

> '*Frequent trials of the James Stevens [No.14] . . . have been made at Harwich since her arrival there. The tests have been carried out in company with the Newhaven motor lifeboat . . . Several minor improvements have been found practicable and been added. The engineers and inspectors appear to be of the opinion that the behaviour of the James Stevens [No.14] under the new conditions is very satisfactory. The trials have proceeded under most of the conditions of sea and weather that may reasonably be expected to prevail on the occasion of a lifeboat call. Under favourable conditions for sailing, the motor may be dispensed with,*

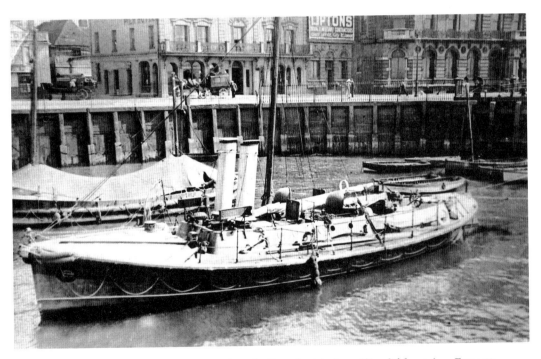

The second City of Glasgow moored in the Pound with the sailing lifeboat Ann Fawcett alongside. (By courtesy of Ken Brand)

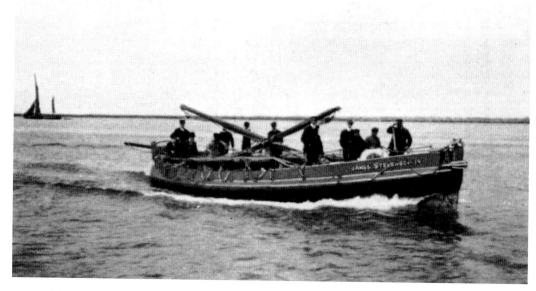

The converted motor lifeboat James Stevens No.14 was one of several early motor lifeboats that were based at Harwich for trials in 1906 and 1907.

and the sails only used, thus effecting an economy in fuel. Members of the crew are qualifying to take charge of the motor, and will . . . be entirely independent of professional aid from the engineers who have hitherto acted on behalf of the London firm.'

The trials out of Harwich continued throughout November and December 1906, and *James Stevens No.14* was even used, before Christmas, 'in conveying literature and other seasonable gifts to the men of the Cork, Shipwash, and other lightships', according to the *Clacton Graphic and East Coast News* of 29 December 1906. On one of the runs, the lifeboat was at sea for ten hours and her motor ran throughout without breaking down.

In early 1907 the converted motor lifeboats were joined off the Essex coast by another of the conversions, the 1893-built 42ft self-righter *Bradford*, originally stationed at Ramsgate, which had been motorised in 1906 when fitted with a single 30bhp Briton petrol engine, but re-engined in 1907 after the first engine proved unsatisfactory with a 30bhp Tylor four-cylinder model. In February 1907 the Newhaven and Ramsgate boats, escorted by *James Stevens No.14*, were taken out in hurricane force winds, rough seas, rain and snow, going fifteen miles off the coast, and returning safely, having 'successfully stood the severe test'. Numerous problems had been experienced in the various boats during these trials, with the seas and sands off Harwich providing a stern test for the experimental craft, but these early motor lifeboats set the scene for future lifeboat building. All the converted motor lifeboats served their various stations for a number of years, with *James Stevens No.14* staying at Walton until 1928 and *Albert Edward* operating from Clacton until March 1929, followed by a further three years at the Arranmore station on Ireland's north-west coast.

Despite the motor lifeboats being trialled out of Harwich, the steam lifeboat remained on station and in fact Harwich did not get its own motor lifeboat for another sixty years. But *City of Glasgow* continued to give good service, and on 7 April 1908 she performed what proved to be her most notable service. She put out in the early morning after a telephone message from the Kentish Knock lightvessel reported that the three-masted schooner *Notre Dame de Toutes Aides*, of Nantes, bound from Dordrecht to Brazil, had stranded on the sands in gale force winds. The Margate lifeboat had attempted to launch, but had been damaged in the heavy seas so was unable to offer any assistance and had returned to station. As soon as the information reached Harwich, *City of Glasgow* put out. In the meantime, an attempt by HMS *Dreadnought*, which was in the neighbourhood, to effect a rescue failed as the ship's small cutter proved too small to get alongside the casualty in the heavy seas, although it then stood by until the lifeboat arrived.

When the lifeboat arrived, the seas were so heavy that it was impossible to get alongside the schooner for long, and after two attempts to get a rope across, with it snapping on each occasion, Coxswain Matthew Scarlett realised he would have to get to the vessel without a line. He steamed straight towards the vessel, taking the lifeboat as close as he dared, thus enabling the crew to jump to safety. This manoeuvre had to be repeated five times before the survivors of the crew, nine in number, were aboard the lifeboat. They were completely exhausted by their ordeal and, had the rescue not been effected when it was, would probably have lost their lives. One man had been washed overboard early in the morning, and another, who tried to leave the schooner in the small ship's boat, was drowned when the boat capsized. As soon as the lifeboat was safely clear of the wreck, the rescued men were given biscuits and hot coffee and made as comfortable as possible for the return trip. They reached Harwich at 4.10pm, where the shipwrecked men were landed and taken to the Hanover Square Dining Rooms where, according to the *East Anglian Daily Times'* report in the 8 April 1908 edition,

> '*the men were very kindly treated. Hot tea and a hot meal were provided, and with a good fire and dry clothes, the poor fellows were made very comfortable. They appeared dreadfully downcast over the loss of their ship. Not one of the men was able to speak English, and through an interpreter, the skipper declined to say anything as to the experience through which they had passed. He merely remarked that he was tired, and preferred to say nothing.*'

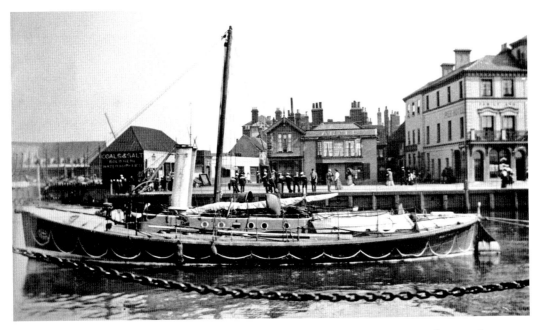

A fine profile view of the second City of Glasgow at her usual moorings in the Pound. She was the last steam lifeboat to be built by the RNLI. (By courtesy of Ken Brand)

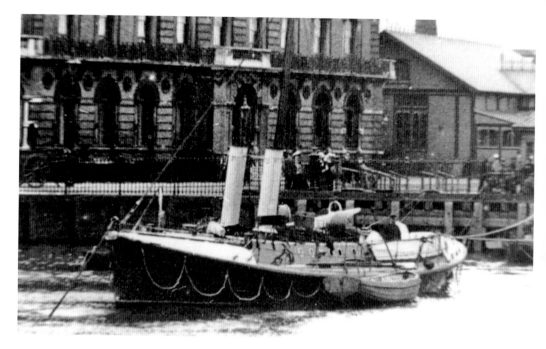

City of Glasgow at moorings in the Pount. (By courtesy of Harwich RNLI)

The newspaper added that: 'Coxswain [Scarlett] had been out many times, and could recall many experiences, but he will doubtless rank Tuesday's as the most important and the most successful launch with which he has ever been concerned. 'It was a lucky thing it did not happen in the night,' said the Coxswain.' The RNLI concluded the official account by stating, 'The service of the Harwich boat was a good one and splendidly performed, dogged determination playing a conspicuous part in it.' The Committee of Management, in recognition of the efforts of the Coxswain and crew during the very difficult service, provided the crew and engine-room staff with additional monetary rewards in the form of a special grant of £1 in addition to what was also sent.

Meanwhile, the captain of the schooner wrote to the press to express his gratitude, saying 'I also thank the men of the lifeboat *City of Glasgow*, of Harwich, who, at the risk of a thousand dangers, did not shrink or hesitate in face of the perils before them. Ten times they came to us and were repulsed by the force of the waves, which were really waves of sand saturated with water. When once on board, our saviours gave us every possible care, going so far as to divest themselves of their own clothes to cover us. I am looking forward, on my return to France, to tell my compatriots how again has been proved the great courage and self-sacrifice of the English sailors when engaged in trying to save life.' Further rewards were forthcoming in August 1908 at the International Conference on Life-Saving held at St Nazaire and Nantes. Members of the Conference conferred diplomas upon the Coxswain, crew and engineers, and each diploma was accompanied by the silver medal of the Society of the Hospitaliers Sauveteurs Bretons. The awards were forwarded to the British Government delegate, who forwarded them to the RNLI for presentation to the recipients.

On 9 September 1908 *City of Glasgow* was called out again, launching just after 4pm in a fierce gale after a wireless message had been intercepted at Felixstowe from the South Light to the North Foreland stating that a small two-masted iron-built ketch, *San Pedro*, of Rio de Janeiro, was in difficulty. The steam lifeboat launched made her way through very heavy seas and had a very rough passage to the scene. On the way out of the harbour onlookers from the shore saw the boat being completely enveloped in the seas. The lifeboat found the vessel in a poor condition, dragging her anchor, her sails torn, and she was unmanageable. While the lifeboat was alongside the casualty, Coxswain Ben Dale slipped and fell into the sea, but was quickly rescued, and 'appeared little the worse for his immersion', according to subsequent reports. The vessel was towed into Harwich, where she was anchored in the Pound at about 10pm. Large numbers of people watched the arrival of the lifeboat, and much curiosity was displayed over the queer shaped vessel, which bore unmistakable signs of having had a very rough time. The vessel was bound from Stockton to Brazil with coal and pig-iron and was manned by four crew, one of whom remarked when they were safely alongside that his ship was 'only fit for the river and ought not to cross the sea'.

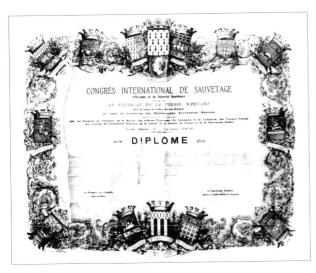

One of the Diplomas awarded by Congrès International de Sauvetage to the Harwich crew for the service to the schooner Notre Dame de Toutes Aides. This one was presented to William Dale. (By courtesy of Ken Brand)

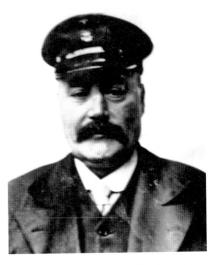

George Armstrong was Chief Engineer on the second City of Glasgow for twenty-five years and lived in West Street. (By courtesy of Ken Brand)

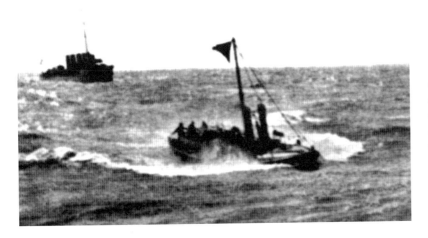

City of Glasgow on service to the schooner Notre Dame de Toutes Aides, of Nantes, on 7 April 1908, as depicted in The Lifeboat journal. (By courtesy of the RNLI)

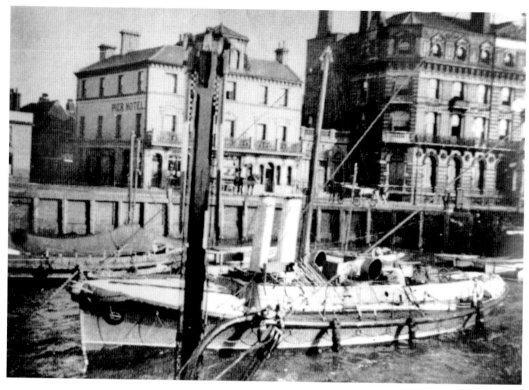

The twin-funnelled City of Glasgow served at Harwich from 1901 to 1917, during whcih time she launched ninety-nine times on service and is credited with saving eighty-seven lives. (By courtesy of Ken Brand)

The next services by *City of Glasgow* were of a somewhat more mundane nature, starting on 14 May 1909 when she went to the local smack *Tripper*, which was aground on the south-west corner of the Gunfleet Sands. The lifeboat put out at 12.50pm and was taken as close to the sands as possible, standing by until the tide flowed enabling the smack to float off. A further seven launches were undertaken during the rest of the year, none of which resulted in effective services being carried out.

During 1910 *City of Glasgow* was launched another seven times on service, helping a number of different vessels that had got into difficulties on the sands. On 19 August she stood by the barque *Fox*, of Arundel for more than twelve hours, returning to station at 3.10am on 20 August after the vessel had floated off. She stood by the Liverpool steamer *Hurricane* during the morning of 14 October and late at night on 27 October went to the steamship *Baltzar von Platen*, of Hamburg, assisting the vessel until 8.50am on 28 October. The final service of the year saw *City of Glasgow* standing by the barge *Baltic*, of London.

On 5 April 1911 *City of Glasgow* was called out twice, first in the morning to the small steamer *Humber*, of London, but she managed to get off the Sands unaided, and again in the afternoon. Just after 2pm the Coastguard reported another vessel in distress, and the lifeboat found the brigantine *Volant*, of Hull, with a crew of six, bound from London to Hull, in difficulty in the rough seas and gale force winds. The lifeboat men managed to assist the vessel into Brightlingsea. Another routine service was completed later the same year, on 30 October, when *City of Glasgow* went to the barge *Antje*, which was bringing coal from Hull to Harwich and had gone ashore on Felixstowe beach.

Seas were breaking over the vessel, and the master decided to abandon her, so he and the two crew, together with their dog, were taken into the lifeboat, and landed at Harwich Pier. The lifeboat later managed to get the barge afloat, but she sunk a few minutes after being pulled off the beach.

In 1913 *City of Glasgow* rendered two effective services, the first on 21 August to the schooner *Christabel*, of Whitstable, which was bringing coals from Hartlepool to Whitstable. She went aground on the Sands, a mile and a half south-west of the Gunfleet lighthouse. The lifeboat crew found her there, and five of them went on board to help jettison part of the cargo so that, early in the morning of 22 August, the vessel floated off on the tide. As no further assistance was required, the lifeboat returned to her station. Just over two months later, on 25 October, *City of Glasgow* saved the Trinity House pilot cutter *Will o' the Wisp*, of London, which was suffered a broken mast, so the lifeboat towed the vessel to harbour.

Over three days in March 1914 *City of Glasgow* went to help no fewer than three different vessels. The first of these was assisted on 18 March 1914 when, shortly before 10am, a telephone message was received by the Coastguard reporting a vessel in trouble east of Woodbridge Haven showing signals of distress. *City of Glasgow* launched immediately, battling with strong southerly winds as she 'ploughed her way through the heavy seas, at times burying her nose into the waves and throwing huge volumes of spray over herself', according to the *East Anglian Daily Times*' account. She soon found the 112-ton ketch *Malvoisin*, of London, labouring heavily, while on a voyage from Lynn to Rainham Creek with 100 tons of potatoes. The ketch's master requested help from the tug *Revenge*, which had also gone to assist, and the tug brought the ketch and her five crew into Harwich, escorted by the lifeboat, through very rough seas and a south-westerly gale.

The lifeboat crew helped *Malvoisin's* crew clear up their vessel once it had been secured, but before the lifeboat could get back to her moorings reports were received that another vessel was in difficulty

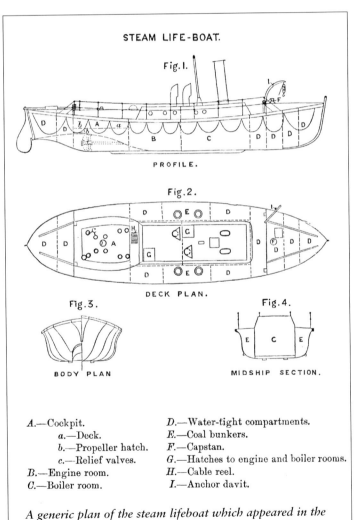

STEAM LIFE-BOAT.

Fig. 1.

PROFILE.

Fig. 2.

DECK PLAN.

Fig. 3.

BODY PLAN

Fig. 4.

MIDSHIP SECTION.

A.—Cockpit.
    a.—Deck.
    b.—Propeller hatch.
    c.—Relief valves.
B.—Engine room.
C.—Boiler room.

D.—Water-tight compartments.
E.—Coal bunkers.
F.—Capstan.
G.—Hatches to engine and boiler rooms.
H.—Cable reel.
I.—Anchor davit.

A generic plan of the steam lifeboat which appeared in the RNLI's Annual Reports circa 1900-1927 showing the mast after the funnel as on the second City of Glasgow.

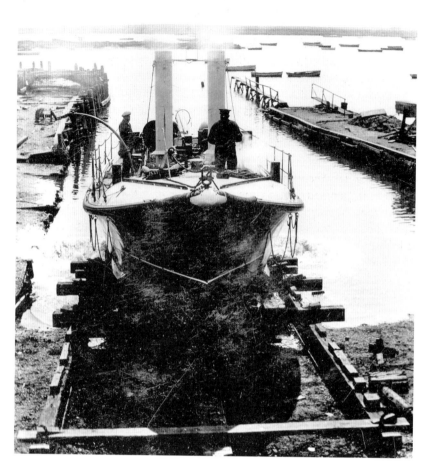

An unusual photo of the second City of Glasgow, with, on the port side, George Armstrong (chief engineer). It is not known where or when this photo was taken. (From an old postcard supplied by Ken Brand)

close to the Shipwash, so the lifeboat immediately set off, leaving harbour at 4.45pm in conditions that were better than earlier. This second launch proved to be unnecessary, however, as the vessel needed tug assistance, so the lifeboat returned to her station. But at 9.56pm the following day, 19 March 1914, *City of Glasgow* was called out again with some of the crew having to leave their seats in the Harwich Picture Palace to answer the call. This time the sea was calm, although a fresh westerly breeze was blowing as the lifeboat made for the Cork lightship to find out what assistance was required. The lightship had picked up an SOS message via its wireless from the barque *Matador*, of Bremen, which had gone ashore on the Kentish Knock with a cargo of wood. The lifeboat men assisted the barque's crew in getting rid of the cargo, with the lifeboat remaining alongside for two hours, and returned to station at 4.40am having been at sea for nine hours.

When war broke out in July 1914 Harwich harbour became an important base by the Royal Navy, and although initially the lifeboat remained operational, the conflict eventually resulted in the station's closure in 1917. Before that, however, *City of Glasgow* completed a few more services, including one on the first day of 1915 when she launched to the Norwegian steamship *Obediance*, which was aground on the Shipwash Sands. As the lifeboat headed out to the casualty, she came across the collier *Harriet*, of Leith, which had twenty-six of the steamer's crew on board, all of whom had been saved. So the lifeboat returned to port, but as the crew were mooring the lifeboat, they received a message, via the Coastguard, from the destroyer *Acheron*, which had brought in fourteen of the steamer's crew, that the captain and chief mate were still on the vessel. So, at 9.28pm, the lifeboat went out to the steamer for a second time, arriving on the scene to find huge seas breaking over and battering the ship. The lifeboat had great difficulty approaching the wrecked vessel but, after going round it three times to enable the Coxswain to assess the best approach, she was taken alongside. As it was impossible to moor to the ship, with the heavy seas repeatedly striking the vessel and completely covering the lifeboat, *City of Glasgow* had to be held in position so that the captain and mate could safely get on board the lifeboat. The lifeboat men afterwards took the twenty-six men from the collier and arrived back at Harwich at 8.30am on 2 January.

Soon, *City of Glasgow* was going to casualties of the war, launching at 5.35pm on 17 January 1915 to the minesweeper *Eaton*, which was in difficulty on the Barrow Sands, and not returning to station until 2.30am the following day. She went to another war casualty on 22 September 1915, this time the Nederland Steamship Company's 9,181-ton steamer *Koningin Emma*, of Amsterdam, which had struck a mine and gone aground near the Shipwash Sands with about 150 passengers on board and a crew of fifty, bound from Java to Amsterdam. *City of Glasgow* stood by all night as the vessel was listing badly, and when the tide rose she floated and began to heel over. The lifeboat remained close by, steaming round the vessel, until about 8.20pm. Once it was realised that the vessel would become a total wreck, most of the crew were taken off and put aboard *Batavia*, another steamer, and the lifeboat saved a further twenty.

The final service undertaken by *City of Glasgow* was another long one. She launched at 4.45pm on 7 January 1916 to the steamship *Zeeland*, of Rotterdam, which was carrying coal from Blyth to London, and had gone aground near the Longsand lightship at about midnight in gale force winds and very heavy seas. The lifeboat stood by all night and in the early morning, together with the tug *Thames*, assisted to refloat the vessel, which was able to resume its voyage unaided. The lifeboat returned to Harwich at 5.15am on 8 January. Not only did this prove to be *City of Glasgow*'s last service at Harwich, but it was also the last service for Coxswain Matthew Scarlett, who 'died in tragically sudden circumstances' on 12 April 1916. He had been on the crew for forty years, the last twelve as Coxswain, and according to the *East Anglian Daily Times* 'is said to have possessed a wonderful knowledge of every sandbank in the vicinity, and in every respect he may be said to be an expert and accomplished lifeboat man.'

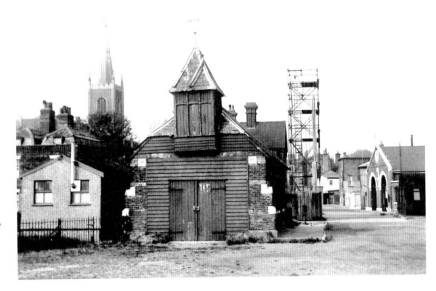

During the era of the steam lifeboat, the 1876 lifeboat house, which had been unused since 1881, was divided in two and half of it used as a coal store. This photo shows the building in 1957 with the ornamental turret intact. (Grahame Farr, by courtesy of the RNLI)

None of the launches by *City of Glasgow* during the remainder of 1916 and 1917 resulted in her rendering any more effective services, and in October 1917 the Admiralty wrote to the RNLI requesting her use. Their letter stated that, while they were not seeking to take over the Institution's lifeboats, the Harwich steam lifeboat was an exception. As a result, the RNLI suggested they purchase the lifeboat with the option for the Institution to reacquire her at the end of the war. In December 1917 the Admiralty decided to go ahead with the acquisition and bought the boat and her equipment for £4,290. With this, the Harwich station was closed as the RNLI did not to send a pulling and sailing lifeboat to the station in place of the steam boat as no tug was available to tow her, and the Institution's Committee stated that getting to the sands unaided was too difficult for a sailing craft. In February 1918 a pension of £3 16s 3d per annum was granted to Adam Garnett, who had been Coxswain for the previous twenty months. Fireman Charles Knight and Donald Wood, the second fireman, were no longer needed, so the former was given a gratuity of £74 6s 0d and a pension of £27 17s 3d per annum, while the latter was transferred to the steam lifeboat then in service at Dover.

At the end of the war the question of reopening the Harwich station was raised and in July 1919 Commander Innes, RN, Deputy Chief Inspector of Lifeboats, visited Harwich and Walton-on-the-Naze to discuss with the two local committees whether Harwich should have a lifeboat and the future of the Walton station. The Harwich committee passed a resolution that, in view of amount of shipping using the harbour, most of which came from the north, a lifeboat at Harwich would be in a better position than one at Walton to render assistance should it be needed. Meanwhile, the Walton committee, with twenty-five members in addition to the Honorary Secretary, unanimously agreed that both Harwich and Walton lifeboats should be retained, but, unsurprisingly, if one boat was to be taken off station the Walton lifeboat should be retained, 'not only on account of its record but on account of its geographical position'. The Inspector reported back to the RNLI's Committee of Management, which then decided that the Walton motor lifeboat would be retained, as that was already on station, but no lifeboat would be stationed at Harwich, although the boathouse would be retained in case the station was reopened.

The boathouse had been used for a number of years as a coal store for the steam lifeboat, and the RNLI had spent money maintaining it. In July 1917 eight wire guards were fixed over the windows of the boathouse at a cost of £5 6s as they were 'being constantly broken by boys throwing stones'. In September 1917 local painter G. H. Green received £15 5s for repairing and painting the building, even though the station's closure was imminent. And although in 1919 the RNLI intended to retain the boathouse, in 1922 it was surrendered to the War Office.

Meanwhile, the station's closure was formalised by the end of 1919, even though, in December, letters were sent by the Corporation of Harwich and the local Trades Council and Labour Party expressing regret at the decision by the Committee of Management to close the station and hoping that such a decision might be reversed. But the decision stood, and in July 1920 a Thanks on Vellum was voted by the RNLI's Committee to John Paterson to mark his retirement as the station's Honorary Secretary. Paterson was manager of Lloyd's Bank, as well as a JP in the borough and secretary of the Royal Harwich Yacht Club.

The station's last lifeboat *City of Glasgow*, after being sold to the Admiralty, was converted into a patrol boat and renamed *Patrick*. As such, she carried out a service, on 26 June 1918, to a German submarine *UC-11*, a minelayer, which hit one of its own mines off the Sunk Lightship. A huge explosion was seen by the crew of Patrick who, when they arrived at the scene, saw a lone survivor floating nearby. He was Lieut Kurt Utke, skipper of *UC-11*, which had mistakenly hit its own mine while at periscope depth. After serving the Admiralty in the UK, it is believed that *Patrick* went to the Nile, but further information about her whereabouts is lacking.

Reopening the Station

D uring the 1950s and 1960s Harwich harbour became increasingly busy with pleasure boats, leisure users and small craft. Felixstowe Dock started to expand its commercial operations with additional berths constructed, including a tanker jetty. Parkeston Quay continued as a passenger ferry port, with a greater frequency of ferry sailings to Europe while the ferries themselves got ever larger, carrying more passengers and vehicles. As well as commercial shipping, yachts and pleasure boats were increasing in numbers as more and more people used the picturesque and sheltered harbour for leisure pursuits afloat.

The need for a lifeboat to cover this increasingly busy area became acute in the early 1960s and the reopening of the station was the result of several drownings in the harbour and off Dovercourt. In the winter of 1961 a boy who had lost his model aeroplane in the sea used a canoe from the

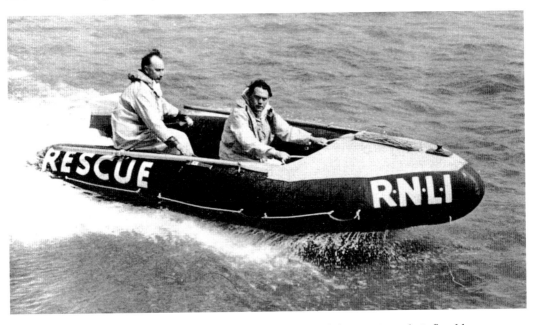

The first inshore lifeboat to serve at Harwich was one of the RNLI's early inflatables, powered by a single outboard engine and fitted with just basic equipment.

boating lake to retrieve it. This capsized, and before the boy could be rescued he had drowned, affected by the cold. This led to the formation of the RNLI Harwich Branch Committee in 1962 and a Harwich Harbour Rescue Fund was instigated. On 17 September 1964 another tragic accident occurred when Graham Bunn, a fourteen-year-old schoolboy, drowned off Angel Gate, Harwich. Following this tragedy, a public meeting was called and representatives from yacht clubs and local organisations attended, as well as and members of the public, who were understandably concerned about the safety of the beaches in the area.

The Harwich RNLI Branch Committee was by now well established and a campaign was started with the backing of the mayor, S. Simmons, to establish a harbour rescue boat. In 1963 the concept of an inflatable rescue boat was being evaluated by the RNLI. Ray Wood, Chairman of the Harwich Inshore Rescue Boat Committee, participated in trials of the RNLI's inflatable ILBs at Gorleston on 19 February 1964, arguing that such a boat should also be stationed at Harwich. In 1965 the RNLI agreed to provide an inshore rescue boat (IRB) at Harwich for the summer season of 1965. The

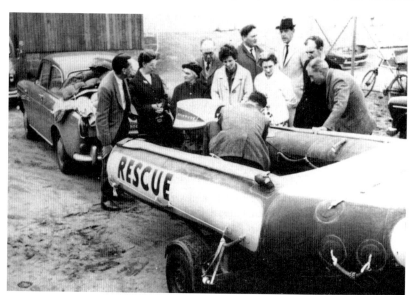

The first Harwich inshore rescue boat, No.71, arrived by road from Littlehampton on 28 May 1965. (By courtesy of Harwich RNLI)

The first crew members for the inshore rescue boat examine the new craft shortly after it arrived in May 1965. It was declared operational on 11 June. Pictured are, left to right, Les Smith, Jeff Sallows, Doug Jennings, Richard Jordan, Terry Bennett, Aubrey Seaman, Ray Wood and Don Mudd. (By courtesy of Harwich RNLI)

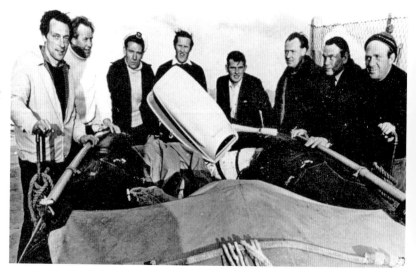

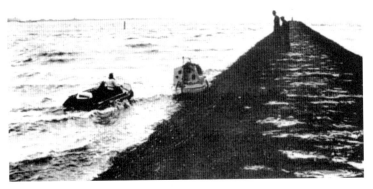

The first IRB on service to the motor boat Scimitar, which was being pounded against the harbour breakwater, 10 October 1965. (By courtesy of Harwich RNLI)

Inshore Rescue Boat No.71 returned from her first service which involved bringing in a dinghy with one occupant on 18 June 1965. (By courtesy of Harwich RNLI)

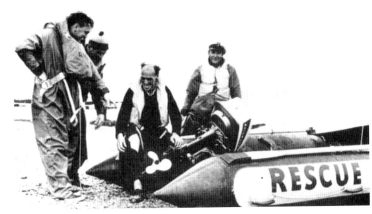

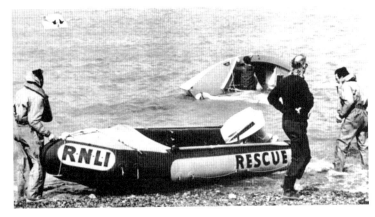

The IRB on service to a sailing dinghy, with four boys on board, which capsized off Wrabness on 8 May 1966. (By courtesy of Harwich RNLI)

Graham Bunn Harwich Harbour Rescue Fund contributed £250 to the IRB Fund, which donated the money to the RNLI to defray the £750 cost of the boat. The new craft, no.71, arrived on 28 May 1965, having been brought by road from Littlehampton. Following tests, launching trials and crew training, the boat was declared operational on 11 June 1965 and the Harwich lifeboat station had been re-established. The D class inflatable lifeboats on station from 1965 to 1978 were housed in a former army garage, since demolished, at Angelgate (now called Timberfields), close to the 1876 boathouse, which was occupied by a further education sailing club at the time. The ILB was launched off a trolley which was pushed over the beach by the crew.

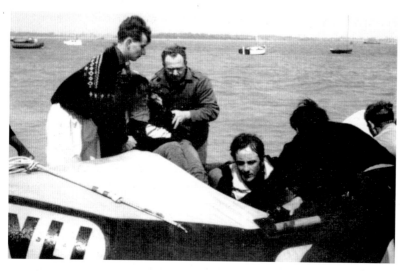

The inshore rescue boat (IRB), later known as the inshore lifeboat (ILB), is the smallest lifeboat in the RNLI fleet. Since being introduced in 1963, the design has been refined and developed and the ILB has become an efficient, effective and essential life-saving tool. The 16ft inflatable lifeboats, made from nylon coated with hypalon, are usually crewed by two or three, powered by a 40hp outboard engine, and can be launched quickly and easily. They are equipped with VHF radio, GPS, flexible fuel tanks, flares, an anchor, a spare propeller, a compass, first aid kit and knife. The ILB's advantage over the conventional lifeboat was its speed which, at twenty knots, was considerably faster than any lifeboat in service during the 1960s. The ILB also has the advantage of being able to go alongside other craft easily, or pick up persons in the water, without causing or suffering damage.

The first service by the new IRB was carried out on 18 June when she went to a man who was drifting out to sea in a dinghy. He was landed ashore at Harwich uninjured, with nothing worse than a pair of torn trousers. She helped a yacht on 29 July and the cabin cruiser *Taifung* on 2 September, and then undertook two services in October, the first on 10 October when the 20ft motor boat *Scimitar* was reported to be pounding on the breakwater at the harbour entrance. The lifeboat crew found the craft empty apart from some fishing gear as the boat had broken from moorings at Shotley. The last service of the year came was performed on 31 October, just an hour before the ILB was due to be taken out of service for the winter. She launched to assist the 30ft motor ketch *Pandora* from the Orwell Yacht Club, which was in difficulty about a mile off Felixstowe Pier. The yacht, with three fishermen on board, was towed into the river Deben with her engine out of action and steering gear damaged. When the IRB was withdrawn at the end of the 1965 summer season she had undertaken six services. Summer-only operation of inshore rescue boats was usual at the time, and the RNLI continued to operate summer-only stations well into the 1990s. However, on 18 September 1966 the RNLI decided that the Harwich station should remain operational throughout the year and so the ILB remained on station.

In 1966 the IRB returned for the summer season and on 8 May was required to assist six schoolboys and a teacher from Derbyshire, whose sailing dinghy had capsized off Wrabness. They had tried unsuccessfully to right the dinghy, and the IRB assisted in getting the craft to the shore. As a fourteen-year-old-boy was suffering from exhaustion and exposure, they were all sent to hospital for a check-up. At 2.43pm on 30 May 1966 a small sailing dinghy was reported to have capsized one mile off Dovercourt beach. The IRB launched at 2.48pm in a moderate east-north-easterly breeze and moderate sea, with an ebbing tide. The dinghy was found waterlogged with her two-man crew in the water alongside. After taking them on board, the IRB crew anchored the dinghy before returning to station at 3.06pm. The rescued people were supplied with dry clothing by the crew on arrival at Harwich.

With the success of the inshore rescue boat, the continued expansion of boating activities in and around the harbour, and the considerable growth in shipping at both Harwich and Felixstowe, the RNLI decided to re-establish the offshore lifeboat station at the port. At the time, a new fast 44ft self-righting lifeboat was being developed, and Harwich was seen as an ideal place for one of the new craft. The design was based on a United States Coast Guard (USCG) steel-hulled rescue cutter and could reach speeds in excess of fifteen knots, considerably faster than any British lifeboat then in service. The RNLI purchased one of these boats from the USCG in 1963. Given the operational number 44-001, she was taken on a tour of lifeboat stations in Britain and Ireland in 1964 to assess the suitability and ascertain crew opinions of the new design.

44-001 represented a radical departure from the traditional motor designs then used by the RNLI, but as none of these had seen service at Harwich the crews there had no preconceived ideas and many were keen to operate the new design. After gaining a favourable reception from lifeboat crews during trials and from the tour by 44-001, the RNLI embarked upon a construction programme of six boats, with various additions and modifications incorporated. The design was self-righting by virtue of its inherent buoyancy, and was designated the class name Waveney after the river close to the Brooke Marine boatyard at Lowestoft where the first six were built for the RNLI. The boat allocated to Harwich was the fifth of the class and, powered by twin 215hp Cummins V6 diesel engines, she had a top speed of fifteen knots. She arrived at Harwich on 19 September 1967, and the original intention was for her to be stationed in the harbour for an experimental period of two years. Peter Burwood, who was originally from Clacton-on-Sea, was appointed as Coxswain/Mechanic of the new boat. He had been on board the prototype boat 44-001 during her tour round the coast having been employed as a full-time mechanic by the RNLI.

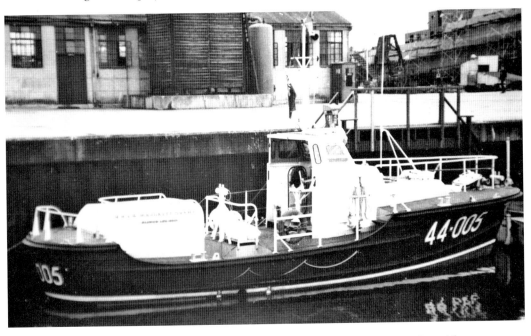

The 44ft Waveney Margaret Graham, operational number 44-005, moored outside Brooke Marine at Lowestoft shortly after being built. (By courtesy of Harwich RNLI)

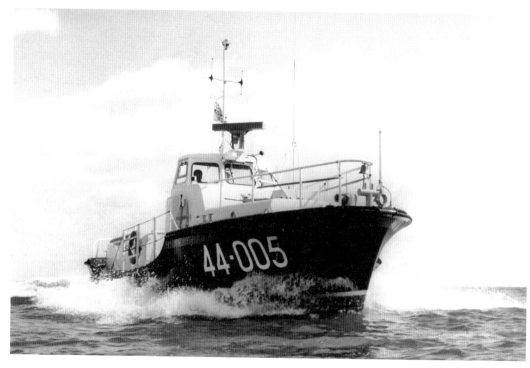

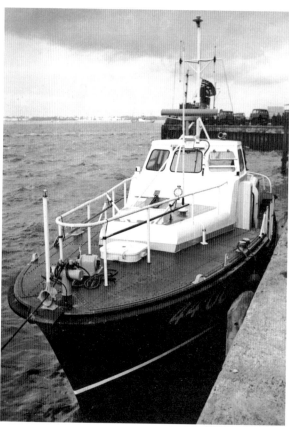

The first 44ft Waveney to serve at Harwich was Margaret Graham. She was one of six Waveneys built for the RNLI by Brooke Marine at Lowestoft in the late 1960s, and served at Harwich until 1980. (By courtesy of the RNLI).

(Below) Margaret Graham alongside Harwich Quay in 1967 on the day she arrived. (By courtesy of Ken Brand)

The new lifeboat was named *Margaret Graham* having been funded by a gift from an anonymous donor. She was formally named and dedicated at a ceremony on 27 September 1967 at Trinity Pier attended by hundreds of people. The ceremony was opened by the Mayor, Councillor L. E. Hostler, who welcomed the arrival of the new boat, which reflected an increased level of shipping in the area, and said: 'May I thank the RNLI for conferring this honour upon us and thank the crew of local men who we know we shall be very proud of.' Lieut Commander D. J.

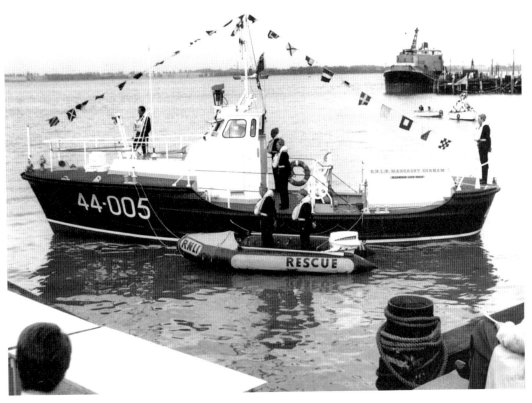

The scene during the naming ceremony of 44ft Waveney Margaret Graham at Harwich on 27 September 1967. (By courtesy of Harwich RNLI)

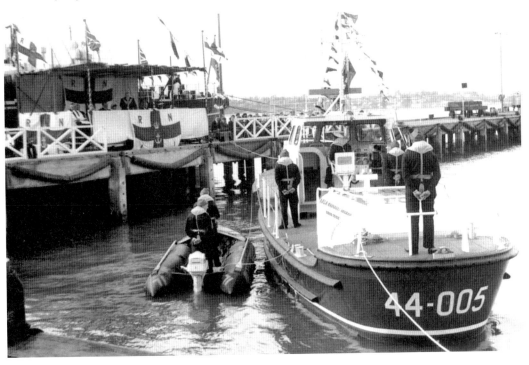

Wilford RNR, the RNLI District Inspector, then described the new lifeboat, after which Stirling Whorlow, RNLI Secretary, formally delivered her into the care of the branch. She was accepted by the President, T. H. F. Bernard. The service of dedication was conducted by the Rev D. Noel Thomas, vicar of St Nicholas Church, assisted by Canon A. H. Johnson, vicar of All Saints' Church, Dovercourt, and the Rev A. J. Herring, of the Dovercourt Congregational Church. At the end of proceedings, the boat was named by the Deputy Master of Trinity House, Captain G. E. Barnard, who cut the cord which released the bottle of champagne against the boat's deck.

The first call for the new lifeboat came on 30 September 1967, just three days after her naming ceremony. *Margaret Graham* and her crew searched an area twenty square miles from late at night until 2am on 1 October but found nothing and returned to station having been at sea for nearly three and a half hours. Two girls, Irene Newman and Annette Boelyn, who were working backstage on a Felixstowe Amateur Dramatic and Operatic Society production saw what appeared to be a rocket with white stars fired out to sea off Cobbold's Point. The girls called the coastguards at Felixstowe and Honorary Secretary Captain D. Gibson decided to launch the new boat.

A more testing service came just over two weeks later, on 17 October 1967, when the lifeboat launched to the 6,000-ton tanker *Astrid Elizabeth*, of Bergen, in gale force nine winds, gusting to force ten. The tanker had a leak in her engine room twenty-two miles out to sea. The lifeboat spent two and a half hours to reach the casualty, and found her at anchor. She stood by in the heavy weather until the German tug *Heros* arrived from Dover, and then circled the casualty until the tug had a line aboard and the tanker could weigh anchor. The lifeboat was then released from the scene and headed back to Harwich. Afterwards, Coxswain Peter Burwood said: 'The crew took everything in their stride as though they had been on the boat all their lives'.

During 1968, *Margaret Graham's* first full year on station, she performed a number of rescues,

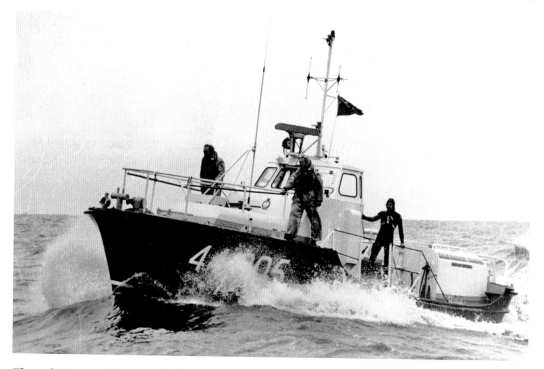

The 44ft Waveney Margaret Graham pictured in 1967 shortly after she had arrived on station. (By courtesy of Ken Brand)

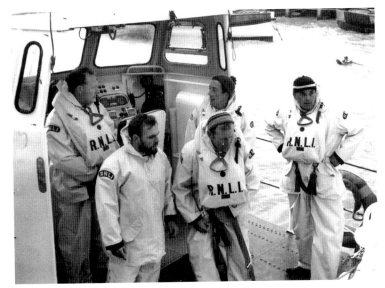

Some of the first Harwich lifeboat crew on board *Margaret Graham*, possibly taken on the day she arrived at Harwich, 19 September 1967. They are, left to right, Aubrey Seaman, Coxswain Peter Burwood, Doug Jennings, Les Smith and Ray Allen. (By courtesy of Harwich RNLI)

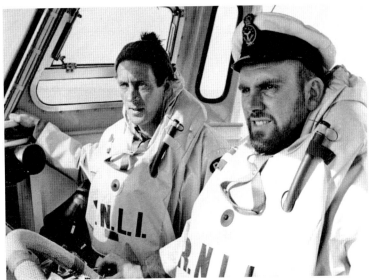

Les Smith and (on right) Coxswain Peter Burwood on board *Margaret Graham* in 1967. Les Smith served on the ILB from 1965 to 1976 and was also the first Second Coxswain on the *Waveney*. (By courtesy of Ken Brand)

proving the need for a lifeboat at Harwich. Having helped commercial vessels earlier in the year, on 22 August both the Waveney and inshore lifeboat were launched after the yacht *Sandora* went aground on the Millbay Rocks off Dovercourt seafront. The yacht's crew of six teenagers, who were on holiday at Walton, had spent three hours in the sea trying to keep the yacht on an even keel after she had gone on the rocks, and were found by the lifeboat crew using the lifeboat's radar equipment, with visibility down to just fifty yards due to fog. The lifeboat was unable to get close enough to take the yacht in tow due to the shallow water, but the ILB transferred three girls from the yacht to the lifeboat. *Margaret Graham* then stood by until 8pm, by when there was enough water to get close enough to take the three boys off. One of the lifeboat crew was transferred onto the yacht, a tow was rigged, and the vessel was brought into harbour.

At 5.23pm on 3 February 1969 the duty pilot informed the honorary secretary that a catamaran with two people on board was adrift near Platter's buoy. *Margaret Graham* slipped her moorings at

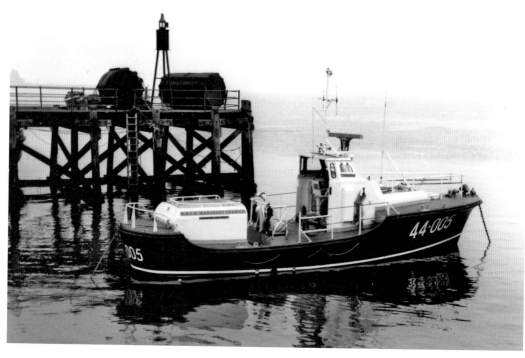

44ft Waveney Margaret Graham ar moorings in the Pound, June 1968, during her first year on station. (Grahame Farr, by courtesy of RNLI)

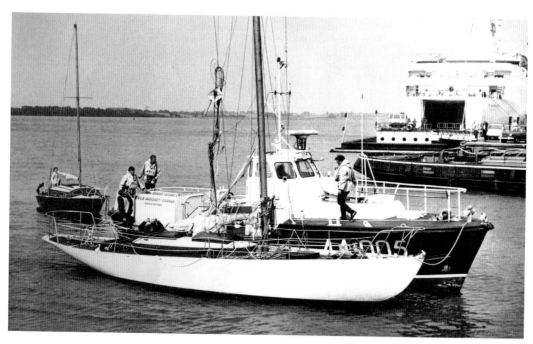

Margaret Graham bringing in the yacht Viola, which had a damaged mast after being struck by lightning, on 27 June 1970. The other yacht in tow was also being brought in by the lifeboat. (By courtesy of Ken Brand)

5.30pm in a light north westerly breeze with a slight sea, three hours after high water. A Dutch ferry stood by the drifting boat until relieved by the motor vessel *Essex Ferry* of Harwich. The catamaran continued to drift and was a mile east of the Cork Spit buoy when the lifeboat reached it at 5.50pm. The lifeboat got a line on board the catamaran and started to tow. This was made difficult by the unusual construction of the drifting boat coupled with a freshening wind and a choppy sea. The casualty was berthed at Harwich, and the lifeboat returned to station at 7.10pm.

After this service the reserve lifeboat 44-001 came to the station for a short stint lasting from April and August 1969, during which time she performed one service, helping the trimaran *Three Wishes*. *Margaret Graham* went away for refit, returning towards the end of the summer and was soon in action. She launched at 11.10am on 28 September 1969 to the yacht *Jacaranda*, which had got into difficulties 500 yards off the Sunk light vessel. The crew of the light vessel had floated a line to the yacht and this had been secured, but the weather conditions made it impossible to haul the yacht closer to the light vessel. *Margaret Graham* faced a strong south-westerly wind and rough seas as she made her way to the casualty. At 12.30pm she reached the yacht, which had two crew aboard, and passed across another towline. At 12.47pm, in rough conditions, the tow back to Harwich began and, after an uneventful trip, the lifeboat was back on station at 2.55pm.

The reserve lifeboat 44-001 was on duty again towards the end of 1970, from September to November, and undertook four services. On 10 October 1970 she went out , with the ILB, to the 35ft ketch *Starstream*, which was stranded aground on the Cork Sands half a mile west of the Cork Sands Buoy. By the time the lifeboat reached the scene, the ketch had refloated on the rising tide and was under her own power. The ILB had been rerouted to *Starstream* after the dinghy she had launched to assist had reached Felixstowe beach unaided. Both lifeboats returned to station without their help needed. On 18 November 1970 44-001 was launched to save a man marooned on a rig in Dovercourt Bay in gale force winds and driving rain. The ILB was also launched and managed to take the man off the rig and transfer him to 44-001, which was standing by.

Margaret Graham returned to station on 20 November 1970 and had a busy year in 1971, launching a total of eighteen times and saving fifteen lives, all of which were largely routine services. On 30 January 1971 a new inshore lifeboat was sent to the station, D-201, to replace No.71 which had been at Harwich since the station was reopened. The new boat was a 16ft Avon A360 type, one of just four craft of this type to see service with the RNLI, and she only stayed for three years, leaving at the end of 1973.

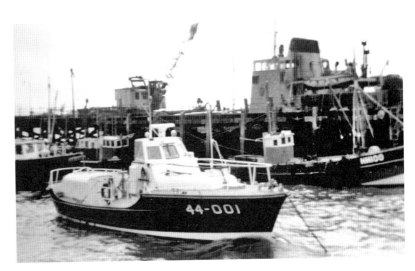

Relief lifeboat 44-001 on station at Harwich, 1972. The boat was completed in 1964 at the USCG Yard and shipped to the UK for evaluation trials. She served in the Relief Fleet for thirty years and is now on display at the Historic Lifeboat Collection in Chatham. (By courtesy of Ken Brand)

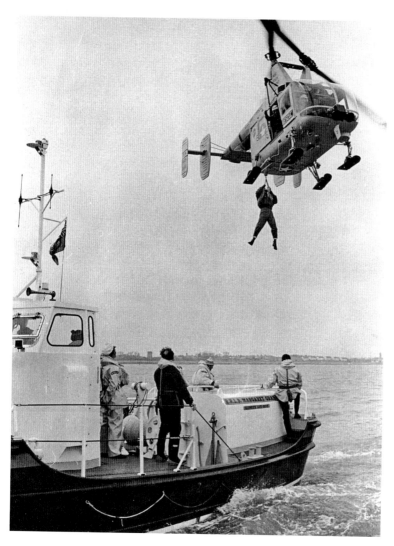

An unusual helicopter exercise for Margaret Graham and the Harwich lifeboat crew as a Husky type helicopter from the United States Air Force base at Woodbridge undertakes winching operations. The USAF's 67th Squadron, the Aerospace and Recovery Squadron, occasionally exercised with Harwich lifeboat. (By courtesy of Ken Brand)

On 31 May 1971 *Margaret Graham* spent the night at sea searching after mystery voices were heard by someone on board the passenger ferry *Avalon*. Shouts were heard from the sea at the after end of the ferry and it was assumed that someone had gone overboard. Lists of the crew and passengers showed all were present, but further reports of voices being heard resulted a nine-hour search for the lifeboat and her crew, but nothing was found. On 14 September *Margaret Graham* launched to the 20ft lobster boat *Joan L*, which had broken down eleven miles out to sea having got a rope caught round her propeller. The lifeboat soon reached the casualty, with the crew finding the skipper was Les Smith, the station's Second Coxswain.

In August 1971 *Margaret Graham* went to Lowestoft for a refit and the reserve lifeboat 44-001 was again on station, staying until February 1972 and launching three times on service. On 17 February 1972 she was involved in a major search operation after two Lightning jet aircraft, on a training flight from RAF Wattisham, collided in mid-air thirty miles out to sea. The Dutch trawler *Wiljo*, which was in the area, picked up one of the pilots, Flight Lieut Paul Reynolds, an hour after the collision. He was later transferred to 44-001 once she arrived on scene, and, after he had been landed at Harwich, the lifeboat returned to the search area. Gorleston, Aldeburgh and Lowestoft

The yacht Viola being brought to Harwich by Margaret Graham on 27 June 1970. The yacht was caught out by a violent summer storm and the mast was struck by lightning. (By courtesy of Ken Brand)

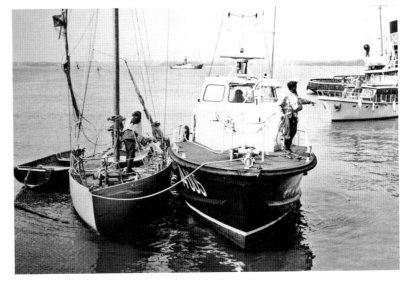

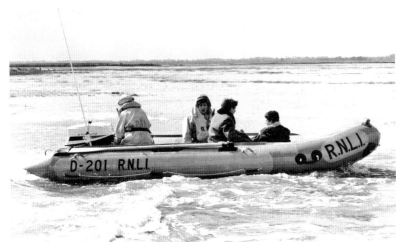

D-201, the second inshore lifeboat to serve at Harwich, returning from service on 27 March 1971. The boat was an unusual design, a 16ft Avon 650, of which only four were used by the RNLI. (By courtesy of Harwich RNLI)

D-201, the second inshore lifeboat to serve at Harwich, returning from service on 27 March 1971 having picked up two men cut off by the tide and brought them back to the beach. The lifeboat crew are Ken Brand (on left) and Barry Scase. (By courtesy of Harwich RNLI)

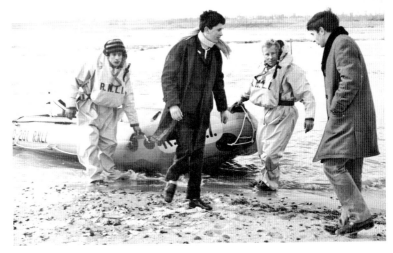

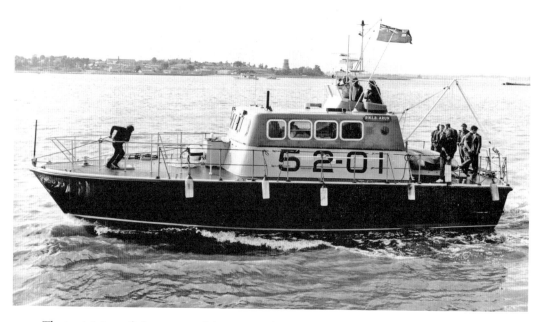

The prototype 52ft Arun, named Arun, visited Harwich on 26 June 1971 during her evaluation trials around the country. While in the harbour, she took part in a search for the occupant of a small speedboat, which had capsized. A helicopter, the ILB, a pilot boat and other craft joined the search, but nothing was found. (By courtesy of Harwich RNLI)

lifeboats were also involved, aided by an RAF Shackleton aircraft and USAF helicopter, but the search was terminated during the night with one pilot still missing, presumed dead.

A few days after this service, on 23 February 1972, *Margaret Graham* returned from Lowestoft having completed her refit and was involved in a long service on 18 June, spending twelve hours chasing the 40ft ketch-rigged yacht *Golden Miller*. The yacht had fired a distress flare because she had engine trouble and was unable to slow down or turn into the wind when forty miles off Harwich. The lifeboat was called out, while two ferries stood by, and a dredger, coaster and tug also went to help, but none could get alongside the yacht because it was making seven knots and could not slow down in the strong winds. *Margaret Graham* crashed through the heavy seas but was unable to make much more than eleven knots in her pursuit of the yacht, so did not gain ground on the casualty. The Gorleston lifeboat *Khami* was also launched and she eventually reached the yacht and brought it into Lowestoft. *Margaret Graham* returned to Harwich after a round trip of 140 miles with two of the crew from *Golden Miller* being taken to hospital suffering severe seasickness.

A number of incidents during 1973 involved evacuating and landing sick or injured crew members from ships off Harwich. On 27 April 1973 *Margaret Graham* landed a crewman from the tanker *British Fulmar* who was suffering from chest pains and required medical attention. On 9 June 1973 the lifeboat landed an injured man, who had fallen while undertaking engine repairs, from the gravel dredger *Pen Stour*. On 18 July 1973 ten survivors from the oil rig supply ship *Nordic Service* were landed at Harwich by *Margaret Graham* after the ship sank forty miles off the Suffolk coast following a collision with the 4,022-ton motor vessel *Finntrader*. The survivors were picked up by *Finntrader* and transferred from there to the lifeboat. On 14 August 1973 *Margaret*

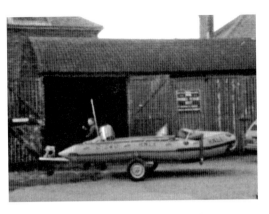

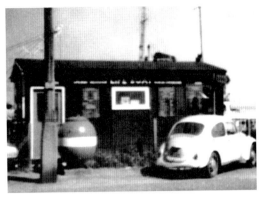

D class inflatable D-240 outside the shed that was used to house the first ILB. (By courtesy of Ken Brand)

The small crew facility on Ha'penny Pier used from 1967 to 1977. (By courtesy of Ken Brand)

Graham landed an injured crew member from the Finnish cargo ship *Finnseal*, having taken out a doctor to the ship to treat the crewman, who had a suspected perforated ulcer.

The lifeboat crew had a busy day on 28 September 1973 going to two casualties. The first call came in the morning with *Margaret Graham* putting out at 10.20am to help a lobster boat in trouble in Dovercourt Bay. A rope fouled the boat's propeller, and it was being swept towards the stone pier when the lifeboat arrived on scene fifteen minutes after launching. The casualty was taken in tow at 10.40am and brought to Harwich half an hour later. Five minutes after being

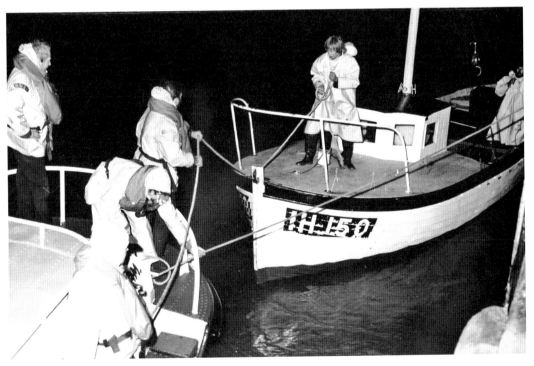

The 31ft fishing vessel Lode Star being brought alongside Harwich Quay after Margaret Graham had towed it to safety on 9 November 1972. (By courtesy of Ken Brand)

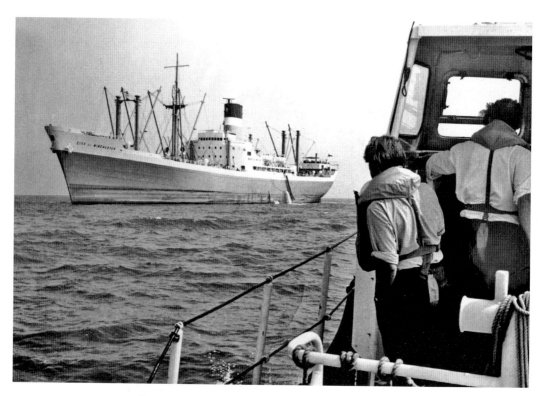

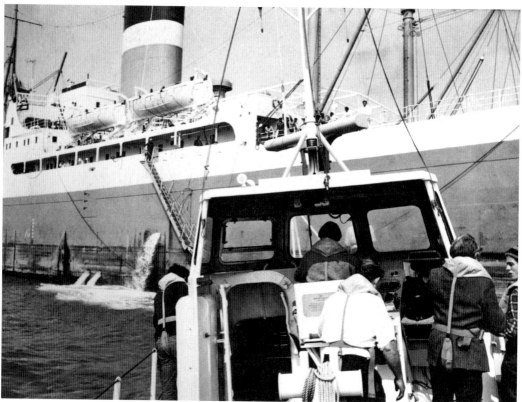

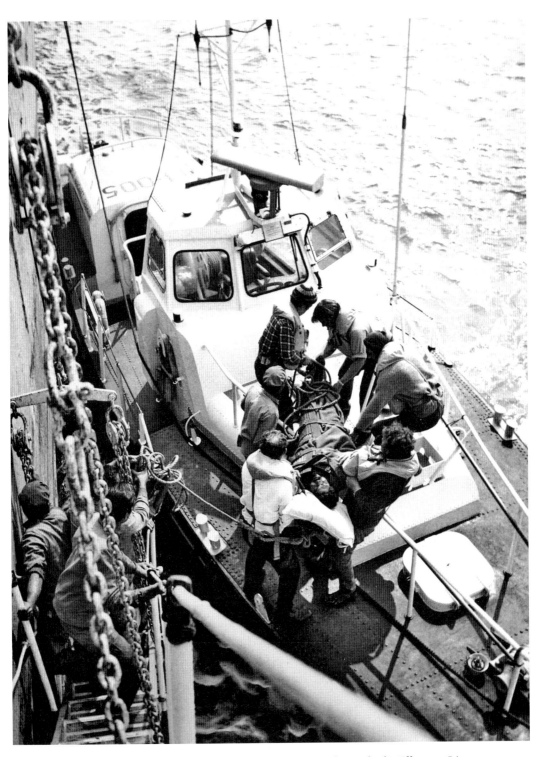

Three photographs showing Margaret Graham coming alongside the Ellerman Line cargo vessel City of Winchester to take off an injured man on 25 September 1970. (By courtesy of Ken Brand)

85

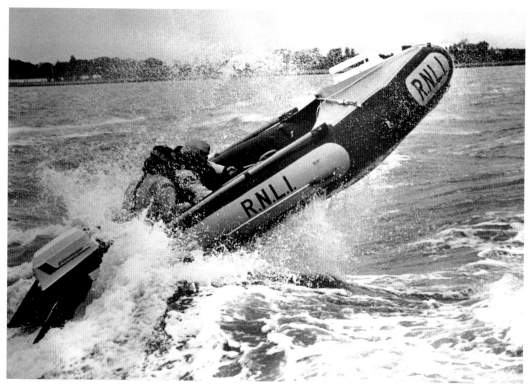

The relief inshore lifeboat D-150 on exercise in December 1972 crewed by Ken Brand and Bob Ramplin. (By courtesy of Ken Brand)

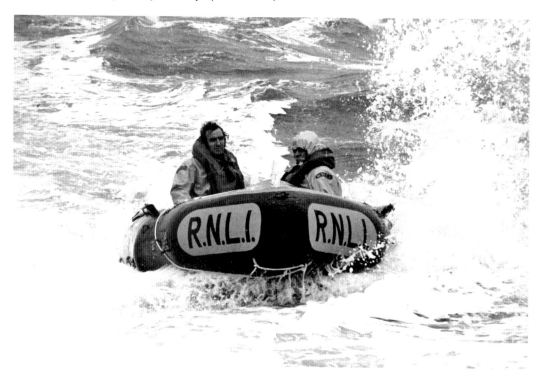

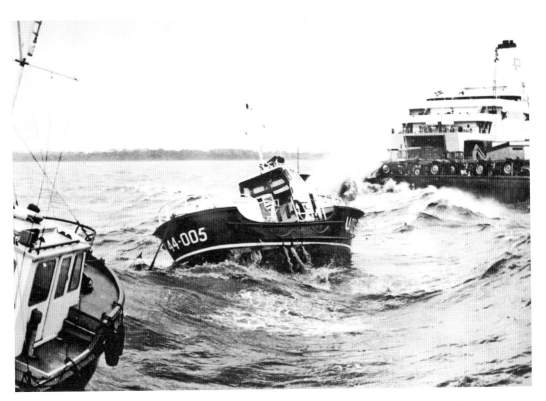

Margaret Graham at moorings in the Pound on 4 April 1973 when north-westerly storm force ten winds hit the harbour. When blowing from this direction, the wind is funnelled down the river causing heavy seas in the Pound. (By courtesy of Harwich RNLI)

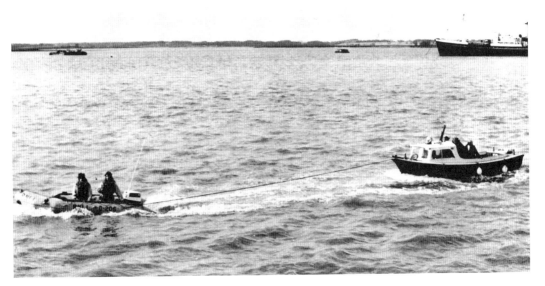

Inshore lifeboat D-208, manned by Ken Brand and C. Moll, towing a customs launch and two customs officers into harbour on 24 April 1974. The launch's engine had broken down and the vessel began drifting before the ILB arrived. (By courtesy of Ken Brand)

refuelled, *Margaret Graham* and her crew were called out again, this time to the 25ft yacht *Boxer*, of Burnham, which had a broken rudder and was caught in force six to seven winds and rough seas. After a passage of an hour, the lifeboat reached the casualty at 12.20pm at the Shipwash Sands, and a tow was rigged. Lifeboat and yacht reached harbour at 2pm, with the couple on board the yacht later commenting they were lucky to have made it safely.

In December 1973 it was announced by Honorary Secretary Captain Richard Coolen that Harwich was to get a new and faster inshore lifeboat. The new lifeboat was an Atlantic 21 rigid-inflatable, a new type developed by the RNLI during the early 1970s, capable of night operation, manned by a crew of three and faster than the smaller inflatable ILBs that had served Harwich since the station had been reopened. The intention was to supply an Atlantic to the station in summer 1974, with the boat to be launched by a davit from a boathouse on Ha'penny Pier. Negotiations were at the time under way between British Rail and Trinity House, who wanted to take over of the pier. However, the new ILB did not arrive at the station until 1978, with the RNLI announcing in 1976 that plans for the new Atlantic had been shelved because, according to Captain Coolen, 'of the escalating costs and the Institution's efforts to modernise and replace other lifeboats around the coast'. So, in the meantime, a series of Zodiac Mk.II type inflatable inshore lifeboats served the station, starting in January 1974 with D-206, funded by Lady D. E. G. Hunt. The relief ILB D-94 was also on station in 1974 from 6 June until 12 September. D-206 stayed until January 1976 when she was replaced by D-240. The last of the inflatables, D-225, came in November 1977 and only stayed for three months.

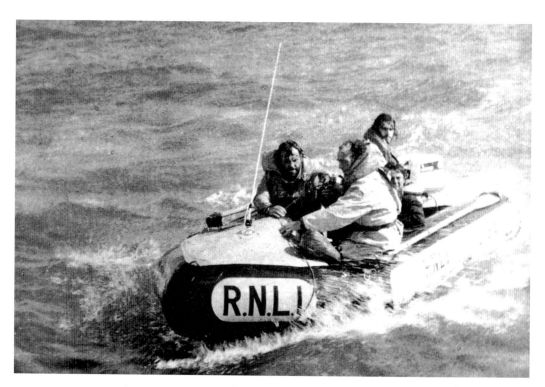

The relief D class inflatable D-94, crewed by Peter Burwood, Aubrey Seaman and Charlie Moll, transferring women and children from the ketch Irene to the relief lifeboat 44-001. The ketch had gone aground on Cork Sand on 10 August 1974 and the lifeboats worked together to save nine people from the vessel. (By courtesy of Ken Brand)

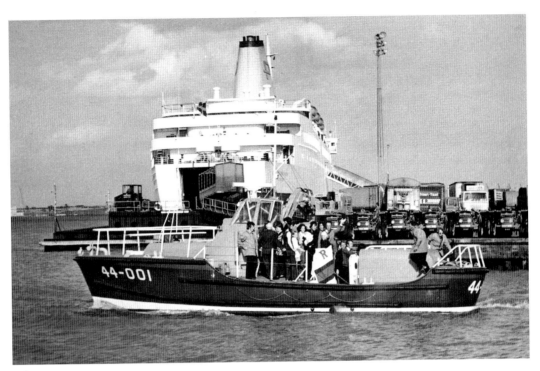

The prototype Waveney 44-001 served as a relief lifeboat at Harwich on several occasions. She is pictured on 8 September 1974 after Helen Brand and Craig Moll had been christened on board her by the Rev Noel Thomas. (By courtesy of Ken Brand)

During the latter half of 1974, the relief lifeboat 44-001 was again on duty, serving the station from 13 June until 31 January 1975, while *Margaret Graham* was taken to Lowestoft for refit. The relief lifeboat launched nine times during this latest stint and saved nineteen lives. Her most notable rescue during this period came on 10 August 1974, when she launched to the ninety-eight-ton ketch *Irene*, which had gone aground on the Cork Sands in force five to six winds and moderate to rough seas. 44-001 went to the casualty but could not get close enough to get alongside because the water was too shallow, so the inshore lifeboat D-98 was used to provide a shuttle service to transfer nine people, including an expectant mother and five children, to the lifeboat. After landing all but four men, who stayed aboard the 1907-built vessel, the lifeboat was able to return to the Sands and tow the vessel to harbour.

Margaret Graham, back on station in January 1975, performed a number of routine services landing sick or injured crew members from ships and in August 1975 completed a fine rescue which Honorary Secretary Captain Richard Coolen later described as 'potentially disastrous'. The lifeboat crew were alerted at 10.30pm on 1 August after five Sea Scouts in canoes were reported missing. Two of their canoes had capsized in the river Deben at 9pm and a third had reached the shore safely, raising the alarm. The Scouts then clung to their craft for two and a half hours before being found by the lifeboat. *Margaret Graham*, searching with other lifeboats, found them two miles from the point at which their canoes had overturned after almost an hour of searching. The crew stopped the engines during the search to listen for shouts and eventually spotted the Scouts 150 yards away. 'It was the crew's initiative which found them,' said Captain Coolen later, adding 'It was terribly dangerous because the boys could have been dead within minutes.'

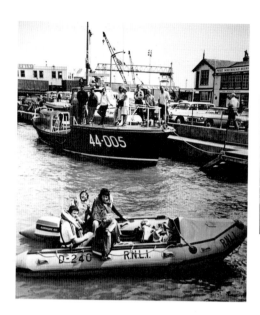

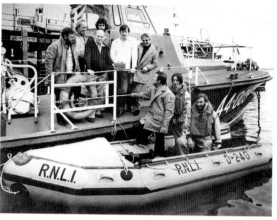

D class inflatable D-240 with Margaret Graham during a public relations trip on 6 June 1976. (By courtesy of Ken Brand)

Just over a month later, on 8 September 1975, *Margaret Graham* was called out four times, bringing in three yachts, a cabin cruiser and fourteen people in total. The first call, at about 8.30pm, was to the yacht *Eipararon*, which had gone aground off Dovercourt with engine trouble. The craft was refloated and as the lifeboat towed the casualty back to Harwich, she came across the twenty-ton cabin cruiser *Gloriette*, which was taking in water and in danger of sinking. The craft was also taken in tow while a salvage pump was being prepared ashore to pump the boat out immediately upon arrival. Before *Margaret Graham* had moored up, red flares were reported being sighted from the Sunk lightvessel so the lifeboat put out again. She soon found the 25ft yacht *Bella Pais*, which had steering trouble. As the yacht was being towed into Harwich, a red flare was sighted off the Stone Pier where another yacht, *Tusquar*, was being pounded against the pier. The police helped the owner ashore while the lifeboat dragged the yacht off and into Harwich harbour. The lifeboat crew eventually finished their work at 3.20am on 9 September having been on service for almost six hours.

On 13 November 1975 relief lifeboat 44-001 came to Harwich again for another spell of duty and on 1 December 1975 the relief lifeboat and her crew were involved in a tragic search for two fishermen whose boat sank the previous day. The 28ft inshore fishing boat *Lilian J* was crossing the bar at the entrance to the river Deben in heavy seas and a gale force southerly wind when she was overwhelmed and sank. The lifeboat and an RAF rescue helicopter from Manston were called out to help search for the two missing men, but after a long search nothing was found.

In January 1976 a new inshore lifeboat was sent to the station, number D-240. She was another D class inflatable, while the Atlantic 21, which the station personnel and crew were hoping for, was delayed. The new boat, funded by the Rotary Club of Snaresbrook, was a standard Zodiac Mk.II boat and stayed at Harwich until November 1977. Her first service was undertaken on 1 April 1976 when she launched at 10.26pm to investigate reports of red flares in Dovercourt Bay, but nothing was found. She was out again the following day and assisted a 15ft motor boat with two persons on board, taking the craft to the entrance to the river Deben where Felixstowe Coastguard Mobile met the ILB. Further service launches followed during the month, with calls on 11 April to a capsized angling boat, on 15 April to a capsized sailing dinghy and on 18 April to another capsized sailing dinghy.

On 23 April 1976 *Margaret Graham* was called out to help the Gorleston lifeboat *Khami*, which was standing by the British coaster *Manta*, bound from Rotterdam to Boston with a cargo of maize. In a north-easterly force seven wind, with rough seas, the coaster started to list after her cargo shifted when she was thirty miles off the Norfolk coast. The Gorleston lifeboat launched to stand by the coaster, whose captain altered course for Harwich, as the ship was rolling heavily with a thirty-degree list, while the lifeboat remained in attendance. *Margaret Graham* put out at 11am and reached the casualty an hour and a half later, allowing the Gorleston lifeboat, which had been out all night, to leave the scene and go to Harwich to refuel before returning to station; she was out for about eighteen hours in all and covered 150 miles during this testing service. In the rough seas, *Margaret Graham* finished escorting the coaster to harbour at 3pm, and half an hour later was back on station.

The seventy-year-old former Swedish customs cutter *L'Atlanta*, with four adults and two children on board, required the assistance of *Margaret Graham* on 9 July 1977 after running aground on the Cork Sands. The 38ft vessel started taking on water so her crew sent out a mayday message , which saw *Margaret Graham* putting out at 12.20pm in a north-easterly force four to five winds and moderate seas. Reaching the scene at 1pm, the lifeboat was unable to get close to the casualty due to the sands, so the lifeboat's inflatable dinghy was used to transfer a tow rope across. The dinghy, manned by two crew, encountered heavy seas in order to reach the casualty, but at 1.10pm the tow line had been secured. The ketch was then towed off the sands but, as she was taking in

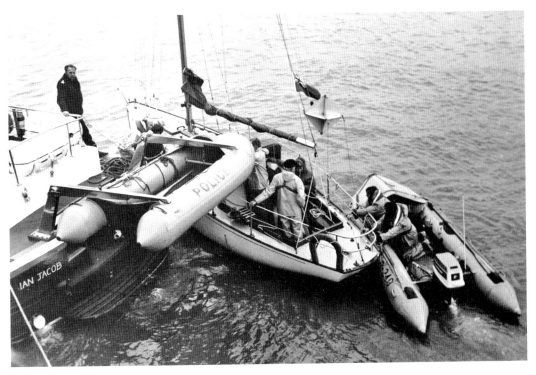

Inshore lifeboat D-240 assisting the 25ft yacht Sea Gem III on 24 August 1977. The yacht was caught out in rough seas and strong winds when its engine failed and the wind started blowing it onto the Stone Pier. The ILB managed to get a line aboard and attempted to hold the yacht off the rocks. The line was then transferred to the police launch, which was also on scene and managed to tow the yacht clear, with Margaret Graham also on scene standing by. (By courtesy of Ken Brand)

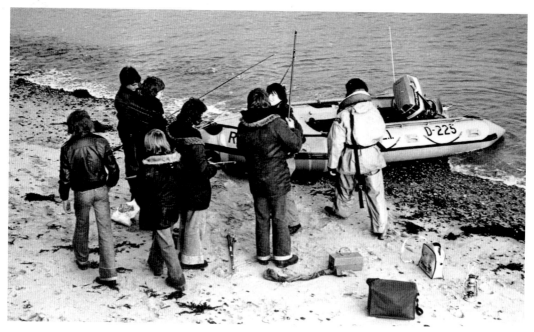

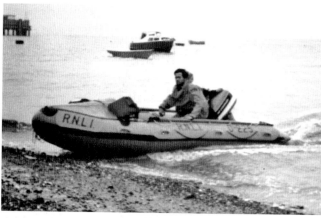

The last service launch by a D class inflatable at Harwich, as D-225 lands children on Dovercourt Beach having taken them off the disused Dovercourt lighthouse on 14 February 1978. (By courtesy of Ken Brand)

D class inflatable D-255 returns to Harwich beach on 12 March 1978 after the last exercise launch of a D class ILB at the station. D-255 served at Harwich from October 1977 to April 1978. (Ken Brand)

water, the two lifeboat men stayed aboard to help bail. The two children were transferred to the lifeboat, and the ketch was towed to Harwich where she was berthed alongside Ha'penny Pier so that a pump could be put aboard to stop her sinking.

On 16 October 1977 the relief lifeboat 44-001 arrived on station with *Margaret Graham* going to Ian Brown's yard at Rowhedge for refit. On 29 October a relief ILB arrived on station, D-225, to replace D-240 which had been damaged and punctured while launching the previous day. So Harwich had two relief boats and both carried out a number of rescues. The ILB was launched on 12 November but was not needed, but was out again two days later after a small dinghy with three men aboard was seen drifting out of the harbour on a strong ebb tide and offshore wind. The wind was force eight but the sea in the harbour was moderate, and after launching at 2.37pm the ILB had reached the casualty within five minutes. The three men were taken out of their dinghy, which was recovered by the Trinity House launch *Thamesis* and taken to Harwich Quay.

Just over a week before these incidents involving the relief ILB, the relief Waveney was involved in a fine service on 2 November 1977 after violent sea had smashed the bridge windows on the coaster *Frederick Hughes* while the vessel was on passage from Rotterdam to Great Yarmouth. The incident occurred about ten miles north of the Outer Gabbard light vessel. The skipper was able to send out a mayday message at 2am just before water put the electronics out of action. The lifeboat put out at 2.45pm and reached the casualty at 7.15am and found the ferries *Gaelic Ferry* and *Stena Normandica* standing by. The master of *Gaelic Ferry* had realised the situation could deteriorate and so manoeuvred his vessel to within 200 yards of the stricken coaster to shield the casualty from the worst of the weather. *Stena Normandica* shone powerful searchlights on the coaster, whose crew

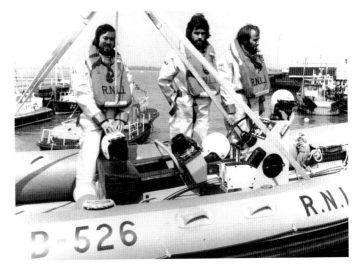

Peter Brand, Charlie Moll and Bob Ramplin on board the Atlantic 21 B-526 shortly after the boat had arrived on station.

The station's first Atlantic 21 rigid inflatable lifeboat B-526 on a publicity launch in 1978 with Bob Ramplin on helm and John Teatheredge crewing. She served at Harwich until October 1987. (Both photos courtesy of Ken Brand)

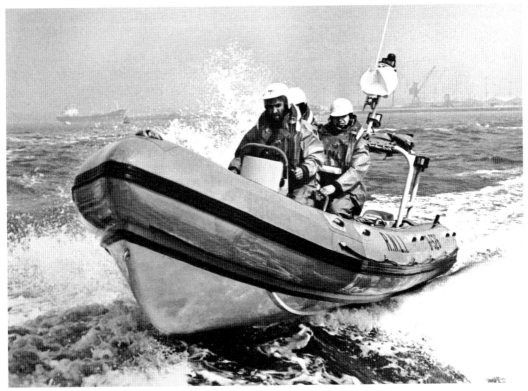

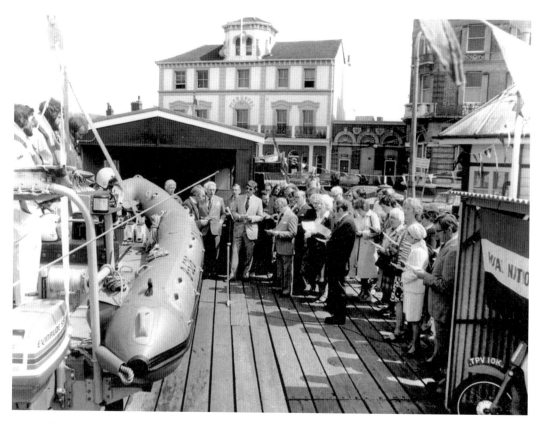

The scene during the dedication ceremony for Atlantic 21 B-526 outside the ILB house on Ha'penny Pier, 27 May 1978. (By courtesy of Ken Brand)

were then able to start pumping fuel by hand and steering was reverted to manual operation. Once the lifeboat had arrived, and still shielded by *Gaelic Ferry*, the coaster began the slow journey back to harbour, escorted by 44-001. The passage took eight hours, and the lifeboat was not back on station until 2.45pm.

In 1978, after five years of waiting, the new Atlantic 21 inshore lifeboat was placed on station at Harwich. The Atlantic rigid-inflatable design had been developed at Atlantic College in South Wales and provided the RNLI with a new dimension in inshore rescue. The Harwich boat, number B-526, had been built in 1974 and used in the Relief Fleet initially, as well as being shown at the Lifeboat Exhibition in Plymouth in July 1974 to mark the RNLI's 150th anniversary. The boat was sent to the station initially in December 1977 to test the newly-installed launching davit on Ha'penny Pier, under the watchful eye of RNLI divisional inspector Mike Pennell, and was then returned to the RNLI Depot at Poole for a refit, before returning to Harwich the following March. The davit was designed by Paddy O'Grady of Cobramold Ltd, Stansted. Meanwhile, the D class remained on station, and the last service by D-225 was performed on 14 February 1978 when she brought ashore six youths who were fishing off the lighthouse at Dovercourt. Although the youths were not in trouble, and the call for help proved unfounded, they were ordered to be taken off by local police.

The new Atlantic 21 returned to Harwich on 19 March 1978 and underwent final trials and testing. The new boat, built at a cost of £15,000, was crewed by three, powered by twin 55hp Evinrude outboards giving her a top speed of almost thirty knots and with two twelve-gallon petrol tanks had a cruising range of ninety miles, considerably enhancing the rescue capabilities of the station. The boat carried VHF radio, a drogue and a radar reflector, and was fitted with air-bags which could be inflated to right the boat in the event of a capsize. The boathouse on the Pier was extended to accommodate the new ILB, and a purpose-designed trolley on rails was installed to get the boat from the house to the davit, which was used to launch the boat. Three crew members, Terry Bennett, Peter Brand and Charlie Moll, had been on an Atlantic 21 training course on the Isle of Wight, and crew training at the station was supervised by Mike Pennell.

The first service by the Atlantic 21 came on 25 March 1978, a week after she arrived, when she was launched to an inflatable shaped as a whale which was swept off Felixstowe pier by a freak gust of wind, with two children on board. The lifeboat was not needed as the inflatable was blown ashore, but the children needed hospital attention. B-526 was out again on service on 29 and 30 March, but on neither occasion was she needed as the casualty got ashore unaided. On 19 April she was taken out on exercise with RNLI divisional inspector Tom Nutman and, after the crew had successfully passed the necessary tests, B-526 was officially placed on station. D-225 was withdrawn from service, and on 18 April left for the Isle of Wight. Two days earlier, B-526 had towed in an angling boat, which had broken down a mile north of the North Cork Buoy.

On 1 May the Atlantic was launched after a sixteen-year-old boy, who had broken into a cabin cruiser moored in the river near Parkeston and was sleeping rough, tried to light the boat's gas stove to keep warm and it blew up. The explosion ripped the boat apart, but the boy survived. The lifeboat found the boy waist deep in mud, with his face and arms badly burned, and suffering from shock and exposure. The lifeboat crew had great difficulty in keeping him conscious until he was landed at Parkeston Quay where an ambulance was waiting to take him to hospital. The lifeboat then undertook a further search of the area and found the 27ft cabin cruiser *Joncla* badly damaged.

The Atlantic 21 had not been purchased by a specific donor, and was never named but was referred to by its number, B-526. So the formal entry into service for the boat consisted of a service of dedication held on 27 May 1978, during which the new lifeboat house was also officially opened. During the ceremony, Lady Norton, MBE, a member of the RNLI's Committee of Management, handed over the boat to the Harwich station, and it was accepted by Howard Bell, Chairman of

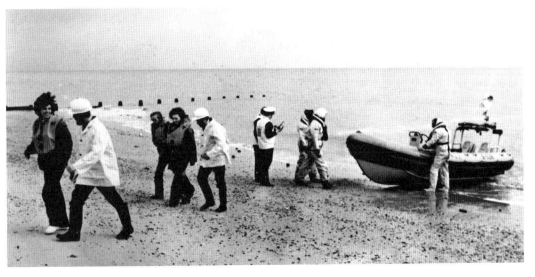

Atlantic 21 B-526 is beached at Walton during an exercise to land the mock survivors, 21 November 1978. (By courtesy of Ken Brand)

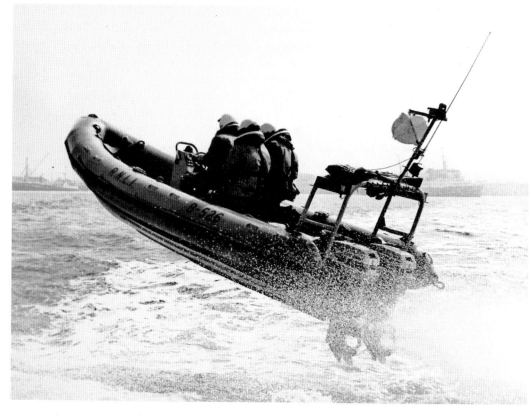

A dramatic photo of the Atlantic 21 B-526 on exercise. This image was later used extensively by the RNLI in publicity material. (By courtesy of Ken Brand)

the Harwich and Dovercourt Branch. The service of dedication was led by the Rev J. Chelton, vicar of St Nicholas Church. The boat was launched for a demonstration run at the end of proceedings, with Lady Norton donning a life-jacket and going afloat for a short trip round the harbour.

While the changes to the ILB service were being made, *Margaret Graham* continued rescue work, returning from refit on 21 January 1978 and then completing a series of services during the year to land sick or injured crewmen from ships. Some of the medical calls were largely routine, while others were more challenging, and on one in September 1978 speed was of the essence. On 24 September a Greek seaman on the cargo ship *Nadina* suffered a severe facial injury when he was hit by a piece of flying metal. *Margaret Graham* put out at 10.45am with Dr Collins on board, and helicopter assistance from RAF Manston was requested as reports were coming from the ship to say the seaman was bleeding very badly. Once the helicopter was airborne, and with time against the rescuers, it was agreed that Dr Collins would be lifted from the lifeboat and winched aboard the cargo ship. The first lift was completed at 11am, and the doctor was transferred to the cargo ship where he treated the injured man, who was then airlifted off and taken by helicopter direct to Canterbury Hospital. Meanwhile, the lifeboat returned to Harwich within an hour of launching.

In 1979 the RNLI announced that a new 44ft Waveney lifeboat was being built for Harwich to replace *Margaret Graham*. Her last full year of service proved to be an eventful one, starting with a dramatic service on 19 January 1979 to the 350-ton motor vessel *Mi Amigo*, which was host to the pop pirate station Radio Caroline. The lifeboat launched at 3.30pm and faced huge seas in force

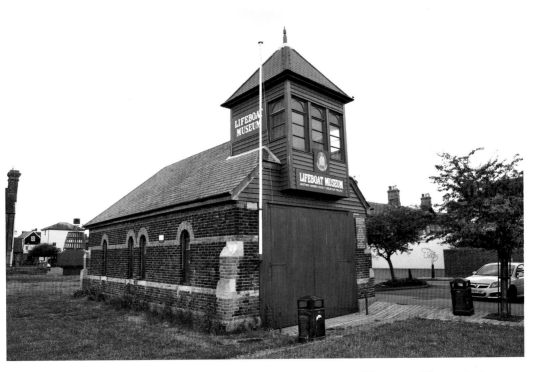

1. *The lifeboat house built at the East Beach in 1876 at a cost of £247 10s. The original ornamental turret was removed in the 1950s but restored in the 1990s when the building became a lifeboat museum. (Nicholas Leach)*

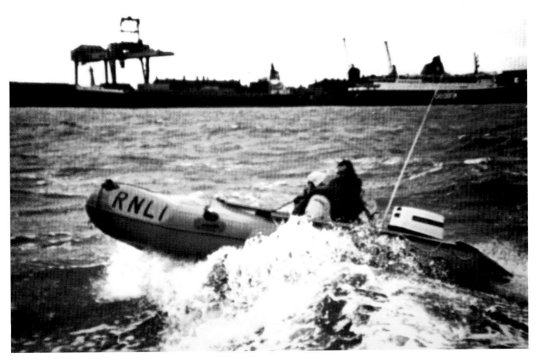

2. *The D class inflatable inshore lifeboat D-206, on exercise in April 1974, was a 15ft 6in Zodiac Mk.II type. She served from 1974 to 1975. (Ken Brand)*

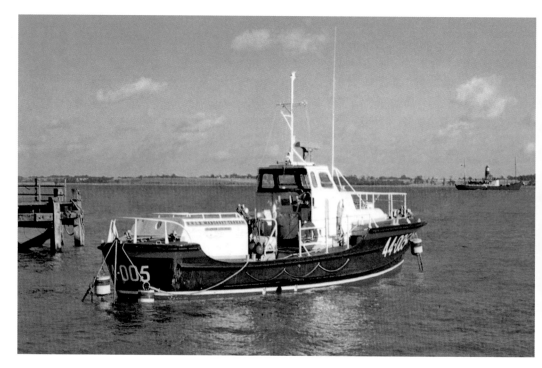

3. *44ft Waveney* Margaret Graham *at moorings in the Pound. During her first years on station her upperworks were painted white, a livery developed by the RNLI during the 1960s prior to high-visibility orange. (From a postcard supplied by Nicholas Leach)*

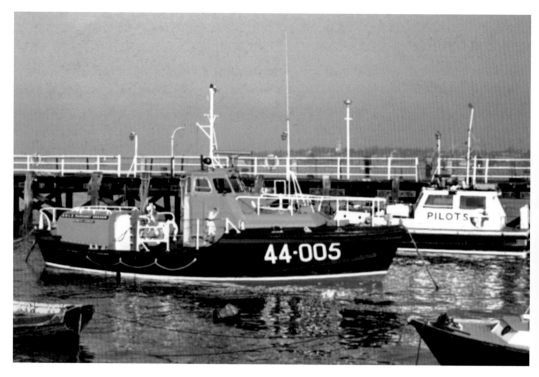

4. Margaret Graham, *close to the pilot launches, at moorings in the Pound after her upperworks had been painted orange. (By courtesy of Harwich RNLI)*

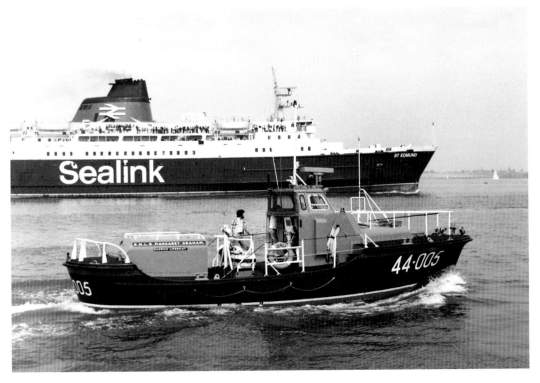

5. *Margaret Graham afloat in Harwich harbour, passing the Sealink ferry St Edmund, which operated between Harwich and the Hook of Holland from 1975 until 1982. (By courtesy of Harwich RNLI)*

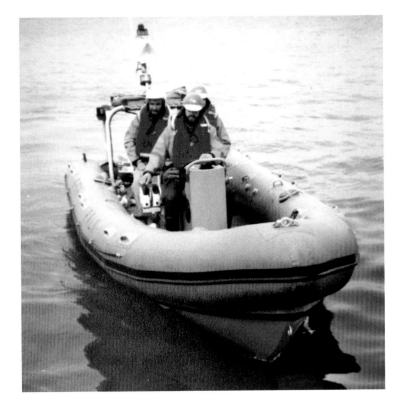

6. *The first Atlantic 21 on station, B-526, putting out from Harwich for a publicity launch in April 1978. (Ken Brand)*

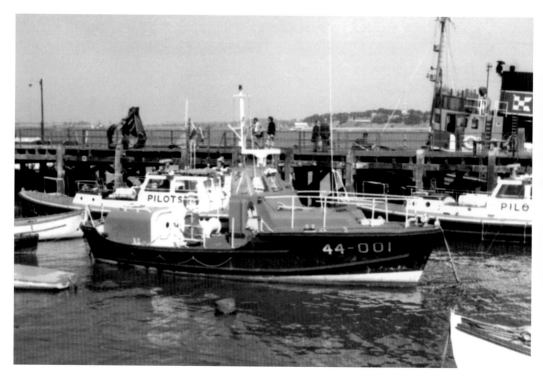

7. The relief 44ft Waveney 44-001, the prototype boat of the class. This boat served at Harwich on a number of occasions during the 1960s and 1970s.

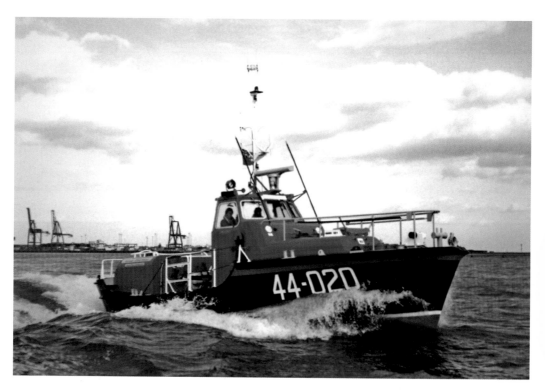

8. John Fison was the second 44ft Waveney to be built for Harwich, and served the station from March 1980 to October 1996. (Ken Brand)

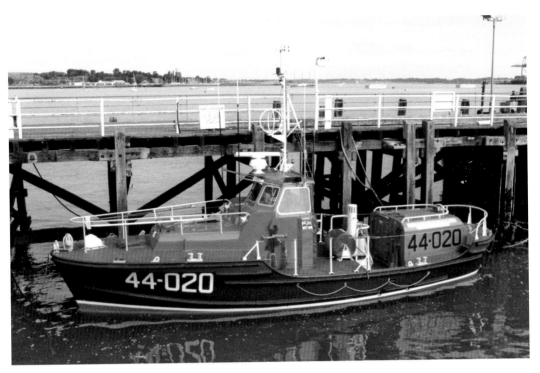

9. *John Fison at moorings in the Pound close to Ha'penny Pier, August 1996. The Waveneys occupied two different mooring locations in the Pound. (Andrew Cooke)*

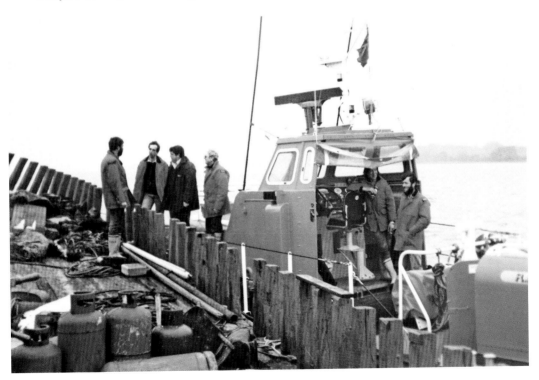

10. *John Fison alongside the former trawler Mary La after the vessel was seen on fire on 14 June 1987. The lifeboat crew went aboard to extinguish the blaze on the vessel, which was anchored in the river Orwell. (By courtesy of Harwich RNLI)*

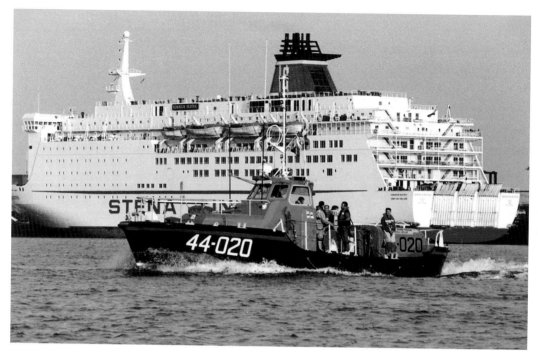

11. *The 44ft Waveney John Fison on exercise in the harbour for the local newspaper, with the Stena Line ferry Koningin Beatrix in the background. (By courtesy of Harwich RNLI)*

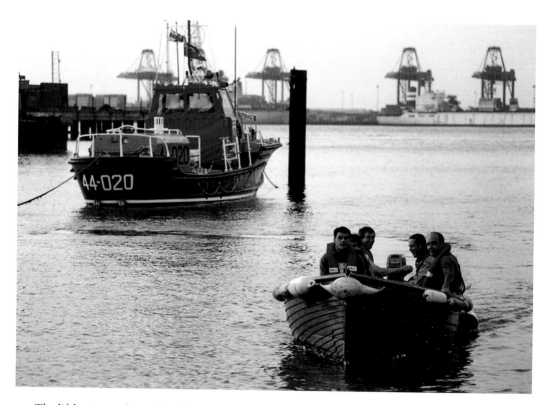

12. *The lifeboat crew leave John Fison at moorings in the Harbour Master's Pound and return to shore in the wooden boarding boat. (By courtesy of Harwich RNLI)*

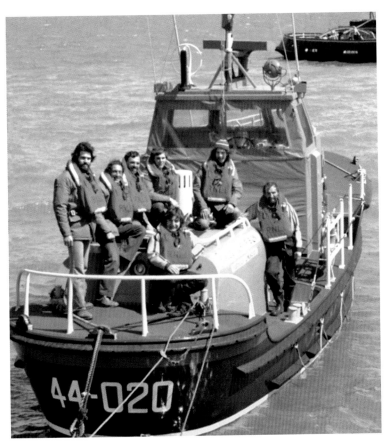

(Left) 13. Lifeboat crew on board John Fison, from left to right, are Charlie Moll, Les Smith, Peter Burwood, Martin Burwood, Ken Brand, Bob Ramplin, with John Teatheredge at front.

(Below) 14. Retired and serving crew: on the pier, left to right, Kevin Smith, Les Smith, Don Mudd, Aubrey Seaman, David Gilders, Bob Ramplin and Peter Burwood. On the Waveney: Douglas Good, Alan Sharp, Andrew Moors, Bob Barton, John Teatheredge, Peter Brand, Andrew Webb, Peter Dawson, Jon Rudd, Ken Brand, Captain Rod Shaw, and Paul Smith. On the ILB: Brendon Shaw, Simon Benham, Peter Bull, Glen Davis, Jason Davis and John Reason.

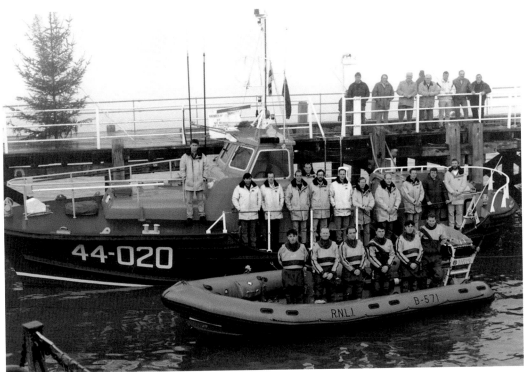

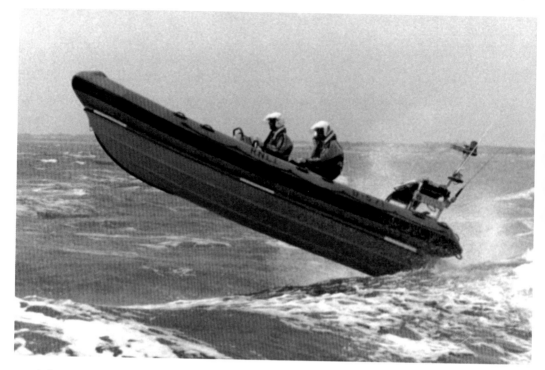

15. *A dramatic photograph of Atlantic 21 B-571 British Diver II in rough seas. The second Atlantic 21 at Harwich, B-571 served from October 1987 to October 2002.*

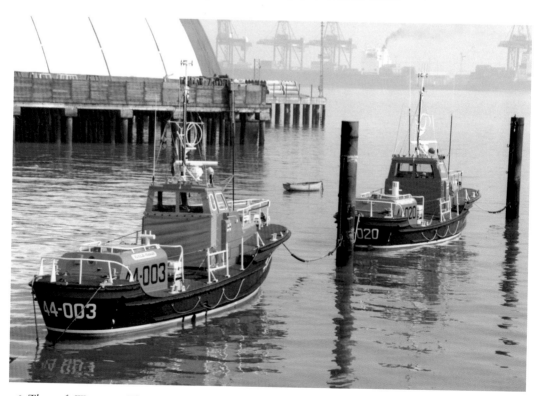

16. *The 44ft Waveneys Khami (on left) and John Fison in the Harbour Master's Pound on 7 May 1995. Khami undertook a relief duty from 4 March to 11 May 1995. (Nicholas Leach)*

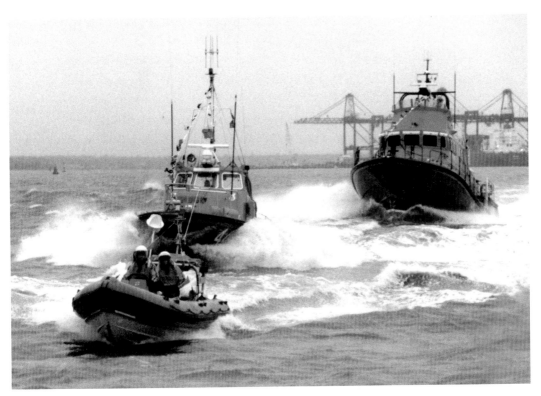

17. The 17m Severn *Albert Brown* arrives on station, escorted home by *John Fison* and *B-571 British Diver II*, December 1995. (Orwell Photography, by courtesy of Harwich RNLI)

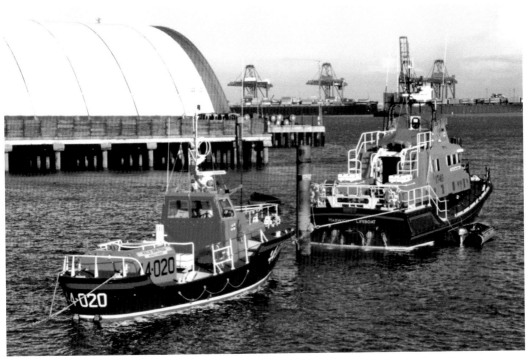

18. *John Fison* and *Albert Brown* at moorings in the Harbour Master's Pound in October 1996, when crew training on the Severn was being completed. (Peter Edey)

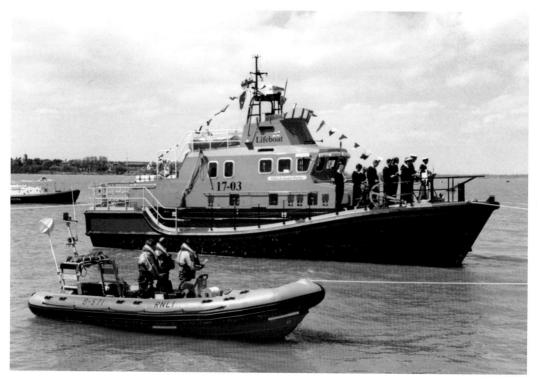

19. *The scene during the naming ceremony of 17m Severn Albert Brown at Navyard Wharf on 25 May 1997, with Atlantic 21 B-571 British Diver II in attendance. The lifeboat was named by Terry Waite CBE. (Nicholas Leach)*

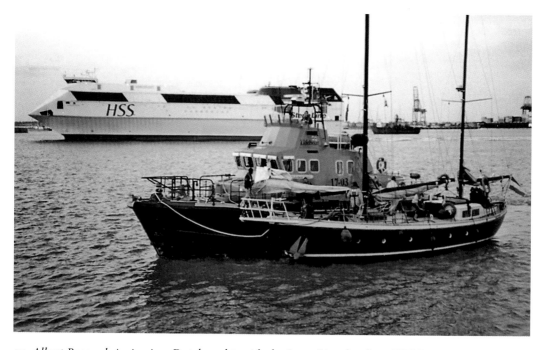

20. *Albert Brown bringing in a Dutch yacht, with the Stena Line fast ferry HSS Discovery arriving in port. (By courtesy of Harwich RNLI)*

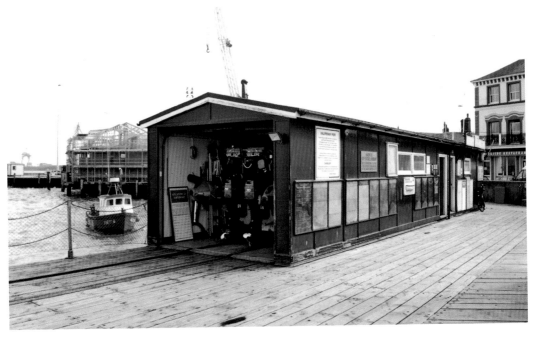

21. The ILB house and crew room on Ha'penny Pier with Atlantic 21 B-571 on her trolley. The house was built in 1977 having been funded through the 1974 Rotary Fete held by the Harwich and District Rotary Club. In this photograph, taken in September 2001, the new lifeboat station can be seen under construction to the left. (Nicholas Leach)

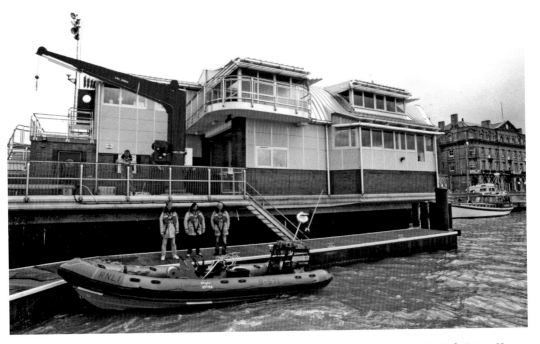

22. The lifeboat station building completed in 2002 with Atlantic 21 B-571 British Diver II in the water, July 2002. Captain Rod Shaw is standing by the davit with, left to right on the pontoon, Peter Dawson (Coxswain), Alan Sharp and John Rudd. Note the former lifeboat Albert Edward on the right. Built in 1901, she served at Clacton-on-Sea from 1901 to 1929 and was sold out of service in 1932. (Peter Edey)

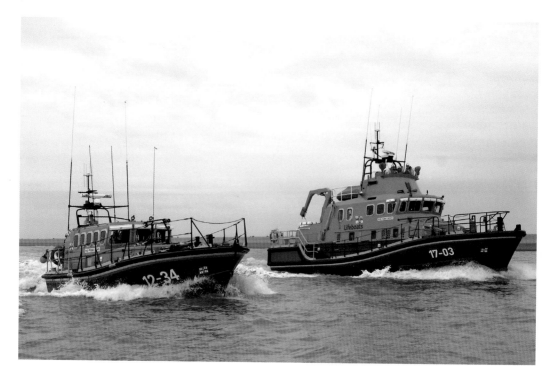

23. *Albert Brown on exercise off the Suffolk coast with Aldeburgh's 12m Mersey lifeboat Freddie Cooper, June 2004. (Nicholas Leach)*

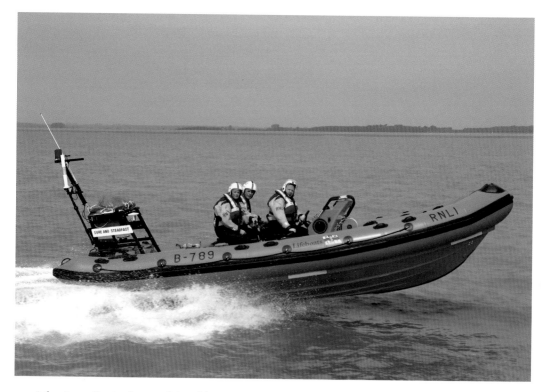

24. *Atlantic 75 B-789 Sure and Steadfast on exercise off the Suffolk coast in June 2004. B-789 was placed on station in October 2002. (Nicholas Leach)*

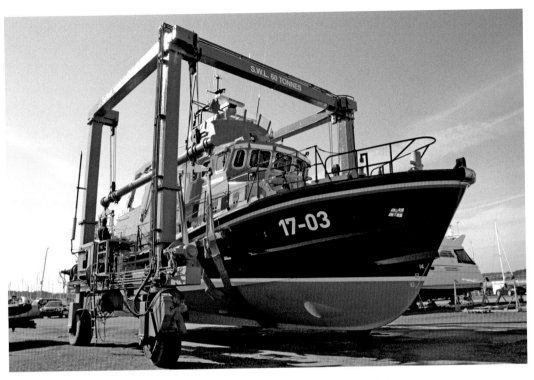

25. *Albert Brown out of the water at Levington Marina. (Peter Edey)*

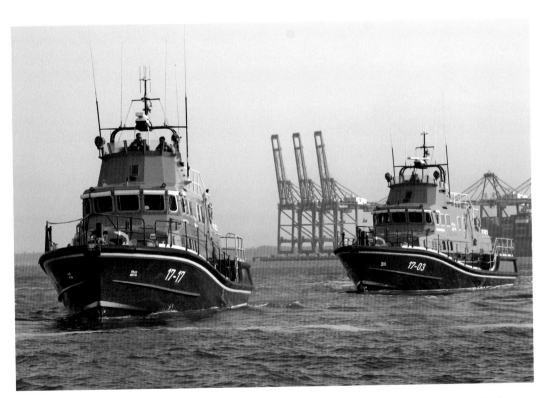

26. *Relief 17m Severn Fraser Flyer with Albert Brown in May 2008. The station boat had returned to station the previous day after maintenance work at Poole. (Graeme Ewens)*

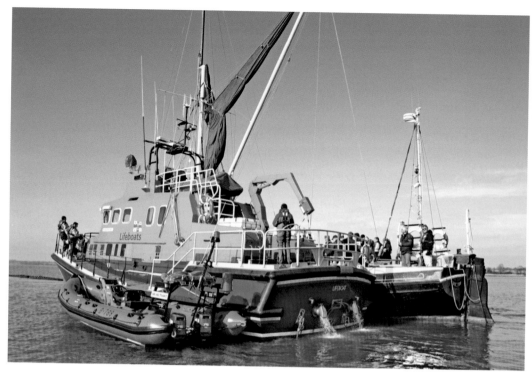

27. Relief 17m Severn The Will and Atlantic 75 B-789 alongside the barge Victor during a *medical exercise involving the local Coastguard, police and RAF search and rescue helicopter in February 2009. (Nicholas Leach)*

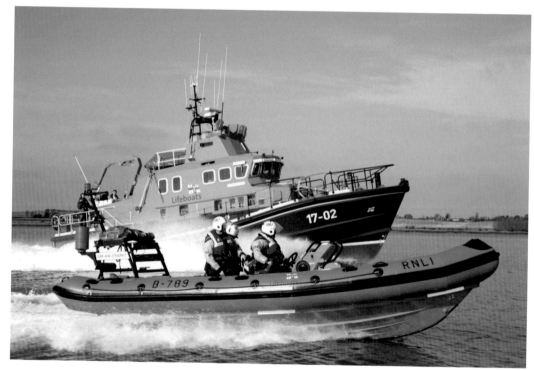

28. Relief 17m Severn The Will and Atlantic 75 B-789 Sure and Steadfast at speed in the river *Stour returning to station after exercise. (Nicholas Leach)*

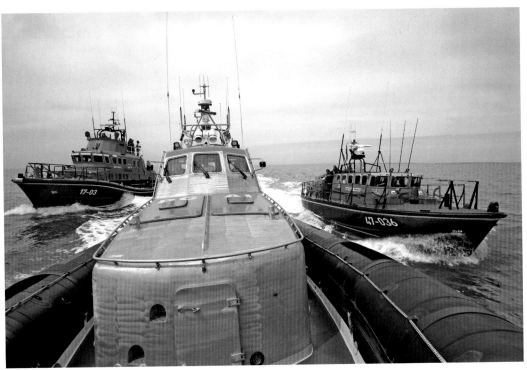

29. *Albert Brown and Walton and Frinton lifeboat Kenneth Thelwall II exercise with the KNRM lifeboat Jeanine Parqui from Hook of Holland, July 2010. (Nicholas Leach)*

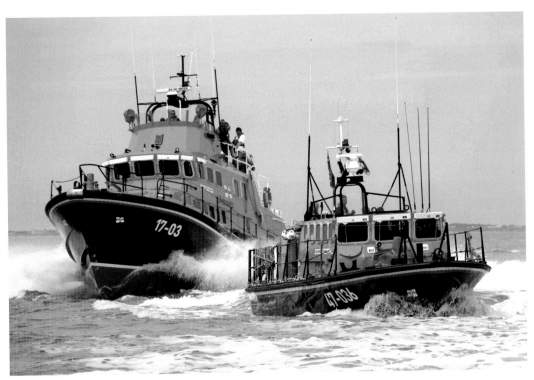

30. *Albert Brown with Walton and Frinton's 47ft Tyne lifeboat Kenneth Thelwall II. Joint exercises with Harwich's neighbouring lifeboats are regularly held. (Nicholas Leach)*

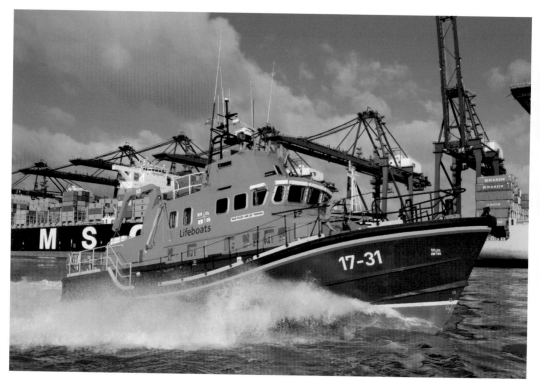

31. *Relief 17m Severn* Roger and Joy Freeman *on engine trials off the Trinity Terminal at Felixstowe container port, January 2011. (Nicholas Leach)*

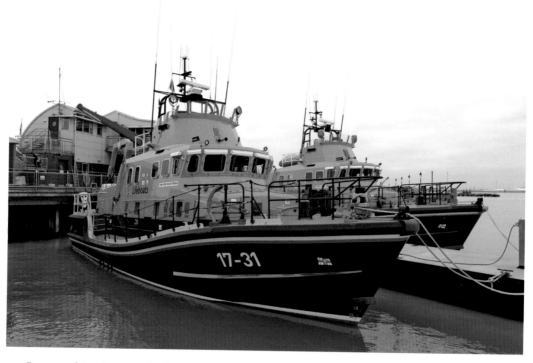

32. Roger and Joy Freeman *in the mooring pen with* Albert Brown, *which had returned from Poole the previous day, also alongside, 31 January 2011. (Nicholas Leach)*

eight to nine gale force winds to reach the casualty, which was moored fourteen miles off Walton and had started to take on water in the engine room. Both electric and petrol pumps on board the ship had failed and so a mayday was sent out. Harwich lifeboat made a round trip of fifty-five miles in five and a half hours, battling with 25ft waves and storm force winds to reach the casualty. *Mi Amigo* was expected to sink, but the storm abated in time and she was able to be repaired. The five on board, three disc jockeys and two crew, were taken off by the lifeboat, and landed at Harwich just after 9pm.

Bad weather proved very nasty for two Ipswich fishermen, who were rescued by *Margaret Graham* just in time on 28 January. The men, suffering from cold and exposure were adrift off Felixstowe in a snowstorm in their 16ft angling boat. The lifeboat put out at 11.05pm and reached the casualty within fifteen minutes, and several attempts were made to tow the boat to safety, but because of the rough conditions the anglers were taken aboard the lifeboat. They had become delirious because of the cold and the lifeboat crew had to force them to leave their boat, which was subsequently abandoned. The men were landed at Harwich and taken by ambulance to Harwich and District Hospital.

Two more notable rescues took place in May 1979, the first on 5 May to the Spanish cargo vessel *Isle Del Atlantico*, which was listing eleven miles off Walton. *Margaret Graham* put out at 7.45pm and stood by for four hours until the list had been corrected, returning to station at 3.10am on 6 May. The lifeboat was called out again on 26 May after 200-ton coaster *Queenford*, bound for Mistley, was reported to be sinking fifteen miles off the coast in south-westerly force six to eight

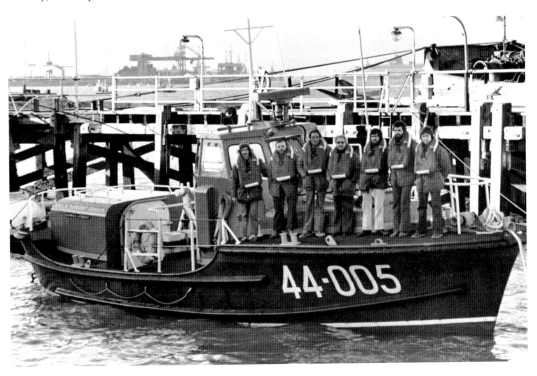

Lifeboat crew on board Margaret Graham in January 1980. They are, left to right, Ken Brand, Peter Burwood (Coxswain/Mechanic), Les Smith (Second Coxswain), Howard Bell (Branch Chairman), Peter Brand, Charlie Moll, and John Teatheredge. She departed Harwich two months after this photo was taken, having launched 173 times on service. (By courtesy of Ken Brand)

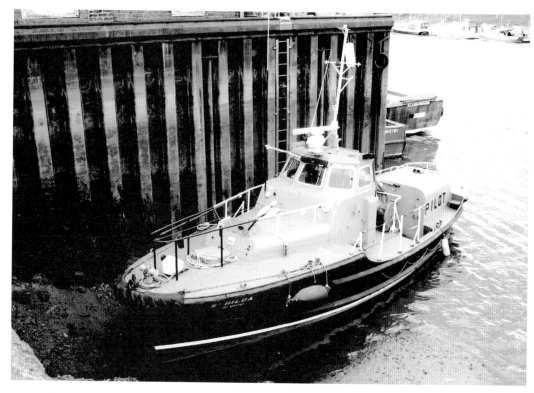

After service Margaret Graham was sold out of service to become the Whitby Harbour Board's pilot boat St Hilda of Whitby. (Nicholas Leach)

winds. *Margaret Graham* and two ships stood by while an RAF helicopter lifted off the two crew members and landed them on the beach. The skipper stayed on board to try to steer the crippled vessel into either Harwich or Felixstowe but, as conditions worsened, he too abandoned ship. The list was so pronounced that he was able to slide down the vessel onto the rubbing strake and then step to the lifeboat. The coaster eventually beached a mile south of the Orfordness lighthouse.

The last service performed by *Margaret Graham* was to the 4,000-ton cargo vessel *Arlington* on 25 January 1980, which had a fire in her engine room. Both Harwich and Aldeburgh lifeboats reached the casualty at the same time, and *Margaret Graham* stood by while the tug *Hibernia* made fast a tow line. The lifeboat returned to Harwich at 9.25am having been away from station for almost six hours. This was the last of 173 service launches undertaken by *Margaret Graham* in her twelve and a half years on station at Harwich, during which time she saved seventy-seven lives and this outstanding record of service saw Harwich become one of the RNLI's key stations.

After leaving Harwich in March 1980, *Margaret Graham* served as a Relief lifeboat for six years, and then went to Amble in Northumberland for a further thirteen years. She was sold out of RNLI service in August 1999 having served the Institution for a remarkable thirty-three years, saving almost 100 lives in the process. She was bought by Scarborough Borough Council who sent her to Whitby where she became the local pilot boat *St Hilda of Whitby*, operating under the auspices of the Whitby Harbour Board.

John Fison

The replacement for *Margaret Graham* was a new 44ft Waveney named *John Fison*. Built by Fairey Marine at Cowes, she had cost £243,487 and had been funded by gifts from Mrs D. E. Fison, in memory of her husband, Mrs D. Knowles, and the John Jarrold Trust, as well as the bequest of Mrs Annie Sutcliffe and a gift from Fisons Ltd. She was named after the late John Fison, the former manager of Fisons Fertilizers' South African operations. She arrived at Harwich on 10 March 1980, and was placed on station the following day, after a three-day passage from the RNLI headquarters in Poole during which she was crewed by Coxswain/Mechanic Peter Burwood, crew members Ken Brand and Bob Ramplin, and district inspector Tom Nutman. The final stage of the passage, from Ramsgate, was undertaken in heavy seas whipped up by force six winds. She was

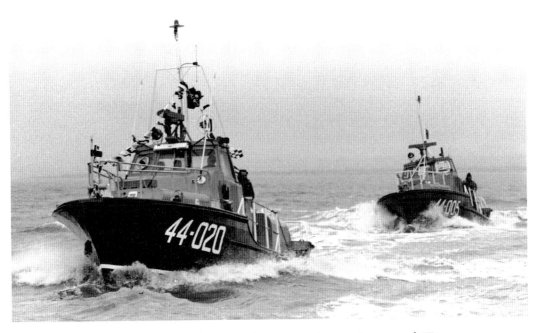

John Fison leads Margaret Graham into harbour on the day the new 44ft Waveney arrived on station, 10 March 1980. (By courtesy of Harwich RNLI)

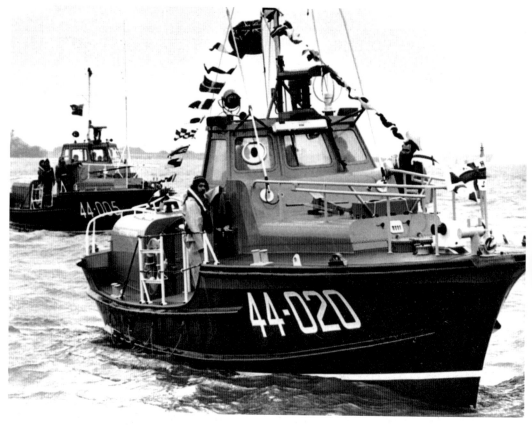

John Fison makes her debut at Harwich in March 1980. (By courtesy of Harwich RNLI)

escorted into harbour by *Margaret Graham* on the final stage of her journey to arrive on schedule. There to greet her were station personnel and crew members, including honorary secretary Captain Richard Coolen, vice-chairman Howard Bell and two other committee members, the Rev James Chelton, lifeboat chaplain, and Dr James Corbett, representing the town's doctors. The new Waveney was more than three knots faster than her predecessor, with a top speed of around sixteen knots, and was fitted with twin 250hp Caterpillar 3208T diesel engines.

Before she had performed a rescue, *John Fison* was taken to Oulton Broad boatyard on 31 May 1980 for painting ready for her formal naming ceremony, with relief 44ft Waveney *Khami* arriving in her place. *John Fison* returned on 14 June, and on 28 June undertook her first service. It was a routine medical evacuation and saw the new boat launching at 9.09pm, with Dr Duncan McPherson on board, to the 13,530-ton tanker *British Poplar* to tend to one of the tanker's crew who had suffered a stroke. The lifeboat reached the casualty at 10.15pm, half a mile from the Sunk lightvessel, and the sick man was transferred across on a stretcher and landed at Harwich. He was then taken by ambulance to hospital, while the lifeboat was ready for service again by midnight.

John Fison was out again on 12 July 1980, launching at 7.22pm after reports that a yacht was firing red flares a mile and a half east of the Sunk lightvessel. An hour after putting out, the lifeboat reached the casualty, the 32ft motor yacht *Lady of Longcombe*, and found she had engine failure while on passage to Walton Backwaters from south Wales with three crew aboard. She was taken in tow by the lifeboat and brought to Harwich at 10.35pm. Six days later the lifeboat was out again, this time spending seven hours at sea and having to travel thirty-five miles to assist the 23ft yacht *Snow Goose*, which, with a crew of three, had a broken mast south of the Outer Gabbard lightvessel. The yacht was reached at 3.10pm, and after a five-hour tow was brought in to Harwich.

A few days after this service, on 26 July 1980, the new Waveney was officially named and dedicated at the Trinity House Pier. Among the guests welcomed by Mr T. M. F. Bernard, president of the branch, were the Mayor and Mayoress of Harwich, Mr and Mrs Lindsey Glenn, the MP for Harwich and his wife, Mr and Mrs Julian Ridsdale, the High Steward of Harwich and his wife, Mr and Mrs William Bleakley, and Tendring Council chairman, Mr F. Good. The new Waveney was handed over to the RNLI on behalf of Mrs Dorothy E. Fison by Mr A. A. D. Phillips. The lifeboat was received by Captain J. B. Leworthy, a member of the Committee of Management, who in turn delivered her into the care of Captain Richard Coolen. The service of dedication was led by the Rev J. H. Chelton, Vicar of St Nicholas' Church, Harwich, and Chaplain of the lifeboat station, assisted by Captain R. Dare of the Salvation Army and Father J. Lindburgh of the Roman Catholic Church,

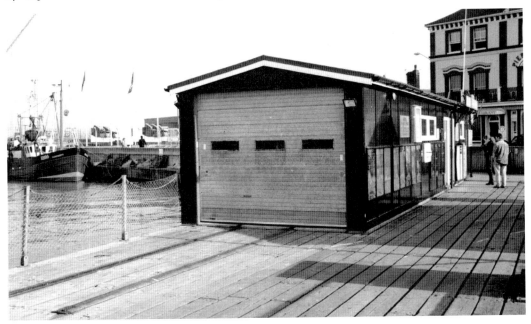

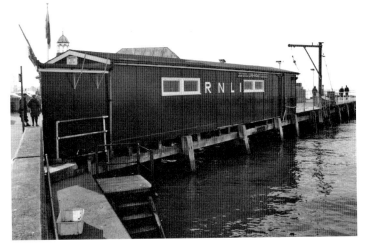

The ILB house was re-sited and rebuilt in 1977 on Ha'penny Pier, and a davit launching facility was constructed for an Atlantic 21. The work was funded from the proceeds of the 1974 Rotary Fete held by Harwich and District Rotary Club; an extension was added in 1990, and a larger crew room provided in 1993. It was used until 2001 and was demolished on completion of new boathouse, and replaced by a café. (Nicholas Leach)

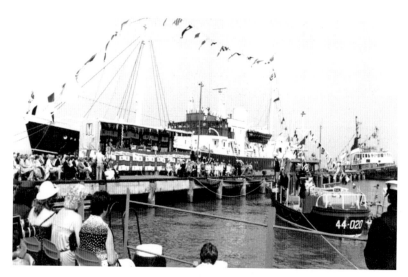

The scene during the naming ceremony of John Fison at Trinity House Pier on 26 July 1980. (By courtesy of Harwich RNLI)

Mrs Dorothy Fison with other guests after the naming of John Fison. (By courtesy of Harwich RNLI)

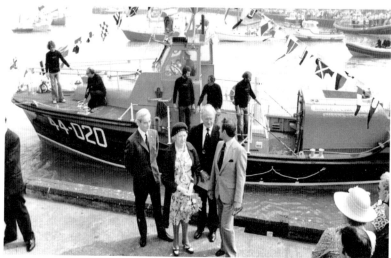

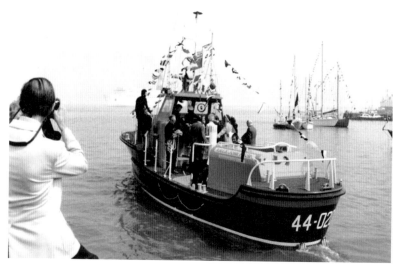

John Fison puts out for a short trip with special guests aboard at the end of her naming ceremony on 26 July 1980. (By courtesy of Harwich RNLI)

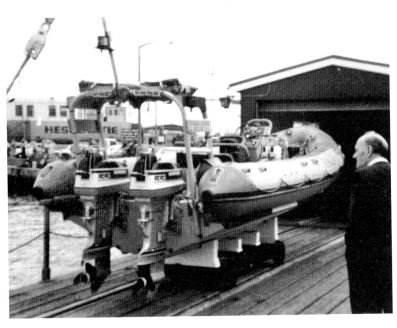

Harwich. After a vote of thanks by Dr B. E. Lovely, president of Harwich and Dovercourt ladies' guild, Shelley Moll, daughter of the lifeboat's assistant mechanic, presented a bouquet to Mrs Fison, who then named the lifeboat *John Fison*. The breaking of the champagne bottle was greeted with a chorus of hooting from Trinity House ships, British Rail ferries, the harbour tugs and yachts which, dressed overall, had attended the ceremony.

John Fison's first full year of service, 1981, proved to be relatively quiet, but the inshore lifeboat was involved in a fine rescue on 17 April. B-526 was launched at 10.13pm, manned by helmsman Robert Ramplin and crew members Peter Brand and Peter Dawson after the sighting of a red flare in Dovercourt Bay had been reported. Walton and Frinton's 48ft 6in Oakley lifeboat *Earl and Countess Howe* also put out, slipping her moorings ten minutes later under the command of Coxswain Frank Bloom to back up the Atlantic. The evening was overcast but clear with a strong breeze to near gale, force six to seven, blowing from the north east and moderate seas. After setting out at full speed the Atlantic had to ease down to half speed when, after clearing Stone Pier to head for Pye Sands, she met the full force of the weather. At 10.20pm the pounding of the boat sheared the pin holding the mast, so a screwdriver was fitted in the pin's place to keep the mast in its position. A search was begun in the Pye Sands area but at first no casualty could be seen through the driven spray in the rough, confused seas. Then, at 10.25pm, a parachute flare was put up and by its light the casualty was sighted near an old blockhouse on the shore.

The ILB approached to within forty yards, from where the casualty could be seen by the white water breaking over her. Helmsman Ramplin could not get alongside the casualty because of underwater obstructions, so he turned the Atlantic's bows into the sea and allowed her to be taken in by the wind and waves until she just touched, when Peter Brand, who had volunteered to investigate, swam and waded to the casualty. The casualty, the 24ft yacht *Dunkit*, was about 20ft from the shore and when Peter Brand reached her he found two people on board, although a third had waded ashore through the surf to seek help. Crew member Brand decided that they should radio for more assistance so signalled to the Atlantic 21 to come closer. Again, Helmsman Ramplin put the Atlantic's bow to sea and let her drift in but, just as crew member Brand boarded, a large breaking wave lifted the ILB and stalled her port engine, and she was driven ashore. Several

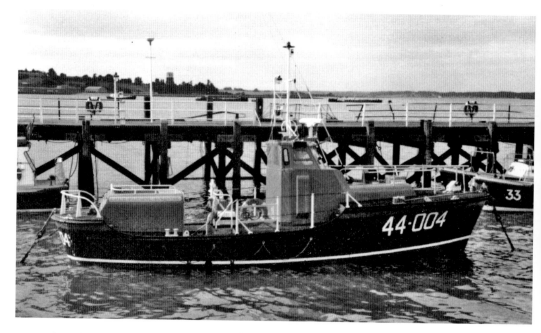

The relief 44ft Waveney Faithful Forester moored in the Pound on 6 August 1981. She temporarily replaced John Fison, which went to Rowhedge the following day for a refit. Faithful Forester was built at the same time as Margaret Graham, and served at Dover from 1967 to 1979 before entering the relief fleet. (Ken Brand)

attempts were made to relaunch the boat by the crew, but although the three together could at times hold the boat into the onshore seas, as soon as helmsman Ramplin boarded to restart the engines the weight proved too much for the other two men to hold and the boat was driven ashore.

By 10.50pm Walton and Frinton lifeboat *Earl and Countess Howe* had arrived and she helped the Atlantic's crew by illuminating the area with her searchlight. At 10.57pm, after ten unsuccessful attempts with all three crew members at times being swept off their feet, the Atlantic was launched with helmsman Ramplin on the controls leaving the other two crew members on the shore. The Atlantic headed for the Walton lifeboat, but just as she approached a large wave lifted her bows on to the lifeboat. At 11.03pm a crew member from Walton lifeboat went aboard the Atlantic as crew and she returned to Harwich to be refuelled and made ready for service. Ashore, the man who had first waded through the surf had returned and he remained at the casualty while crew members Brand and Dawson helped the other two people through the marshes, being met by the police. *Earl and Countess Howe* stood by until everyone was safely ashore and then returned to station. All the people on shore were picked up by car, and the yacht was towed off the beach the next day. For this service framed letters of thanks signed by the Duke of Atholl, chairman of the Institution, were presented to helmsman Ramplin and crew members Brand and Dawson.

On 19 December 1982 the worst incident in the modern history of Harwich harbour occurred. The ferry *European Gateway*, outbound from Felixstowe to Zeebrugge, and the inbound train ferry *Speedlink Vanguard* collided in the harbour approaches. *European Gateway* was hit amidships by the bulbous bow of *Speedlink Vanguard*, started listing, and within a short space of time had capsized. The depth of water in the area was such that half the vessel remained above water. The severity of the situation resulted in a major rescue operation, with all available boats and harbour tugs responding to the call for assistance. *John Fison* launched ay 11pm and proceeded at full speed to the area. On scene within minutes of the collision were two pilot boats, which started to take people off *European Gateway* as she was capsizing, while *Speedlink Vanguard* launched a ship's lifeboat to assist, and Walton and Frinton lifeboat also launching to help.

As *European Gateway* lay capsized, the boats on scene were still picking up people from the water, with many people assisting in the rescue operation. In spite of the extremely difficult conditions, including high winds, pitch darkness and floating debris, sixty-eight survivors were picked up within an hour of the collision occurring. A head count ascertained that six people were unaccounted for, so *Dana Futura*, which was inbound for Parkeston Quay, provided additional lighting with her searchlights to aid the rescue craft searching for the missing persons. Some people who had already been rescued were transferred to *Dana Futura* where, with the aid of the ship's sauna, the survivors were treated for cold and exposure. The search was eventually terminated when five bodies had been recovered, leaving one person unaccounted for. In recognition of their outstanding contribution to the rescue, the crews of the two pilot boats were awarded the RNLI's Bronze medal. Framed letters of appreciation signed by the RNLI Chairman were awarded to the three masters of Alexandra Towing's tugs *Sauria*, *Alfred* and *Ganges*. Coxswain Peter Burwood and the lifeboat crew also received letters of appreciation.

One of the most infamous incidents in the history of Harwich lifeboat station took place on 5 July 1983. The lifeboat committee had chartered the local passenger ferry *Brightlingsea* for an evening cruise to raise funds for the station, but the event ended in the ferry running aground and the ILB being launched to transfer the passengers to the shore. On board the ferry were ninety-nine lifeboat supporters, who were looking forward to a pleasant summer evening cruise up the river Stour to Mistley. The evening was planned so that *Brightlingsea* would arrive at Mistley at high tide and return down river on the ebb tide. Of those on board, seven held Master Mariner certificates, two were local pilots and another was the Commodore Captain of a ferry company. However, mistakes were made when navigating the vessel up river, and she ended up going aground.

Atlantic 21 B-526 was launched at 9.04pm and made her way nine miles upstream towards the casualty, reaching it twenty-five minutes later. The three lifeboat crew were met with gesticulations, the raising of wine glasses by some of those on board, and cheers of appreciation and recognition for family and friends. The tide had fallen considerably in the time that they had been aground, but

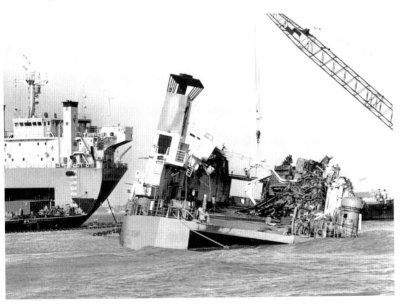

The ferry European Gateway, built in 1975, was salvaged by the Dutch salvage company Wijsmullers after she had been involved in a collision in December 1982. By that time the North Sea had pounded the wreck, the vessel was severely damaged but she was rebuilt as the ferry Flavia and served in the Mediterranean. (By courtesy of Harwich RNLI)

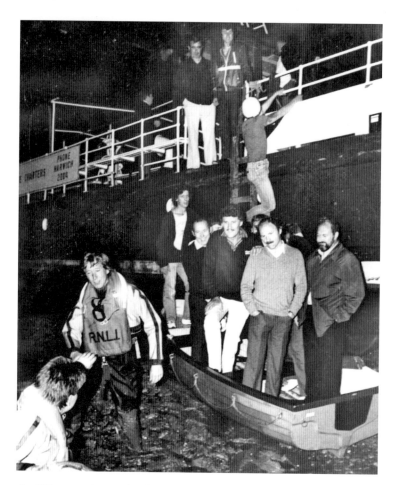

the ILB crew obtained a dinghy for use as a platform across the mud and one by one the committee members and lifeboat supporters were brought ashore via the dinghy and the ILB. As the last passengers were being landed ashore in relays by the ILB, two coaches arrived at Mistley Quay to take them away. The incident led to a certain degree of mirth among the local crew, with Captain Rod Shaw, then the press officer, commenting: 'It was quite a sour point that we had to rely on the service of our own charity to get us home. Although we had elderly people and young children on board nobody made a fuss, and there was no danger. In fact, spirits were exceptionally high!'

The first service of 1984 for *John Fison*, on 3 January, proved to be an arduous one, and was the first of thirteen launches during the year. She put out at 11.35pm on 3 January after the 500-ton cargo vessel *Gladonia*, of Goole, which had engine failure, was reported to be drifting with six persons on board fifty-two miles off the Essex coast in force six winds and rough seas. The lifeboat arrived on scene at 5.45am to find a Dutch tug was already in attendance. At first light, a tow rope was attached, and the lifeboat stood by as the tow commenced, ten miles north-east of the North Hinder Buoy. *John Fison* escorted the vessels for an hour before making for Harwich, arriving back at station at 4pm having been out on service for seventeen hours. The crew were made up of Acting Coxswain Les Smith, Bob Ramplin, John Teatheredge, Peter Brand, David Gilders and Eddie Clifton, and they arrived back at station cold, exhausted and hungry, having had only a cup of coffee since leaving late the previous night. Bob Ramplin said afterwards, 'We only just scraped home . . . We had sixty gallons of fuel left, just enough for another three hours' running.'

Further services followed during May and June 1984, with *John Fison* and B-526 launching to a series of yachts and motor vessels that had got into difficulty. On 22 May the lifeboat landed a man with a badly cut hand from the motor vessel *Tom Grant*. On 31 May she went to the 35ft Belgian yacht *Velleda* with six person on board, which was aground on the Cork Sands in fog. The Walton lifeboat was also called out, and the Harwich boat returned to station having taken off a woman, with the yacht later being refloated and towed to the river Orwell. *John Fison* was called out to the same yacht again on 3 June, which was caught in a south-easterly gale, and towed her to Harwich.

On 6 January 1985 *John Fison* was again tasked to stand by one of the ferries that operate out of Harwich after the train ferry *Speedlink Vanguard* suffered engine failure and began drifting towards the Kentish Knock sandbank. The lifeboat put out at 7.30pm in a north-easterly force seven to nine wind, which later rose to hurricane force ten, accompanied by very rough seas. The lifeboat reached the casualty at 10.15pm five miles south of the Knock Bell Buoy, by which time her engines had been repaired. *John Fison* then escorted the vessel three miles east of the Sunk lightvessel before returning to station, reaching Harwich at 1.20am on 7 January after a very rough trip.

On 9 July 1985 the relief Waveney 44-001 arrived and *John Fison* went to Crescent Shipyard at Rochester for refit. 44-001 was involved in a number of rescues during the summer, the first on 19 July when she launched just before 5pm to the Dutch yacht *Anne Chien*, which was in difficulty twenty-one miles out to sea in force six winds. 44-001 towed the casualty and her four crew back to harbour. On 28 July the lifeboat was again out to a yacht, *Marna Jane*, which needed assistance after its mast broke when a mile off the river Deben. The yacht and its four occupants were towed

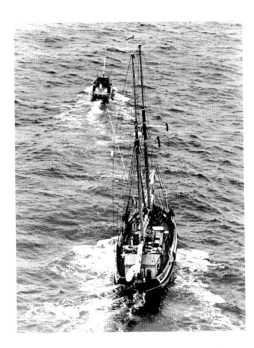

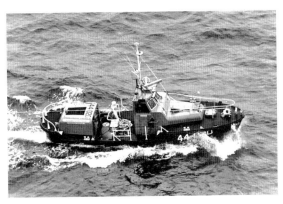

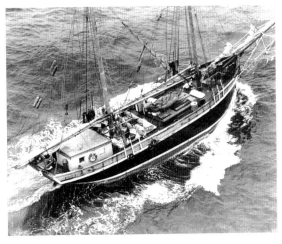

John Fison on service in force five winds to the 107ft twin-masted gaff schooner Stina, of Maldon, on 8 June 1984. The casualty, which was taking in water after hitting a submerged object, was towed by the lifeboat for more than twenty miles. (By courtesy of Harwich RNLI)

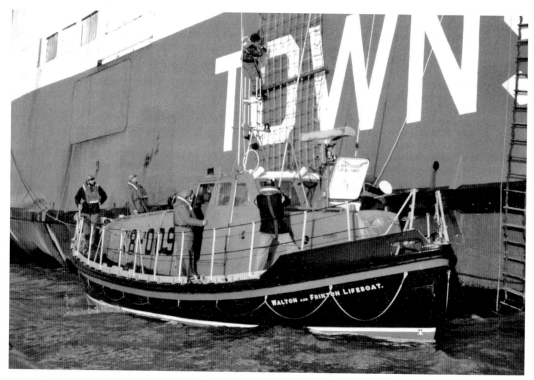

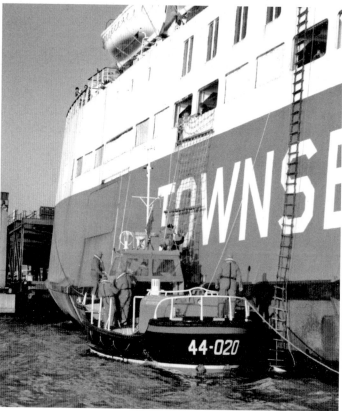

Walton and Frinton lifeboat
City of Birmingham, a 48ft
6in Solent class built in 1970,
and John Fison alongside
the Townsend Thoresen ferry
Viking Viscount during an
exercise on 26 November 1984.
The scenario for the exercise,
organised by the British
Shipping Federation, involved
the ferry sinking and the crew
being evacuated. The lifeboats
were involved in taking the
crew members as they climbed
off the ship. (Ken Brand)

to Harwich Harbour Board jetty. 44-001 went to another yacht on 7 August, the 27ft *Sabre*, whose crew were unsure of their position, and she performed her last effective service of her stint at Harwich on 18 September, when she went to the 40ft motor boat *Moby Dick*, which was the former lifeboat *Alfred and Clara Heath*. *Moby Dick*, on her way from Lowestoft to Gibraltar with three persons on board, hit the Shipwash Sands and so 44-001 towed her to Harwich

John Fison returned to station on 4 November 1985 and on 16 November the station's Atlantic 21 was taken to the RNLI Depot at Cowes for refit, with relief Atlantic B-513 *William McCunn & Broom Church Youth Fellowship* arriving in her place. Meanwhile, on 18 November *John Fison* went out on service, launching to the 932-ton Moroccan coaster *Amina*, with eight persons on board, which was having steering difficulties. The lifeboat escorted the coaster, while the Trinity House vessel *Patricia* was also in attendance. The lifeboat put out just after midnight and returned to station on 5.25am after a difficult service undertaken in force eight winds and rough seas. The relief Atlantic undertook her first service the following day, launching at 2.45pm to the 20ft angling boat *Scorpion* with two people on board, whose outboard engine had broken down.

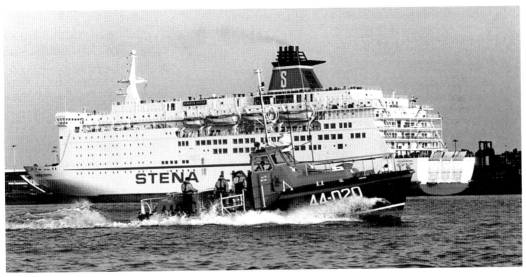

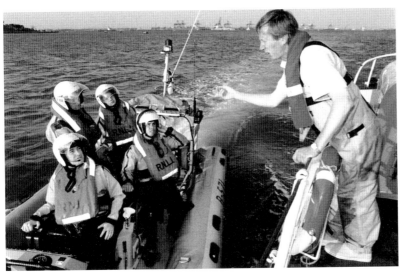

John Fison and Atlantic 21 with an East Anglian Daily Times newspaper reporter on board to feature the lifeboat. Peter Dawson on the Waveney and on the Atlantic are John Teatheredge (on helm), and left to right John Reason, Brendon Shaw, and Jason Davis. (By courtesy of Harwich RNLI)

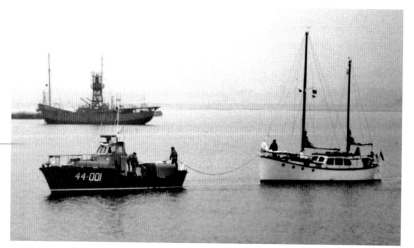

Relief 44ft Waveney bringing in the former lifeboat Moby Dick on 18 September 1985 after the boat, built as Alfred and Clara Heath in 1922 and stationed at Torbay and Salcombe, had drifted onto the Shipwash Sands due to mechanical failure. (By courtesy of Harwich RNLI)

The relief Atlantic B-513 had a very busy day on 24 November 1985, with three casualties needing assistance even though conditions were slight with a north-westerly force three wind blowing. The crew of Paul Smith, Ken Brand and Eddie Clifton were using the boat for a publicity launch when the Coastguard informed them at 11.11am that a windsurfer was in difficulty near Beach End Buoy. The ILB took the board and the surfer on board and landed them at Landguard Point. A few minutes later a 16ft angling boat with two men aboard was seen drifting off Shotley, so the ILB towed the craft to Shotley Pier. The ILB returned to station at 12.10pm, but was out again at 3.33pm after an unmanned fishing boat was reported off Shingle Street, but this proved to be a false alarm and the ILB was recalled.

In June 1986 the station Atlantic 21 B-526 returned from refit, in time to participate in a service of rededication on 6 July 1986 held to mark the twenty-first anniversary of the reopening of the lifeboat station. The service, which saw both lifeboats being dedicated, was led by the Rev Bill Dodd, vicar of Harwich and chaplain of the lifeboat station, assisted by the Rev Brian Tween, Captain John McCombe and Canon Brian Grady. A large number of people were in attendance, and the intention was to raise the profile of the lifeboat and meet the people who support the RNLI. And the following day, B-526 was in action after a man fell into the sea from Parkeston Quay while letting go the mooring ropes from the motor vessel *Belina*. The ILB was not needed on this occasion as the man was pulled from the water by Sealink shore personnel.

The twenty-first anniversary year saw *John Fison* undertake a number of medical evacuations, with the first on 5 April 1986 when she landed a sick man from the DFDS ferry *Dana Anglia*. On 22 July she brought ashore a five-month-old baby from the ferry *Tor Britannia* after the baby had sustained head injuries in a fall on the vessel. The child and two adults were transferred to the lifeboat via the vessel's pilot door, and landed at the Harbour Board jetty where an ambulance was waiting to take them to hospital. On 9 September *John Fison* went to the dredger *Arco Tyne* to take off a sick crew man who had acute appendicitis. And the final medical service of the year came on 13 October when *John Fison* took a doctor to the container ship *Dorothee* to treat two injured crew men, one with a crushed hand and the other with a partially severed finger. The men were taken off the ship and landed at Felixstowe Dock from where they went to hospital.

In April 1987 the relief lifeboat *Khami*, which had originally served at Gorleston, was sent to Harwich while *John Fison* went to Crescent Shipyard for a survey. While at Harwich, the relief lifeboat undertook four services, the most notable of which was undertaken during the afternoon of 14 June after she was returning from a publicity visit to the East Coast Boat Show at Ipswich. Her

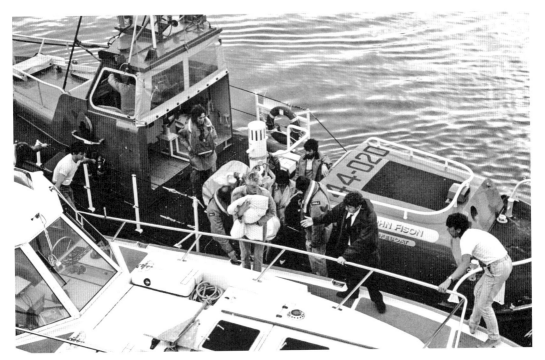

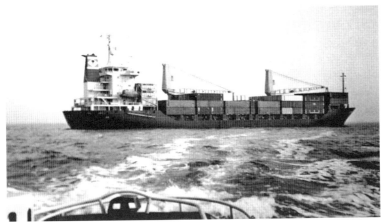

John Fison and her crew land a five-month-old child from the ferry Tor Britannia on 22 July 1986. (By courtesy of Ken Brand)

The German-registered container ship Dorothee, seen from John Fison, from which two injured men were landed, 13 October 1986. (By courtesy of Ken Brand)

five-man crew spotted smoke billowing from the former trawler *Mary La*, at anchor in the river Orwell. The crew, together with Harwich branch chairman Howard Bell and honorary secretary Captain Rod Shaw, were dressed in functional clothing and lifejackets, although they were wearing good clothing beneath in order to appear smartly turned-out at the show. The local fire services had been alerted, while Second Coxswain David Gilders and his crew prepared the extinguishers and fire hose aboard the lifeboat. On arrival alongside the 70ft vessel, the crew saw that a dinghy trailed astern and it was assumed that the three-man crew of the *Mary La* were aboard.

The lifeboat crew shouted to try to locate crew members aboard *Mary La*, but to no effect. Captain Shaw, accompanied by Emergency Mechanic Ken Brand and crew member Paul Smith boarded the burning vessel, despite the emission of heavy acrid smoke from various openings and signs of fire about to break through the deck. While other crew members began work with buckets, extinguishers and fire hose, Captain Shaw decided to open the fore hatch with great care

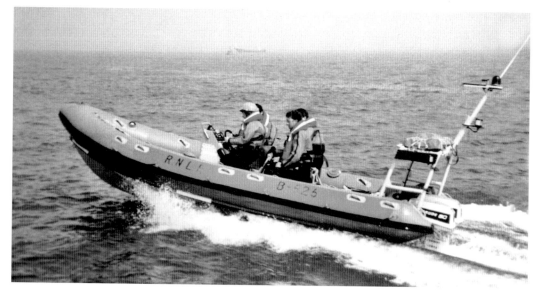

The station's first Atlantic 21 B-526 heads out of harbour on exercise. (Ken Brand)

and covered by the hose. When deemed safe, crew member Smith entered the forward compartment followed by Captain Shaw and began searching. The owner of *Mary La* arrived alongside in a small dinghy at around 2.30pm and was able to confirm that no one else was aboard the former trawler.

As the smoke cleared, once the fire was extinguished, the lifeboat crew found hazardous material below decks including pressurised containers of acetylene, oxygen, propane and butane gas alongside petrol and diesel. With small outbreaks of fire still occurring, the lifeboat crew began moving hazardous items to the upper deck. At 4.10pm the fire service dory *Suffire I*, having returned ashore for more personnel, made fast alongside and took over the completion of the operation. The lifeboat left for Harwich, returning to station at 4.45pm. Following this service, a

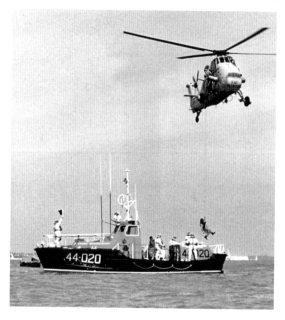

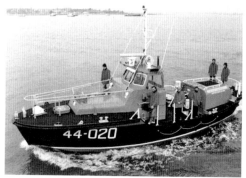

(Above) John Fison returning to station from exercise. (By courtesy of Harwich RNLI)

(Left) John Fison on exercise with an RAF Wessex rescue helicopter. (By courtesy of Harwich RNLI)

framed letter of thanks signed by the Duke of Atholl, the RNLI chairman, was presented to Second Coxswain David Gilders, Emergency Mechanic Kenneth Brand, crew members Peter Dawson, Paul Smith and Robert Barton, and to branch chairman Howard Bell and Captain Rod Shaw.

John Fison returned to station on 19 July 1987 and four days later was boarded by HRH The Duke of Kent, president of the RNLI, during the Duke's visit to lifeboat stations in Essex. His first call was at Harwich, where he was accompanied by the Deputy Lord Lieutenant of Essex, Robert Adcock, and Rear Admiral Wilfred Graham, the RNLI's director. He went aboard *John Fison*, escorted by Coxswain Peter Burwood, and was shown the launching arrangements for the Atlantic 21. Long-serving crew member Ken Brand presented the Duke with a limited edition plate inscribed by the crew, after which he was flown by helicopter to Walton and Frinton. He went on to visit the stations at Clacton-on-Sea, Southend-on-Sea and West Mersea.

On 25 August 1987 the Atlantic 21 B-526 launched in force seven winds to the Ipswich-chartered yacht *Libra* on board which was a man with severe head and face injuries, sustained in a fall which left him unconscious. The ILB arrived alongside the yacht at 2.50am, twenty minutes after launching, and the crew found a man, John Crawshaw, to be in a serious condition. The yacht was aground and so the man was taken aboard the ILB, whose crew attempted resuscitation and heart massage to no avail, landing the man ashore to a waiting ambulance. In the letter of thanks sent by the RNLI Deputy Director, Brian Miles, after this service, he said, 'This was a very unpleasant

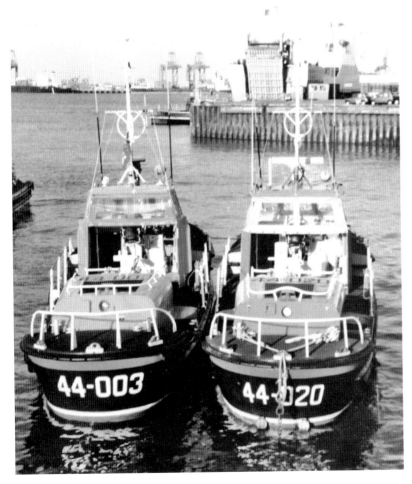

John Fison (on left) with relief 44ft Waveney Khami on 20 July 1987. John Fison had just returned to station following a refit, and Khami was about to leave for a relief duty at Great Yarmouth & Gorleston. (Ken Brand)

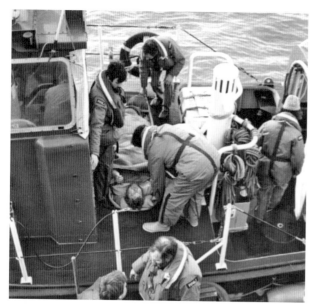

A suspected heart attack victim is brought off the DFDS North Sea ferry Dana Anglia by John Fison on 5 April 1986. The lifeboat met the ferry near the Wadgate Ledge Buoy and the casualty was transferred across on a stretcher and landed at Harwich harbour. (By courtesy of Ken Brand)

(Below) Harwich lifeboat crew on board John Fison, from left to right, are John Teatheredge, Martin Burwood, Charlie Moll, Ken Brand, Peter Burwood, Les Smith, and Bob Ramplin. (By courtesy of Harwich RNLI)

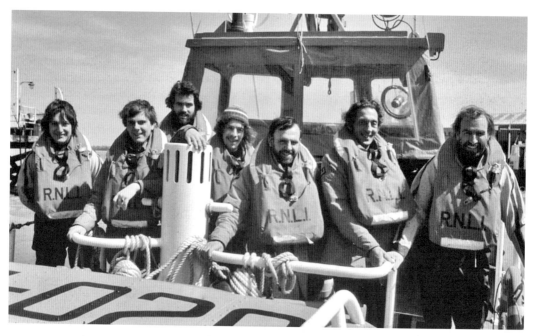

service which was carried out in the best traditions of the lifeboat service, conducted under the most adverse conditions. I would like on behalf of the Institution to commend crew members Charlie Moll, Paul Smith and Eddie Clifton for their exceptional dedication to duty on this occasion.'

This proved to be one of the last services undertaken by B-526, which was replaced on 31 October 1987 by a new Atlantic 21. The new lifeboat, B-571, funded by the British Sub-Aqua Clubs and named *British Diver II*, was fitted out at the RNLI's Inshore Lifeboat base at East Cowes after the hull had been built by Halmatic Ltd, of Havant. Her first effective service was performed on 24 December 1987, when she brought in an angling boat with two men after the boat's engine failed. The naming ceremony of the new Atlantic 21, which cost £35,000, was held on 19 June 1988 at the lifeboat house on The Quay, with C. Crawford, Chairman of the Harwich and Dovercourt Station Branch, opening the proceedings. The boat was handed over by Mr R. L. B. Norgren, Chief Executive of the British Sub-Aqua Clubs, and was passed into the care of the station by Anthony Oliver, head of fund-raising at the RNLI. Captain Rod Shaw, station honorary secretary, accepted the boat and the Rev Bill Dodd, Chaplain of the lifeboat station and vicar of St Nicholas Church conducted the service of dedication. At the end of the ceremony Mr Norgren named the lifeboat.

The new Atlantic 21 was involved in a tragic incident on 16 February 1988. B-571 launched at 1.32pm after a child reported that his father was missing from a yacht in the river Deben. Manned by Ken Brand, Peter Brand and Paul Smith, the ILB reached the 35ft ketch *Tisza*, of Dover, at 2.08pm to find an eleven-year-old on board alone. The boy, Matthew Szegedi, explained that he and his father, Erno, had gone to their boat, which was moored in the river, but when the dinghy was tied up it capsized. The father, who only had one arm, was able to push his son aboard the yacht before being swept downriver by a strong ebb tide. The boy managed to throw him a life ring before breaking into the locked cockpit of the yacht and calling for help. The ILB landed the boy at Waldringfield and then, assisted by an RAF search and rescue helicopter, began to search for the father. His body was found by the helicopter a mile and a half downstream from the ketch. Matthew was later awarded a Royal Humane Society certificate for bravery in recognition of his efforts to pull his father back aboard the yacht before the river proved too much for them both.

Four lifeboats, three helicopters, three tugs and a harbour launch were involved during a major incident on 24 March 1988 after the ferry *Nordic Ferry* became immobilised a mile south-west of the South Bawdsey Light Buoy following a fire in the engine room. The 18,700-ton vessel was en route from Zeebrugge to Felixstowe with 348 passengers and crew on board when Harwich Harbour Operations were first informed of her predicament. No assistance was requested as the fire was believed to be out. However, at 7.10am, with the vessel now anchored, the master reported the bulkheads were still hot, and asked for fire services to attend. A fire tug and patrol launch

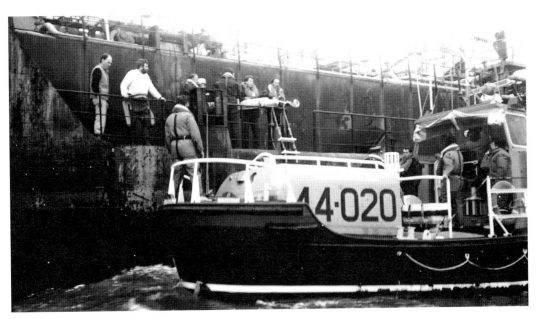

John Fison taking part in an exercise on 13 December 1987 with Essex Ambulance Personnel and the tanker Orionman in the Platters Anchorage. B-571 British Diver II was also involved in the exercise. (By courtesy of Ken Brand)

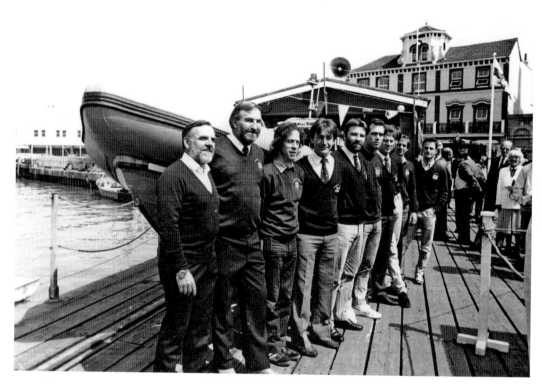

The scene during the naming ceremony for Atlantic 21 B-571 outside the ILB house on Ha'penny Pier, 19 June 1988. The crew (pictured above) are, from left to right, Peter Burwood, Bob Ramplin, Ken Brand, John Teatheredge, Paul Smith, Charlie Moll, Eddie Clifton, Dougie Good, Bob Barton and Andrew Webb. (By courtesy of Harwich RNLI)

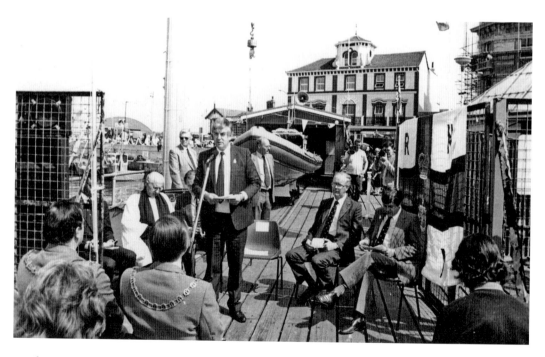

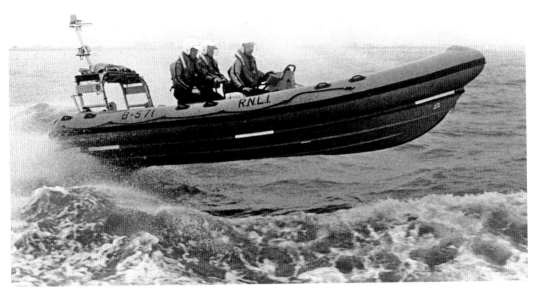

Atlantic 21 B-571 British Diver II served at Harwich from October 1987 to 2002. (By courtesy of Harwich RNLI)

were sent to the casualty, and because of the possibility of a large scale evacuation from the ferry all emergency services were alerted. At 7.38am the Atlantic B-571 and Waveney *John Fison* were launched, followed by Walton and Frinton's 48ft 6in Solent *City of Birmingham* and Aldeburgh's 37ft 6in Rother *James Cable* just after 8am. The lifeboats reached the casualty in a south-westerly gale, and, having received confirmation that the fire was out, stood by while the electrical system and engines were tested. At about 10am the master of *Nordic Ferry* asked for the lifeboats to withdraw to Harwich harbour and stand by as their presence was causing anxiety among the passengers. By 10.22am the ferry was under tow to Felixstowe by tug, berthing safely at midday, when the lifeboats were released, with the Harwich boats reaching station soon afterwards. The last lifeboat did not reach her station until 3.30pm, by when 130 lifeboat crew man-hours had been spent at sea.

The speed of the Atlantic 21 was put to good effect on 1 October 1988 when honorary secretary Captain Rod Shaw tasked the boat and her crew after a mine severely damaged a trawler. At about 7.30pm the trawler *Niblick* sent a mayday saying that a mine had exploded, extensive damaging the vessel, and that she was sinking about four miles north of Shipwash lightvessel. *John Fison* was requested by the coastguard, but Captain Shaw, having assessed the calm weather and force three wind, informed the coastguard that he was also launching the Atlantic for fast response. Nothing further was heard from the casualty and the extent of the damage and injuries was unknown so the Atlantic 21 proceeded at full speed with the Waveney following.

The Atlantic arrived on the scene at about the same time as a helicopter, which placed a winchman on board. Once the Atlantic was alongside, a crewman went aboard to find that the skipper had assessed the damage, which had blown its Lister engine off its mounting, and hoped the ingress of water could be contained. The Atlantic was able to help further by transferring the

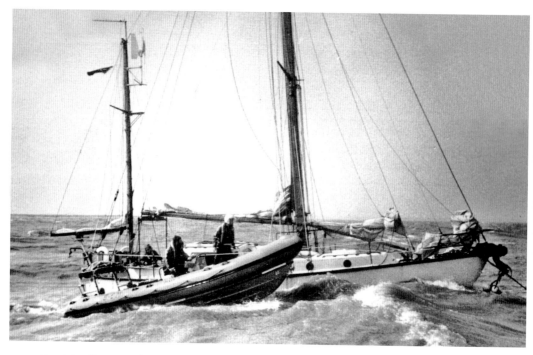

On 6 April 1988 Atlantic 21 B-571 assisted the 40ft yacht Home Spun, with three persons on board,

skipper to a nearby trawler to negotiate a tow, with the trawler already retrieving her gear to assist. The ILB , with the Aldeburgh lifeboat *James Cable* also now in attendance and *John Fison* nearing the scene, all stood by until the tow was passed. With the tow connected, and the trawlers moving towards Lowestoft, the Harwich lifeboats were stood down while Aldeburgh's Rother provided initial escort of the casualty. Following this service, Captain Shaw and the crew members at the station were sent a letter of thanks from the RNLI's chief of operations.

During 1989 two relief lifeboats came to Harwich. The 44ft Waveney *Khami* was on service from February to the end of April, and in the summer the relief Atlantic 21 B-514 *Guide Friendship I* was on duty during July and August while B-571 went for refit at Cowes. The relief Atlantic was in action, together with *John Fison*, on 17 July, launching in the early hours of the morning to the 35ft yacht *Westwind of Stour*, which was aground on the north end of the Cork Sand, and was bumping on the sands. The lifeboat reached the scene first but could not get close enough to effect a rescue so advised the occupants, nine of whom were children, to stay aboard until the ILB arrived. Once the ILB arrived, the yacht's occupants were taken off and transferred to the lifeboat, with the ILB suffering some minor damage while alongside the yacht due to the heavy confused seas on the sands. The yacht was later salvaged by local fishing boats. The teenage sailors and their two instructors were on a training voyage to West Germany when the yacht went aground.

Both *John Fison* and Atlantic 21 B-571 *British Diver II* were called to an incident on the river Orwell on 18 March 1990. A moored power boat had burst into flames, apparently when the engine was started, and after the yacht *Stella Maris* had reported the incident B-571 was launched at 10.41am, reaching the popular anchorage at Pin Mill on the Orwell by 11.20am. The lifeboat crew found that the sole occupant of the power boat, the 20ft *Sum Speed*, had been picked up from the water by a dinghy from the yacht which reported the explosion, and had been taken ashore and to hospital suffering from burns. His condition was later described as satisfactory. The blazing power boat drifted alongside a nearby fishing vessel, which also began to catch fire, but the crew of the Atlantic were able to put out this second fire with their extinguisher. *Sum Speed* was settling in the water and sank shortly afterwards, leaving burning fuel on the surface. *John Fison* was launched to provide back-up, and after the Atlantic had liaised with the fire service and taken a representative aboard the badly damaged fishing vessel to check that the fire was out, both lifeboats remained in the area until the fire on the water was out before returning to their station at 12.30pm.

During the last few months of 1990 *John Fison* was involved in a number of challenging services to yachts in difficulties. On 1 September she went to the 27ft yacht *Ajaia* with a fouled propeller twenty-three miles out, launching at 2am and spending over four hours at sea, towing the casualty to Harwich. On 7 September she went to another yacht, the 30ft *Sujuva II*, which was stranded nineteen miles off the Essex coast with a broken down engine in force seven to eight winds and rough seas. The lifeboat spent almost two hours to reach the casualty, and then a further six hours to bring the boat back to harbour. And on 6 October, in force eight conditions, she brought in the yacht *Morning Glory* in force eight conditions spending almost nine hours at sea during the rescue operation. Captain Rod Shaw summarised the rescue: 'It took about two-and-a-half hours for the lifeboat to reach the casualty, and nearly six hours battling against heavy seas to take the tow into Harwich. The yacht was seriously damaged. Most of the furniture was smashed and scattered all over the place, and she was taking in water.'

The final service of the year came on 28 December 1990 when *John Fison* was launched to the 295-ton coaster *Mill Supplier*, which had three crew on board and was on passage from Antwerp to Colchester carrying bird seed. The vessel began to ship water in rough seas off South Galloper, thirty miles off Harwich and was in danger of sinking. Harwich lifeboat was launched at 7.10pm

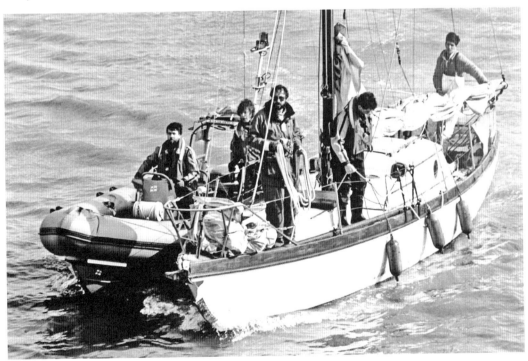

Atlantic 21 B-571 berthing the yacht Prelude at Harwich Harbour Master's jetty, 7 May 1988. (By courtesy of Ken Brand)

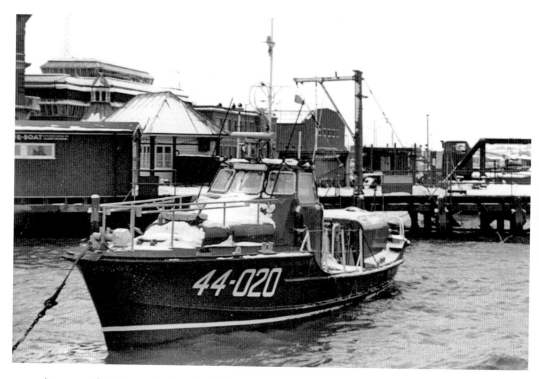

An unusual photograph showing John Fison covered in snow at moorings in the Pound.

with water pumps for *Mill Supplier* and an RAF helicopter from Manston was scrambled. The helicopter and lifeboat arranged a rendezvous at sea, when the pump was exchanged and flown to *Mill Supplier*. It was at first believed that the pump would be sufficient to help the stricken vessel. But when it arrived at the scene, the helicopter found the cargo ship had lost its engines because of the amount of water taken on and its electrical systems were failing. The three-man crew was advised to abandon ship and was airlifted off and back to shore, after which Harwich lifeboat was recalled before arriving on scene. *Mill Supplier* was left to drift with her lights on until it was secured by a tug at about 7am on 29 December, when the vessel was towed to Lowestoft.

During 1990 the two lifeboats at Harwich launched sixty-three times, making the station one of the busiest in the region, and 1991 got off to a hectic start for the lifeboat crew. On 6 January 1991 B-571 *British Diver II* went to the 29ft yacht *Blue Dolphin*, with six persons on board, which had engine failure in force seven winds and towed it to Woolverston's Marina. The next day, 7 January, *John Fison* was out to the Belgian LPG tanker *Foka-Gas I*, which was taking water into her engine room thirty miles out. A helicopter and salvage tug also went to the vessel, and four pumps were eventually put aboard to keep the water level stable. The lifeboat reached the scene at 10pm and stood by for two and a half hours in rough seas during the salvage efforts. When the tug *Anglian Warrior* arrived on scene, a tow was rigged and the tanker was taken to Lowestoft.

The relief Waveney *Khami* was again on station in 1991, from 28 June 1991 to 14 September, undertaking five launches and saving two lives. Her longest service was on 17 August 1991 when she went to the 65ft yacht *Rival II*, with four people on board, which had started taking on water in the engine room. The lifeboat arrived on scene to find water rising in the vessel's engine room, although the RAF Sea King helicopter had lowered a pump to the vessel. Because of the dangerous situation, two of the crew were airlifted off the yacht to safety and landed at Walton-on-the-Naze. The Harwich lifeboat arrived to find the pump from the helicopter would not work and the water level was worryingly high. The boat's engine failed shortly afterwards and so the lifeboat took the vessel in tow, with two people left on board to help two of the lifeboat crew pump the boat out by hand. Four hours later, and by now six miles off the coast, lifeboat men were becoming increasingly worried about the amount of water the vessel was taking on, so the Atlantic was launched to bring a pump from the fire brigade. The ILB crew stood by in case the yacht sank and the crew had to abandon the vessel, but the new pump soon pumped out the water and the lifeboat berthed the old trawler at Ha'penny Pier in Harwich at about 10am having spent more than twelve hours at sea.

On 30 August 1992 *John Fison* went to the 11.5m yacht *Brazilian Legacy* which was caught out in severe weather, force nine winds, over forty miles from Harwich. The lifeboat put out at 12.50am and went through the night to reach the casualty at 4.50am. A tow was connected but due to the severity of the weather and wind direction the craft was taken to Lowestoft. The Lowestoft lifeboat launched to escort the tow, but got diverted to another incident so Gorleston lifeboat came out to take over the tow for the final leg into Lowestoft, enabling Harwich lifeboat to return to station, reaching harbour at 7.10pm after an extremely long service. The honorary secretary Rod Shaw commented afterwards, 'another long service in very rough seas . . . test of endurance for coxswain and crew. Skills and ability of coxswain contributed to very successful service.'

The following day, 1 September 1992 *John Fison* was out again in the gale force winds to help another yacht, the 27ft *Fantasea*, whose crew were unsure of their position and having problems coping with the rough seas and four-metre swells. The lifeboat put out at 10.55am and reached the casualty, which had four people on board, with the help of the SAR helicopter. Once on scene, the lifeboat crew found the yacht's occupants too weak to make the tow fast so a crew member was transferred across to assist. The tow was got under way at slow speed due to the sea conditions and the yacht's construction, with lifeboat and casualty eventually reaching Harwich in the evening. It was another long service for Coxswain Dawson and his crew, who were at sea for fourteen hours.

Towards the end of 1992 the relief lifeboat *Khami* was again on station, serving from 20 October to 6 December while *John Fison* went for refit. *John Fison* returned in December 1992 and in 1993 had one of her busiest years, launching thirty-one times and assisting a wide range of craft. During the summer she helped a number of yachts and pleasure boats that got into difficulty, including the yacht *Mary Josephine* on 14 July. The yacht was aground, and the crew were unsure of their

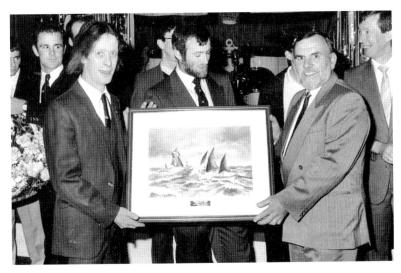

Coxswain Peter Burwood (on right) retired from the post in 1991. A surprise party, attended by colleagues, friends and family, was held on 18 May 1991, at which he was presented with gifts to mark the occasion. He had been in the post since 1967, when the first Waveney arrived on station. (By courtesy of Harwich RNLI)

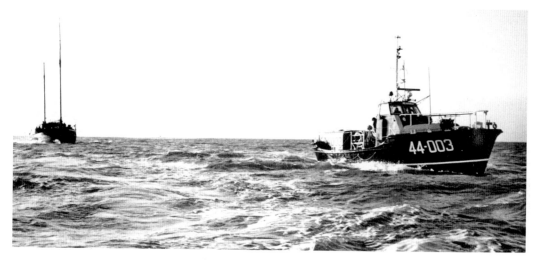

Relief 44ft Waveney Khami towing in the yacht Rival II on 17 August 1991, with the relief Atlantic B-586 Clothworker (out of picture) escorting. (By courtesy of Ken Brand)

position, so both the lifeboat and Atlantic 21 launched to assist. The ILB crew assisted in passing the tow line, and eventually the yacht was eased off the beach into deeper water. The craft was found to be okay so the lifeboat was able to tow it to Harwich. Another yacht, *Bluster*, was helped on 15 August 1993 after it went aground on the river Deben bar and was taking water. The Atlantic 21 was launched and headed straight for the scene, while *John Fison* followed soon afterwards to be ready in case the situation worsened. An ILB crewman went on board to assist the yacht's skipper, whose wife had severed a finger and so was transferred to the yacht club rescue boat to be taken ashore to a waiting ambulance. The ILB and a small local ferry boat took the yacht in tow off the bar and proceeded towards the beach, where *Bluster* was beached to prevent it from sinking.

Between January and March 1994 *Khami* was again on station while *John Fison* went for overhaul, performing only one service during that time. *John Fison* returned on 18 March 1994, and spent the summer assisting yachts and pleasure boats in a series of routine services. On 11 May 1994 she went to the Dutch yacht *Taeke Hadewych*, with the ILB and Aldeburgh lifeboat also responding. The yacht had gone aground, but had refloated before the lifeboats arrived without

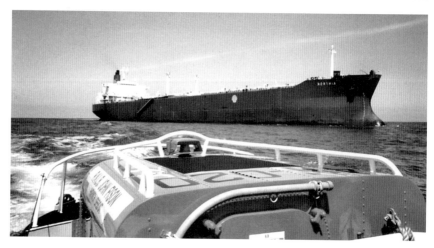

John Fison on service to the 1971-built tanker Northia on 15 June 1993. The lifeboat took out a doctor to an ill crewman, who was landed ashore. (By courtesy of Harwich RNLI)

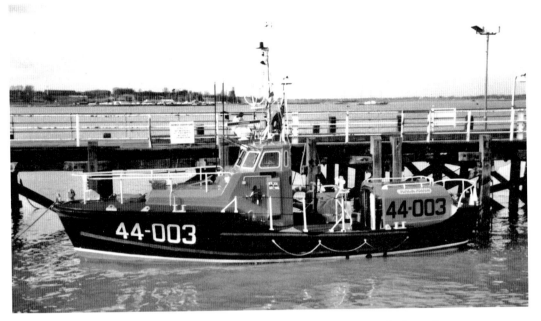

The relief 44ft Waveney at moorings in the Pound. Khami was regularly on duty at Harwich during the 1980s. (By courtesy of Ken Brand)

suffering any damage. On 3 July 1994 *John Fison* went to the cabin cruiser *Mary Rose* which had both engine compartments on fire and required urgent assistance. The ILB, which had been attending a lifeboat day at Felixstowe, was also tasked and arrived on scene to find the fire had been extinguished. The craft had been extensively damaged so *John Fison* towed it in. On 11 July 1994 both lifeboats went to the fishing vessel *Boy Andrew*, which was taking in water and sinking near the Platters Buoy. The ILB took the salvage pump and the local pilot boat was diverted to the scene. Once on scene, with the pilot boat already alongside, the ILB transferred the pump across as water had flooded the engine compartment and the pilot boat commenced a tow. The tow was transferred to *John Fison*, while the salvage pump continued to pump the boat out. The vessel was safely brought in to harbour.

During the first couple of weeks of January 1995, both Harwich lifeboats were launched to the motor boat *Leviathan* on two separate occasions. First, on 6 January *John Fison* brought the boat to safety after launching just before 11pm, with B-571 *British Diver II* also going to help after the boat's engine failed. Then, in the early hours of 15 January both lifeboats were again launched after *Leviathan* was reported to be overdue. The search commenced in the area where the boat was believed to be angling, but when nothing was found the area was expanded. As daylight approached a rescue helicopter was tasked to assist but when reports were received of a craft aground inside the container terminal at Felixstowe the ILB went to investigate. The craft was *Leviathan* and she had been aground since the previous high water, and the occupants stated they were not in need of assistance so the lifeboats returned to station.

Khami was again on station from March to May 1995, but this proved to be her last stint at Harwich. *John Fison* returned from Crescent Shipyard at Otterham Quay on 6 May 1995 and had a relatively quiet summer, although B-571 was called out on numerous occasions throughout August and September. On 1 September 1995 the ILB launched to the 27ft yacht *Prudence* which had a fouled propeller and was aground at the entrance to the river Ore at Shingle Street. The ILB crew arrived to find the craft snagged by a obstruction around the propeller and decided to attempt to tow the craft stern first into deeper water in the hope that the obstruction would clear. As the tow commenced, the obstruction was such that the ILB stern was dragged down and the engines were submerged. All-weather lifeboat support was then requested and *John Fison* put out at 7.55pm to provide support. By this time the ILB crew had got the engines back up and running so a fresh attempt was made to refloat the casualty. Both Aldburgh lifeboats had launched by now, and the inflatable ILB was in the river while both offshore lifeboats stayed outside the river due to lack of water over the bar. B-571 eventually got the craft into deeper water and was able to tow it with the obstruction still on the propeller. The casualty was taken to the nearest safe mooring after which the lifeboats returned to station.

In December 1995 the new 17m Severn class lifeboat *Albert Brown*, which had been built for the station and was one of the first of the new class to be completed, arrived on station, as detailed below. The intention was for her to begin operational service then, and she did perform a service, but due to technical and mechanical problems with the new design, she was taken away again in early January 1996 before crew training had been completed. *John Fison* therefore continued in service and during 1996 performed a number of rescues, which were largely routine in nature, helping a number of yachts during August.

Both lifeboats had to work together during a long a service on 26 August 1996 after the yacht *Pollyanna* went aground on the Cork Sands. The yacht had been returning to harbour, but she sailed south of her intended course and touched the Cork Sands, about six miles offshore, at about 3pm. Unable to get off, her crew informed the Coastguard of her situation and settled down to wait for the tide to rise. For an hour and a half all was well, but as she began to float, and swing

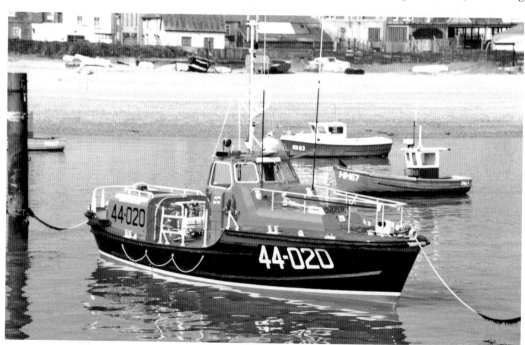

John Fison at moorings in the Harbour Master's Pound, May 1995. Moorings here were taken up in the early 1990s, with the piles installed by the RNLI and built far enough apart to enable a 17m Severn to be moored there. (Nicholas Leach)

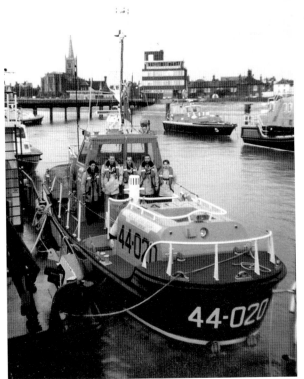

round head to wind, two large swells came behind the sands and dropped her hard on the bottom. Water started to enter the bilge and was rising faster than the pumps could handle, so the crew put out a mayday. By 6.43pm B-571 was on her way, with *John Fison* following five minutes later. The Atlantic reached the scene about fifteen minutes later to find *Pollyanna* with a foot of water in the cabin and the crew inflating their dinghy. Four of them were immediately taken aboard the ILB, while a lifeboat man went aboard the yacht to help stabilise the situation.

A rescue helicopter then arrived on

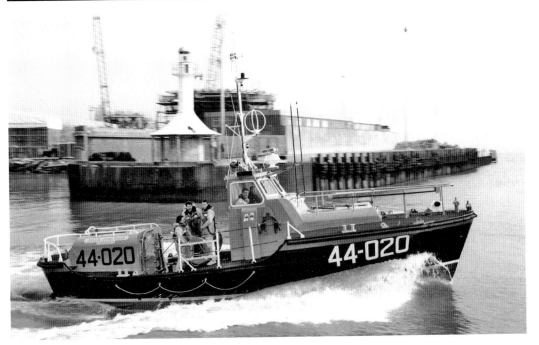

John Fison leaves Lowestoft harbour on exercise in March 1998 while on relief duty at the Suffolk station. (Nicholas Leach)

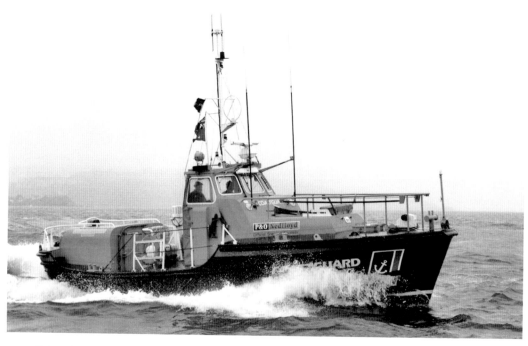

John Fison was sold out of service in August 1999 to Raglan Volunteer Coastguard in New Zealand, where she was renamed Hamilton Rotary Rescue and used as a rescue boat until December 2005. She was then sold by the Coastguard into private ownership, and in 2009 sold again to become a work boat at Fremantle in Australia. She is pictured in October 1999 on trials off Mana, New Zealand. (V. H. Young)

scene with a portable pump, which, together with a helicopter winchman, was lowered onto the lifeboat. It was transferred to the yacht, but before pumping could begin the pilot called down to advise abandoning the vessel immediately as she was rolling over and sinking. The three men on board her – a lifeboat crew member, the helicopter winch man and the yacht's skipper – jumped into the water to keep clear of the mast and rigging as the yacht rolled over, but the Atlantic's radio aerial suffered some damage as the mast descended on her. It was thought that the yacht's keel had become detached as she pounded on the sand, causing her to roll over quickly. The Atlantic picked up the men in the water, transferring the skipper and the four survivors already aboard to the Waveney, before returning to place a marker buoy over the wreck. Both lifeboats then returned to Harwich, the survivors being landed at Suffolk Yacht Harbour.

With the completion of repairs and upgrades to *Albert Brown* nearing completion, *John Fison* undertook her last services as the Harwich lifeboat during August and September 1996. She left Harwich on 6 October 1996 and was taken to Sheerness, where she spent four days before going to Denton Shiprepairers at Otterham Quay for storage and survey. In July 1997 she left Otterham Quay and was taken to Langney Marine at Eastbourne as an emergency relief lifeboat. In October 1997 she went to Lowestoft where she served on relief from 22 October 1997 until 7 November 1998. She was then taken to the RNLI Depot at Poole, via Ramsgate and Newhaven, and was stored as an emergency relief lifeboat until being sold out of service on 24 August 1999 to Raglan Volunteer Coastguard of New Zealand. She was shipped to New Zealand in September 1999 and, renamed *Hamilton Rotary Rescue*, was used as a Coastguard boat-cum-lifeboat based at Raglan.

Albert Brown

In 1995 Harwich was allocated a new lifeboat, which considerably enhanced the station's rescue capabilities. The new craft was one of the first of a new generation of faster all-weather lifeboats being introduced by the RNLI. Two new designs had been developed, the 17m Severn and 14m Trent, each capable of twenty-five knots at full speed and incorporating the latest equipment and technology to make rescue work safer, easier and more efficient. The larger of the two types, the Severn, was deemed suitable for Harwich and the station being the first at which the new class was operational. The Severn, self-righting by virtue of the inherent buoyancy in the watertight

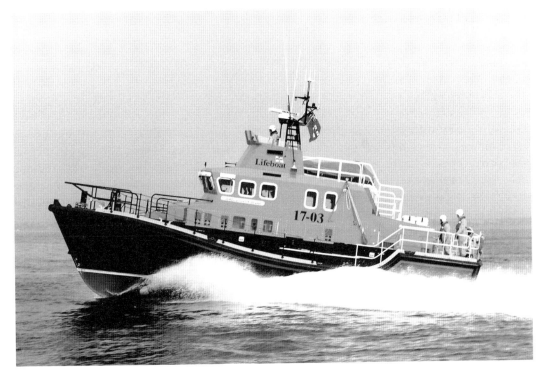

17m Severn Albert Brown during her sea trials in 1995. (By courtesy of RNLI)

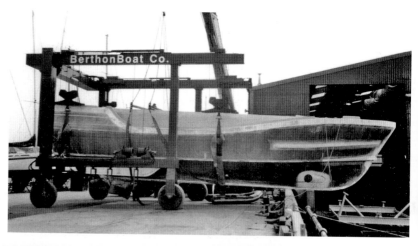

The hull of Albert Brown being brought to Berthon Boatyard, Lymington, for fitting out. (By courtesy of Harwich RNLI)

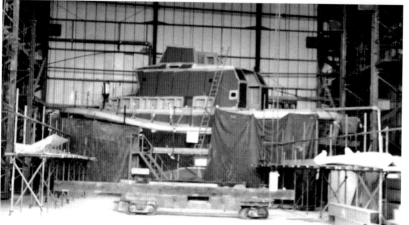

Albert Brown being fitted out at Berthon Boatyard, Lymington, after the hull and superstructure had been moulded by Green Marine, also at Lymington. (Peter Edey)

wheelhouse, was moulded in fibre reinforced composite at Green Marine's Lymington boatyard and the hull was fitted out by Berthon Boat Company, also at Lymington. Work on the hull lasted from early in 1993 to May 1994, with fitting out from May 1994 to August 1995. Her capsize trials were held at Cowes on 26 May 1995, when the boat was deliberately turned over and, within six seconds, had proved her self-righting ability. Twin Caterpillar 3412TA eight-cylinder diesel engines, each of 1,250bhp, were fitted to provide the boat with the necessary top speed.

After fitting out trials had been completed by Berthon in August 1995 the boat was taken to the RNLI Depot at Poole for her forty-hour trials, which were undertaken during the first week of September 1995. She left Poole on 4 September and went to the Channel Islands, staying in St Helier for the first night and St Peter Port for the second night, travelling to Plymouth on 7 September and running trials out of there for a couple of days before returning to Poole on 8 September for further trials. While in the Channel she undertook two services. She was in the vicinity when Plymouth's lifeboat was called to the aid of the fishing vessel *Senex Fidelis* and also escorted the 24ft yacht *Thirst Quencher* in gale force winds and foul weather off Rame Head. Lifeboats on passage report their position to the Coastguard as and can therefore be called on when an incident occurs as they are already at sea and can respond very quickly. The lifeboat was crewed during the trials by, among others, John Rudd (mechanic) and crew members Peter Brand and Ken Brand, as well as staff Coxswain Mike McHugh and Adrian Watling, the mechanic from the RNLI's divisional base.

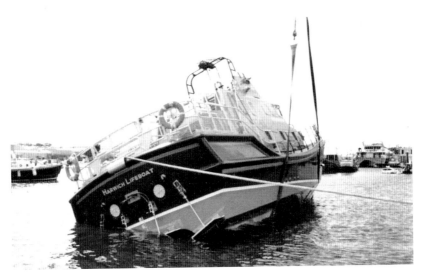

*Self-righting trials
of Albert Brown at
Cowes took place
on 26 May 1995.
(By courtesy of
Harwich RNLI)*

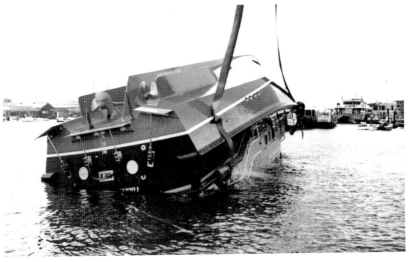

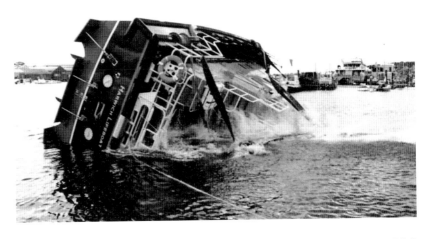

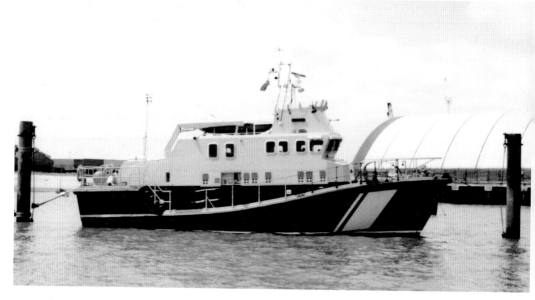

The prototype 17m Severn ON.1179 17-01 visiting Harwich on trials. She had a yellow-painted superstructure, a trials colour scheme which was never used on the boats in service. (By courtesy of Harwich RNLI)

Further trials of the new lifeboat continued throughout October and November 1995, including a passage to Alderney, with extensive crew training on a boat that was effectively the first of her class. Funded from the bequest of Victoria Maisie Brown, of London, the new lifeboat was named *Albert Brown* in memory of the donor's husband. Although she was given the operational number 17-03, indicating she was the third 17m Severn, the first boat was only used for trials and training by the RNLI before being sold to private owners and the second boat was allocated to the Relief Fleet despite being originally earmarked for Stornoway, making *Albert Brown* the first Severn to see operational service.

Albert Brown left Poole for her new station on 19 December, manned by Divisional Inspector Dick Perks, Coxswain Peter Dawson, Mechanic Jon Rudd, and crew members Andrew Moors and Ken Brand. After a two-day passage, with an overnight stop at Ramsgate, she arrived at Harwich on 21 December 1995 to be escorted home by *John Fison* and B-571 *British Diver II*. Additional crew training out of Harwich was undertaken during December 1995 and January 1996, and on 29 December 1995 *Albert Brown* undertook her first service, although she was still on trials with crew training being completed. She went to the motor barge *Sirius*, which was suffering steering problems, and escorted her into harbour from off the Suffolk coast.

A passage to the Hook of Holland was undertaken on 6 January, but during this the boat developed machinery problems with her port engine and so on 13 January she was taken to Langney Marine, at Eastbourne, for repairs. In the event, *Albert Brown* did not return to Harwich after the repairs as expected because problems with Severn class 17-02, *The Will*, the second boat of the class, led to negative press comments on the strength of the new design's hull. So the Harwich boat remained at Langney Marine for much of 1996, where stronger longitudinal ribs were fitted in the hull as the result of the trials programme with 17-02 which showed greater hull strength was required. Once the work had been completed on *Albert Brown* in September 1996, she was sent to Southampton and then on 10 September arrived at the RNLI Depot at Poole for further evaluation. From here, further extended trials were undertaken, including an overnight passage to Salcombe on 16 September and to Plymouth on 17 September. Further engine problems saw the boat visit Pendennis Shipyard at Falmouth on 18 September and she spent over a week there while repairs were undertaken.

With repairs complete, *Albert Brown* returned to Poole on 27 September for one night, setting off the following day for Harwich manned by Divisional Inspector Dick Perks, Second Coxswain Paul Smith, and crew members Ken Brand and Andrew Webb, calling at Ramsgate on the way. She left Ramsgate on 29 September and arrived at Harwich later the same day, and this time was ready for service. Following further crew training, she was officially placed on station on 2 October 1996 and *John Fison* was withdrawn to the Relief Fleet. Her first call came on 17 October 1996, but this proved to be a false alarm. Her first effective service launch came on 6 November 1996 when she spent over two hours escorting the yacht *E. F. Language*, with her eight crew, back to Harwich in

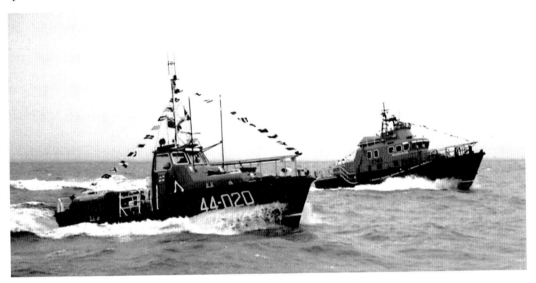

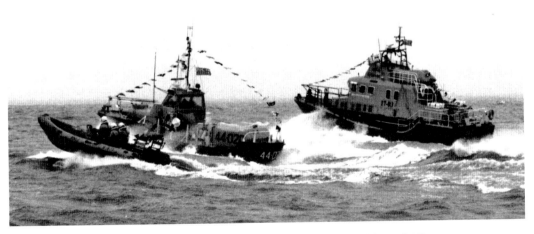

Albert Brown arrives at Harwich on 21 December 1995 escorted by 44ft Waveney John Fison and Atlantic 21 B-571 British Diver II. (Orwell Photography/Harwich RNLI)

131

force nine winds. The yacht was preparing for the Whitbread Round-the-World Yacht Challenge when it got caught out in stormy weather, which split the sail and damaged the navigation and communication equipment.

On 12 November 1996, less than a week after her first service and just over a month after coming on station, *Albert Brown* was called out on a service that put the speed and endurance of the new Severn class to the test. She went to the aid of the 270ft cargo vessel *Union Venus*, which had a fire that had put all the vessel's electrical equipment out of action. Although the cargo vessel was initially thought to be forty miles offshore, *Albert Brown* eventually stood by her fifty-one miles to the east of the station. Launching at 6.28pm, the lifeboat took less than three hours to make the passage to the casualty, despite a force nine ahead of the beam which was producing a very rough sea on top of a six-metre swell. The lifeboat stood by for a further five hours before the casualty was able to restore power and proceed to the river Thames with a tug escort, leaving Albert Brown with the passage back home in the same strong wind and heavy sea conditions. After eleven hours at sea in very testing weather, the Harwich crew reached their station at 4.25am on 13 November and were very pleased with their new lifeboat. In his report, Honorary Secretary Rod Shaw stated: 'Severn class tested for real. Good boat. Long outstanding service in very bad weather. Crew took severe punishment for eleven hours.' Commodore George Cooper, Chief of Operations, wrote to thank the Harwich crew for their efforts on this service, concluding his letter by stating, 'I wish to congratulate the Coxswain and members of the crew on this arduous ten-hour service during which the new Severn class lifeboat proved herself satisfactory to all concerned.'

Albert Brown was officially named and dedicated at a ceremony at Navyard Wharf on 26 May 1997. The event was opened by Colin Crawford, Chairman of the Harwich & Dovercourt Station Branch, with the new boat being formally handed over to the RNLI by Alan Higgs on behalf of the executors of Mrs Victoria Maisie Brown. She had left the money to the RNLI in memory of her husband, Albert, who expressed a wish to help the RNLI. Albert had escaped from Czechoslovakia almost sixty years earlier, and was the only survivor from his family. He married Maisie Victoria, from Newcastle-upon-Tyne, and changed his name so that they became known as the Browns.

Air Vice-Marshal John Tetley CB, Chairman of the RNLI's Search & Rescue Committee, accepted the boat from the donor on behalf of the RNLI, and in turn delivered into the care of the station branch and Honorary Secretary Rod Shaw. The service of dedication, led by the Rev Stephen

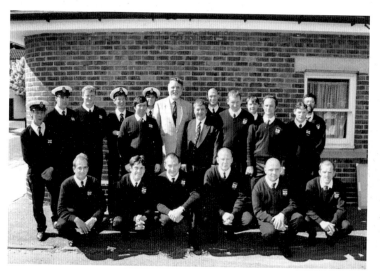

Harwich lifeboat crew after the naming of Albert Brown, left to right: Ken Brand, Jon Rudd, Scott Wiltshire, Peter Dawson, Alan Sharp, Paul Smith, Terry Waite, Rod Shaw, Colin Rotchell, John Reason, Brendan Shaw, Andrew Webb, Stuart Vincent and Peter Brand. Front row, left to right, Bob Barton, Jason Davis, John Teatheredge, Simon Benham, Peter Bull and Andrew Moors. (By courtesy of Harwich RNLI)

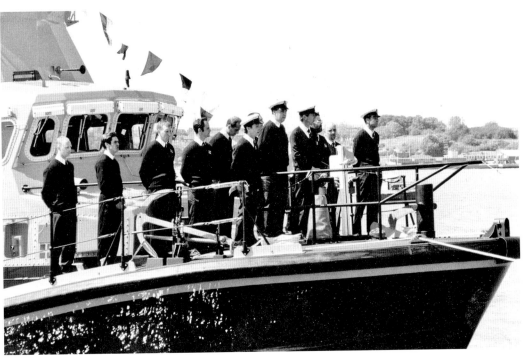

Harwich lifeboat crew on board Albert Brown (above) during her naming ceremony at Navyard Wharf, 26 May 1997. Afterwards, the new lifeboat went out on a short trip (below), with Terry Waite on the flying bridge. (Nicholas Leach)

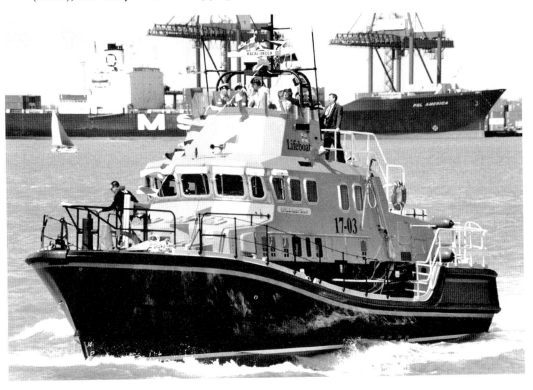

Hardie, vicar of St Nicholas Church, followed. At the end of the service, the boat was officially named by Terry Waite CBE, but before he released the champagne bottle onto the boat passed the kudos of the event onto the late donor of the lifeboat, Mrs Brown, asking her two sisters to stand so that they could receive the acclaim of the crowded quayside. *The Lifeboat* journal reported on the ceremony, concluding its account as follows:

> Terry Waite went on to explain to all those standing outside the gates and along the sea wall that the RNLI was dependent on such public spirited generosity and that they, if they cared to help the lifeboat service in some small way in their turn, could perhaps be sitting inside the guest area, next time that a lifeboat was named. Having joked about the miracle of the button on his podium being able to smash a bottle of champagne on the lifeboat some 100 feet away, Terry proceeded to name the lifeboat and roar with laughter as the said button carried out its work to perfection! The lifeboat surged away from the quayside with Terry waving joyfully to the crowd who, equally pleased and good humoured, waved him and their own quiet heroes into the far distance past huge sprays of water from two harbour tugs – a glorious and fitting finale.

During June 1997 the relief 52ft Arun *Elizabeth Ann*, which had been built in 1979 for the Falmouth station, was on duty because of issues that needed to be resolved with the Severn's engine management system. However, the Arun did not perform any services and by the end of the month *Albert Brown* was back on station and performed a number of services during the rest of the year. On 18 August 1997 she went to the fishing vessel *Yvonne Anne*, which had engine failure

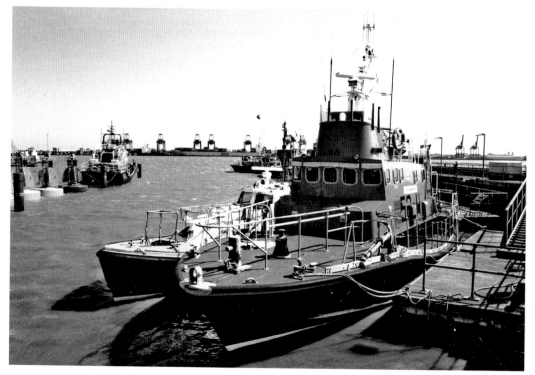

Relief 52ft Arun Elizabeth Ann alongside at the Harwich Haven Authority jetty on 2 June 1997. Stationed at Falmouth for most of her service career, she relieved at Harwich for a few days in June 1997. (Peter Edey)

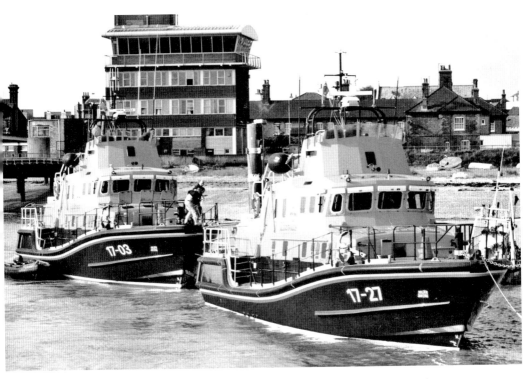

Albert Brown taking over from relief 17m Severn Volunteer Spirit on 4 October 2001. The relief boat had been on station during the summer and Albert Brown is pictured returning to resume her role as Harwich lifeboat. (Peter Edey)

twenty-two miles off the coast, and was involved in a particularly long service five days later when she went to the yacht *Explorer*, which was in difficulty more than forty miles out to sea. In a ten-hour service, the yacht was towed to safety by *Albert Brown*.

Both lifeboats were involved in an incident in the early hours of 10 October 1997 after the small cargo vessel *Ruta*, which was outward bound from the river Orwell, inadvertently left the channel in force eight winds and hit a number of yachts moored in the river. One yacht became fouled on the ship's rudder and was being dragged downriver as the ship failed to stop, and another was also caught by the vessel. The Atlantic 21 B-571 *British Diver II* launched at 6.36am to check the yacht and find out if anyone was on board, with *Albert Brown* putting out an hour later. One yacht was sunk, leaving just its mast visible, and another yacht suffered damage to its mast. The ILB and a rescue helicopter started searching for any persons in water, and *Albert Brown* assisted. After the Harbour Master confirmed that no one was on the sunken yacht and that no other yachts appeared to be missing, the search was terminated and the lifeboats returned to station.

Another relief Arun, the 1990-built *Duke of Atholl*, came to the station a year later, after *Albert Brown* had sustained damage to her bows during a service on 28 May 1998 to the fishing vessel *Wilmar* from which she had brought in an ill crewman. The relief Arun stayed for a fortnight, during which time she performed one effective rescue, on 9 June, going out at 6.36am to the yacht *Ficato*. The vessel, which was in difficulties in force seven winds just over five miles from Harwich, was brought in together with its two crew members.

Albert Brown returned to station on 11 June 1998 and completed a fine service just over a month later, on 26 August. She launched at 1.28pm under the command of Coxswain Peter Dawson into

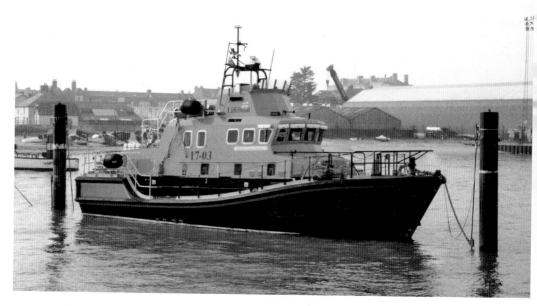

17m Severn Albert Brown at her Harwich Haven Authority moorings, which were installed specifically for the Severn. (Nicholas Leach)

rough seas with a two-metre swell and north-easterly force six to seven winds to the yacht *Pilgrim*, which was in difficulty forty miles from Harwich. The yacht's crew had reported to the Coastguard that they were totally exhausted and their vessel was low on fuel. With the lifeboat making good speed to the casualty, a passing coastal vessel *Raider* had located the yacht and got a tow on board. The lifeboat reached the scene at 3.04pm by when the weather had deteriorated and winds were gusting to force eight and the sea was very rough, with the swell height now almost four metres. Because of the yacht's violent rolling motion, the only way to evacuate the crew was to use the Severn's inflatable Y boat, so this was launched and readied to go alongside. Paul Smith and Brian Hill manned the small boat, but when its engine failed to start they had to row to *Pilgrim* through the swell. Despite this, the two people from the yacht were successfully transferred to *Albert Brown* via the Y boat, and were safely brought to Harwich, arriving at 6.55pm. *Raider* towed the yacht to Queenborough. Following this difficult service, a letter of thanks from the RNLI's Chief of Operations, Michael Vlasto, concluded, 'Although Paul Smith and Brian Hill's contribution to this service deserves special mention, all of the crew are to be thanked for their participation in achieving a satisfactory outcome. Well done everyone!'

On 12 April 1999 both Harwich lifeboats, together with Aldeburgh's 12m Mersey *Freddie Cooper*, were involved in an unusual search. At about 9.30am the container ship *Hyundai General* informed Thames Coastguard they were passing a small yacht, which appeared unmanned. The Coastguard asked the ship to circle the craft to see if anybody was aboard, but no persons appeared on deck even though the yacht's sails were set and the navigation lights were being shown. So the Coastguard tasked Rescue helicopter 125 and Aldeburgh lifeboat *Freddie Cooper*. Both arrived on scene about the same time, and, while the craft was empty, evidence of persons having been on board was found. Meanwhile, both *Albert Brown* and B-571 *British Diver II* has been tasked and took part in a full search, with the Atlantic 21 involved covering the inshore shipping lanes and sandbanks. The offshore lifeboats and helicopter covered the sea area through which the yacht had drifted, searching all day, but to no avail. In the afternoon, a taxi driver informed the Coastguard that he had picked up two persons at Aldeburgh in the early hours of the morning. They were wet and said that their yacht had sunk and they had swum ashore, and on this information the search was terminated. The Aldeburgh crew on board the yacht was replaced by two Harwich crew and *Albert Brown* towed the yacht to Harwich, with the Aldeburgh boat returning to station. Having been out for almost twenty hours, *Albert Brown* arrived at Harwich with the yacht to be met by HM Customs, who searched the yacht and found a quantity of drugs on board.

On 17 July 1999 the local angling boat *Purdy*, based out of Levington Marina on the river Orwell, reported to the coastguard that she had been swamped by a large wave, one person was in the water and the craft was in difficulties, so both Harwich lifeboats were tasked. When the Atlantic 21 B-571 *British Diver II* launched at 9.48am, the casualty's actual position was uncertain so the ILB crew proceeded to the Threshold Wrecks and started searching towards the South Shipwash buoy. *Albert Brown* put out shortly after the Atlantic and the RAF Rescue helicopter 125 was also tasked. As the ILB reached the area, the Rescue 125 located the casualty. A Belgian warship also assisted in the search, and other vessels proceeded to the area. When *Albert Brown* reached the scene, eleven miles from station, she went alongside the casualty to transfer a crew member across to ascertain the situation, with the all-weather boat then coordinating the search for the person washed overboard. Pilot boats and the Walton lifeboat also joined the search, which continued throughout the day, but nobody was found and the incident was terminated at 4.30pm. The skipper on *Purdy* was suffering from shock and generally not feeling well so he was brought ashore and the yacht was towed to Levington Marina and subsequently berthed.

On 5 December 1999 the relief 17m Severn *Fraser Flyer (Civil Service No.43)* came to the station for a six-month stint during which she performed a number of routine services as well as a more challenging one on 28 May 2000. She launched at 10.32am to the Netherlands-registered

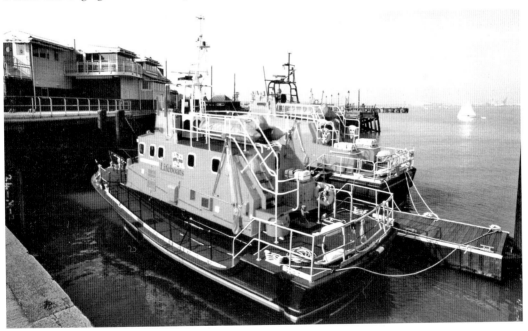

Relief 52ft Arun A. J. R. and L. G. Uridge was on station in February 2002, undertaking one service, while Albert Brown was away for repairs. (By courtesy of Harwich RNLI)

yacht *Rose Bank*. Aldeburgh's 12m Mersey lifeboat *Freddie Cooper* had also launched to the yacht which, with a crew of four, was in difficulty in rough seas and force nine winds seven miles east of Aldeburgh and thirty-four miles from Harwich. In view of the deteriorating weather conditions, the Harwich lifeboat was also requested and *Fraser Flyer* reached the scene at 12.25pm to find that Aldeburgh Coxswain Ian Firman and his crew had tried to establish a tow, but in the atrocious weather conditions had been unsuccessful. The situation was made more difficult by the poor state of the yacht's crew so, after discussion with Coxswain Peter Dawson, it was agreed to abandon the yacht and rescue the crew. The intention was that Aldeburgh lifeboat would recover the yachtsmen, while the Harwich lifeboat kept station behind the yacht to pick up anyone who fell overboard.

Despite the pitching of the yacht and frequent heavy contact between the two vessels, the yacht's crew, including the skipper, was safely hauled aboard the Aldeburgh lifeboat, which had to be taken alongside five times to enable the survivors to be transferred across. The yacht was then abandoned and, having checked the Aldeburgh lifeboat visually for damage, the Harwich lifeboat escorted her to safety. The intention to transfer the four yachtsmen from the Aldeburgh to the Harwich lifeboat in calmer waters was aborted as two of the yachtsmen were suffering from severe seasickness and were too traumatised to be moved, so they were taken ashore at Aldeburgh when the lifeboat was recovered. The rescued crew did not need to go to hospital and were driven to the ferry port after spending some time recovering at Aldeburgh. The Harwich lifeboat returned to station and was refuelled and ready for service at 4.30pm after a difficult rescue.

In the letter of thanks he sent to Harwich station, the Director of the RNLI Andrew Freemantle concluded: 'This was an excellent example of flank station co-operation and Coxswain Peter Dawson and his crew are to be thanked for their contribution to the successful outcome of this service.' Coxswain/Mechanic Ian Firman of Aldeburgh was awarded the Bronze medal for this rescue, and his six-man crew received medal service certificates. The yacht was found the following day still afloat and under way, in the approaches to the Thames Estuary.

On 30 October 2000 work started on a new crew facility, inshore lifeboat house and pontoon berth at Navyard Wharf to provide improved crew facilities and better boarding arrangements for the volunteer crew. The new building, constructed by Tiptree-based firm J. Evers, cost approximately £1.24 million and took six months to complete. The new facility, which was built on piles, provided an ILB house with davit-launching for the Atlantic, a large crew room, an office, spacious changing areas, toilets and a pontoon berth for the all-weather lifeboat. The £50,000 cost of the launch davit was funded by the local East Anglian Daily Times newspaper's Heroes At Sea appeal. The new building was officially opened by Terry Waite in July 2003.

During the twenty-first century the Harwich lifeboat station became one of the busiest in the country, and in 2000 the lifeboats performed ninety-seven services. The most notable of these was on 6 September 2000, when *Albert Brown* and her crew were involved in one of the longest services ever undertaken by an RNLI lifeboat. The lifeboat was on exercise when, at 7.25pm, a call came that the yacht *I Like It* was in difficulty fifty miles off the coast, having lost her rudder. In addition to the crew, the Honorary Secretary Rod Shaw, the Divisional Inspector Martin Smith and Divisional Engineer Adrian Watling were also on board. In north-westerly force six winds, with good visibility and a moderate to rough sea, the lifeboat headed for the casualty, but further into the passage conditions began to deteriorate. Standing by the yacht, whose German crew spoke little English, was the merchant vessel *Baltic Fort*, which offered a lee, provided a communication link and illuminated the scene using the ship's searchlights.

Albert Brown arrived on scene at 9.40pm to find the casualty, even under the lee provided by *Baltic Fort*, pitching and rolling heavily with seas breaking over her deck, and the strong wind, which had risen to force nine, was accompanied by a four-metre swell. On the first approach the

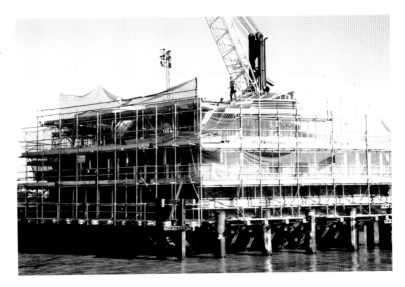

The new lifeboat station under construction at Navyard Wharf, October 2001. (Peter Edey)

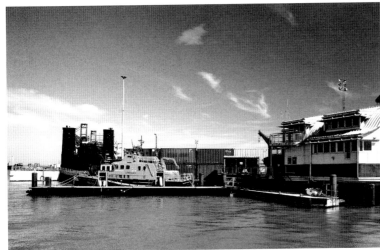

The lifeboat station and mooring pontoons at Navyard Wharf. The Wharf is operated by the Harwich Dock Company Ltd and handles roll on/roll off cargo ships sail to ports in Finland, Sweden, Norway, Denmark and Belgium (Nicholas Leach)

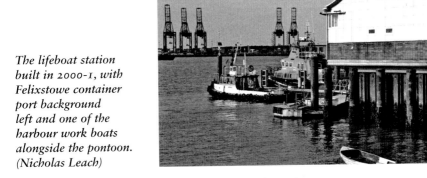

The lifeboat station built in 2000-1, with Felixstowe container port background left and one of the harbour work boats alongside the pontoon. (Nicholas Leach)

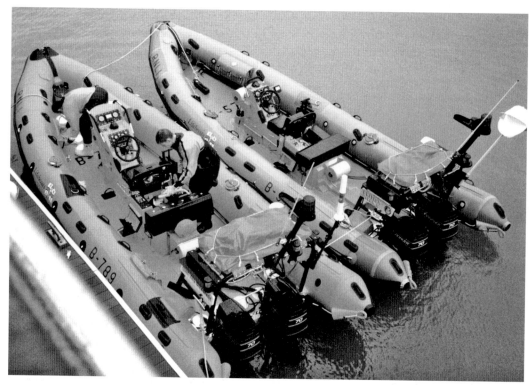

Atlantic 75 B-789 Sure and Steadfast with Atlantic 21 B-571 British Diver II with the former taking over, October 2002. B-571 served at Harwich for fifteen years. (By courtesy of Harwich RNLI)

(Right) The scene during the naming ceremony of B-789 on 18 May 2003 when she was named by Mr John Young MBE, Boys' Brigade Vice-President. (Orwell Photography)

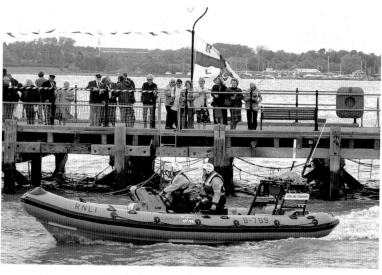

heaving line from the lifeboat landed on the yacht with the tail end in the rigging. The person on the foredeck of the casualty tried to free the heaving line, but failed, with communications to correct this being made through *Baltic Fort*. As the heaving line proved too thick to be made fast, it was released to be retrieved by the lifeboat crew. A second tow rope was then prepared and passed directly to the yachtsman on deck. Although he was extremely tired and in danger of being washed overboard by the heavy seas, he still managed to secure the line before retreating to the safety of the cockpit. During the manoeuvring, the towline came dangerously close under the stern of *Albert*

Brown and at one point snagged on the port trim tab. Meanwhile, *Baltic Fort*, with good intentions, had got close to the casualty and on more than one occasion had to be told to back off in order to give the lifeboat more sea room to manoeuvre.

The weather conditions had not relented as the lifeboat prepared for a long tow back to station, with the position now fifty-eight miles off Harwich. The towline to the yacht was lengthened to ease the strain on the casualty, which was not riding the tow well and frequently careered over about ninety degrees, rolling violently. After half an hour of steering west very slowly into the weather, the lifeboat crew decided to turn about and head east for Zeebrugge as the prevailing conditions were then astern, enabling both a quicker and safer passage. The casualty was broaching at times and there remained the possibility that the yacht could have been lost under tow had the original course been maintained. In the interest of the casualty's safety, this option was the best as the only alternative was to make the fifty-eight mile passage back to Harwich at less than two knots.

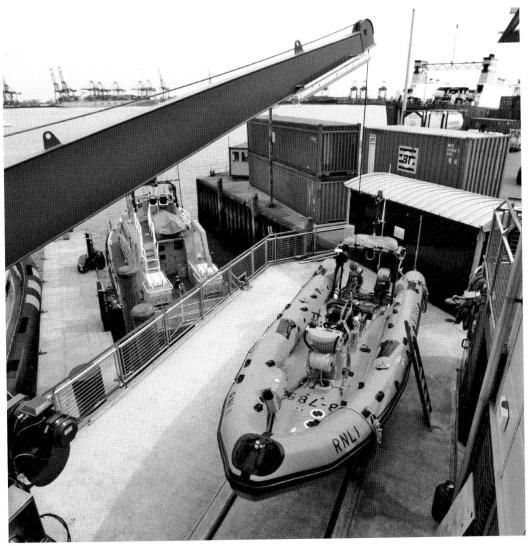

Atlantic 75 B-789 Sure and Steadfast on the cradle beneath the davit outside the lifeboat station, with Albert Brown at moorings. (Nicholas Leach)

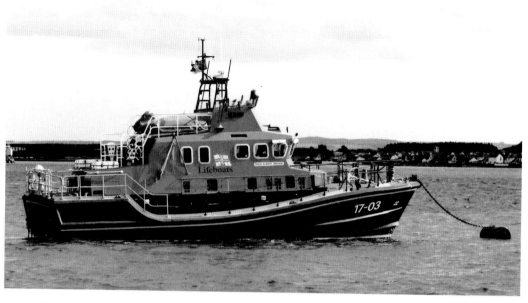

Albert Brown moored in the river Tay close to Broughty Ferry lifeboat station while on passage back to Harwich following a refit at Buckie in August 2003. (Nicholas Leach)

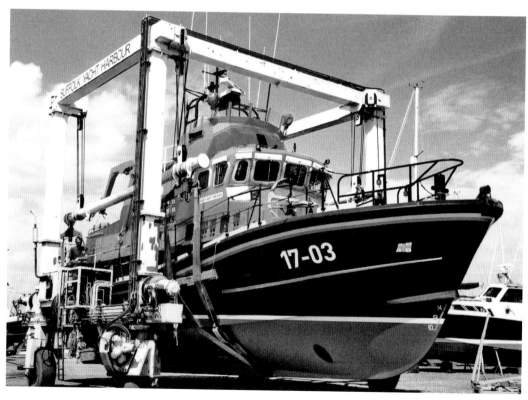

Albert Brown out of the water at Suffolk Yacht Harbour. She is regularly lifted out of the water to have her hull cleaned, or if being overhauled or repaired. (Peter Edey)

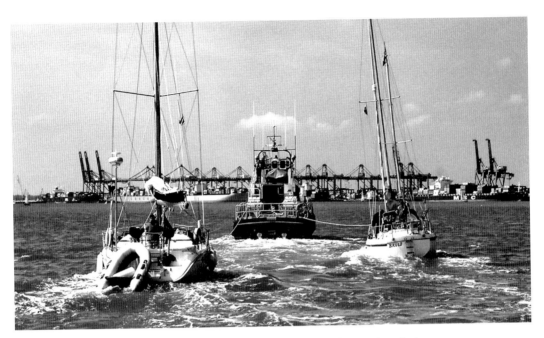

Albert Brown bringing in two yachts on 26 July 2004. (John Teatheredge)

The easterly course took *Albert Brown* and the disabled yacht across busy shipping lanes and considerable shipping in the area of the Noord Hinder Traffic Routing System. They also encountered among numerous sandbanks on the Belgian coast, where the swell was confused causing the lifeboat and casualty to roll violently, but the lifeboat crew was able to negotiate these using the electronic charts. With no charts on board the lifeboat, full use of the electronic charts was made, together with the radar, to make a safe approach to the breakwater moles of the Belgian port. Zeebrugge harbour was reached at 7.30am on 7 September and the casualty was safely berthed in the yacht harbour after the passage throughout the night. The lifeboat left the Belgian port at 11.30pm after taking on board 1,000 litres of fuel, and reached Harwich at 3.15pm. The return passage of eighty-eight miles being undertaken in south-westerly winds of force seven. This very long and arduous service, during which the lifeboat was away from station for twenty-two hours, was completed in appalling weather conditions and resulted in the saving of two lives. In recognition of his leadership skills and for displaying a high level of seamanship, Second Coxswain Paul Smith was accorded the Thanks of the Institution on Vellum. In his letter of thanks, Peter Nicholson, Chairman of the RNLI, concluded, 'I send you the Institution's appreciative thanks for the outstanding seamanship, exemplary team effort and dedication shown by all, which bought this incident to a successful conclusion.'

In 2001 eighty-one services were performed and during the year another relief 17m Severn was on station, *Volunteer Spirit*, while *Albert Brown* went for refit. The relief Atlantic 21 B-590 *Wolverson X-Ray* was also on duty for the first four months of the year, with B-571 *British Diver II* returning in early May. The following year the lifeboats were again very busy, launching more than 100 times on service, with twenty-one launches in July alone. One of the launches in July proved to be a challenging operation for the volunteer crew. *Albert Brown* was called out in the early hours of 8 July 2002 after reports after the Belgian beam trawler *Flamingo* capsized, launching at 12.28am under the command of Coxswain Peter Dawson following. An EPIRB signal had been received by the Coastguard, but the EPIRB belonged to another vessel and this was the vessel that the lifeboat searched for. The search area, more than twenty miles from Harwich, was reached by the lifeboat an hour after launching. On scene the seas were rough, with a two-metre swell and south-westerly winds of force six, gusting to force seven. Shortly after the lifeboat arrived, another vessel located the capsized *Flamingo,* and the lifeboat and other craft spent the night engaged in an intensive search for survivors. A body was recovered by the lifeboat during the night, and a second body was found in the morning, by when Walton lifeboat had joined the search. The Y boat was deployed in the daylight went to *Flamingo's* upturned hull and the crew knocked on it to see if anyone was inside, but it was empty so the Harwich lifeboat was stood down from the search at 12.10pm. After the bodies were landed into the care of the police, the lifeboat was refuelled and ready for service at 2.30pm. Operations Director Michael Vlasto sent a letter of thanks to the station, which concluded: 'This was a long and sad service in which Peter and his crew acquitted themselves well. Please thank each and every one of them for their commitment and efforts. Well done and thank you!'

The Atlantic 21 B-571 *British Diver II* was the busier of the two lifeboats in July 2002, launching twice during the afternoon of 8 July and then again on 11, 13 and 14 July, and twice on 17 July. *Albert Brown* was also out that day, launching at 3.55pm after the motor vessel *Union Gem,* inward bound to Ipswich port and transiting the river Orwell, suffered a steering failure and careered out of the navigation channel and through a number of moored yachts. Three yachts were cast adrift and others were damaged. It was unknown if any people were on board these craft, and whether anyone had been injured or washed overboard. Both Harwich lifeboats launched with the ILB reaching the scene first and immediately beginning a search for persons in the water. *Albert Brown* arrived a few minutes later and went alongside the drifting yachts to ascertain if any had been manned, with the ILB assisted the Severn to place any drifting yachts onto moorings. Meanwhile, the port authority

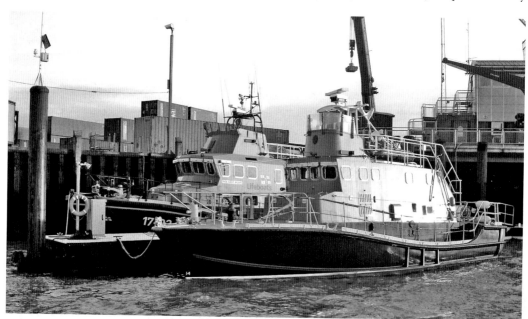

Albert Brown moored in the pen with 52ft Arun Charles Brown, December 2005. Having been sold out of service by the RNLI, the Arun, which served at Buckie for most of her service life, was on her way to China on board the container ship COSCO Shanghai, from Felixstowe container port. Former lifeboats being sold out of service regularly called at Harwich if being transported via a ship out of Felixstowe. (Andrew Moors)

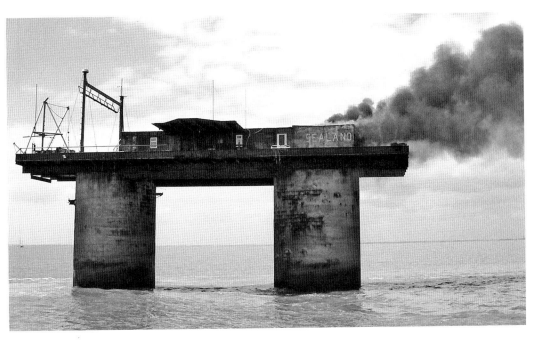

The burnt out Roughs Tower seen from Duke of Kent on 23 June 2006. The lifeboat stood by until a local fire tug extinguished the fire. (Andrew Moors)

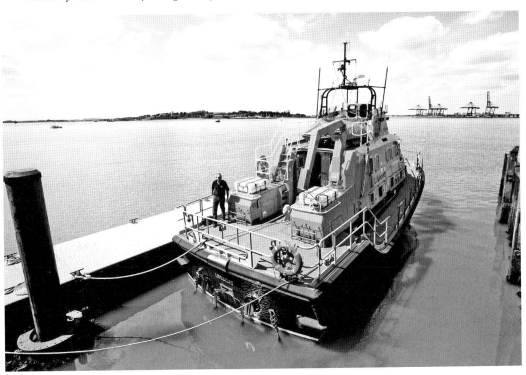

Relief 17m Severn Duke of Kent in the mooring pen, July 2006, with Coxswain Paul Smith on the stern. Duke of Kent, the penultimate Severn to be built, has served at Harwich on numerous occasions. (Nicholas Leach)

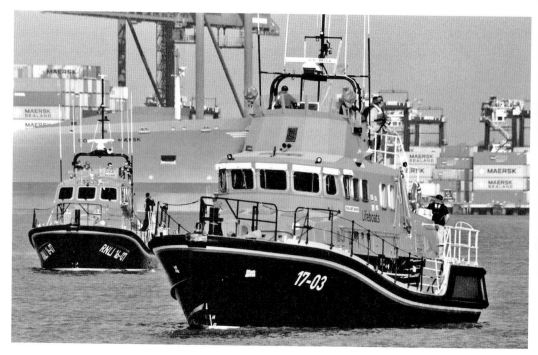

The new 16m Tamar Lester (16-07) is escorted into Harwich by Albert Brown on 14 October 2007. The new lifeboat was on passage from Poole to Cromer. (Peter Edey)

had established that the craft in question were unmanned and, with the area checked, both boats were stood down and returned to station.

On 15 October 2002 a new Atlantic 75 inshore lifeboat, B-789, was placed on station. Named *Sure and Steadfast*, she was funded by the Boys' Brigade, which organised a special appeal to mark the Millennium and chose the RNLI as its special charity. The appeal was launched in early 1999 and concluded in the summer of 2001, during which time a total of almost £160,000 was raised across the UK. This funded two Atlantic 75s, one for Arran Lamlash, named *The Boys' Brigade*, and the other for Harwich. The Harwich boat was named and dedicated at a ceremony on 18 May 2003 at the Ha'penny Pier, with Colin Crawford, Chairman of the Branch, opening proceedings. The service of dedication was led by the Rev Canon Stephen Hardie, Vicar of St Nicholas Church, and at the end of the ceremony the boat was named by John Young, Boys' Brigade Vice-President. The Atlantic 75 was developed in the early 1990s as an improved and enlarged version of the Atlantic 21 and, fitted with twin 70hp outboard motors, had a maximum speed of thirty-two knots. The hull design was revised so that it gave a softer ride than the 21 for the three crew.

On 14 August 2003 both lifeboats were out on exercise when Thames Coastguard reported that the yacht *Wench* was disabled and in difficulty near the Felixstowe Ledge buoy. The Atlantic 75 B-789 *Sure and Steadfast* launched immediately, with *Albert Brown* following. Once on scene, the Atlantic went alongside the casualty and found that the mast shroud had parted and the engine had failed. Of the two children on board, one was very sea sick with the mother concerned as to his well being, so the mother and two children were transferred to *Albert Brown*. A crew member from *Albert Brown* went aboard the casualty and the ILB took the craft in tow, making for the lifeboat berth. *Albert Brown* had landed the persons at the boathouse so that they could get warm and have refreshments, and the ILB eventually arrived and made the casualty fast to the spare pontoon berth.

In 2004, another busy year for the Harwich station, *Albert Brown* was away for the first part of the year and the relief 17m Severn *The Will* was standing in. *Albert Brown* returned from refit in April and had a busy couple of days towards the end of July. On 25 July 2004 the crew of the fishing vessel *Boy Andrew* called for assistance after the craft had become entangled in its own nets, which were also fouled on the seabed. Although the lifeboat got towlines aboard, the vessel, already tilting, capsized alongside the lifeboat. The lines had to be hastily cut by the lifeboat crew, and all three of the fishing boat's crew were picked up by the lifeboat to be landed at Harwich. The following day the lifeboat pulled in two yachts. One of the yachts, *Entropy*, was twenty-five miles east of Harwich, and as the lifeboat took her in tow, another call was received from the yacht *Brulo*, which was six miles further out and unable to sail, so the lifeboat towed the two vessels in together.

In 2005 the lifeboats were called out on 108 services, including no fewer than twenty-eight calls in July , twelve of which came in one week. The incidents ranged from swimmers in difficulty off Earlham's Beach for the ILB to the all-weather lifeboat going nineteen miles on 28 July to the ketch yacht *Paradox* at night. This service was undertaken by the relief 17m Severn *Duke of Kent* which arrived for duty on 15 July 2005 while *Albert Brown* went for refit. The relief boat stayed until November, during which time she undertook fifteen services, the first just three days after arriving. She was also out for five hours during the evening towing in the yacht *Sweet Promise*, which was in difficulties eighteen miles from Harwich in force five winds. After a series of services to help yachts during July and August, the relief lifeboat was called out to back up the Atlantic ILB on

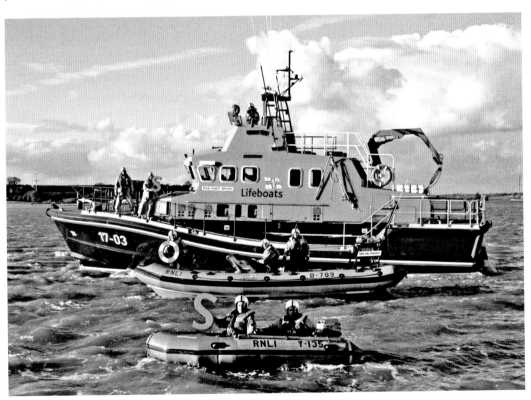

Harwich lifeboats mark the SOS national campaign day on 25 January 2008. The day is intended to allow schools, businesses, pubs, clubs and groups to show their support for the RNLI volunteer crews. Albert Brown, her Y class inflatable Y-135 and Atlantic 75 B-789 Sure and Steadfast put out for a photo opportunity. (Graeme Ewens)

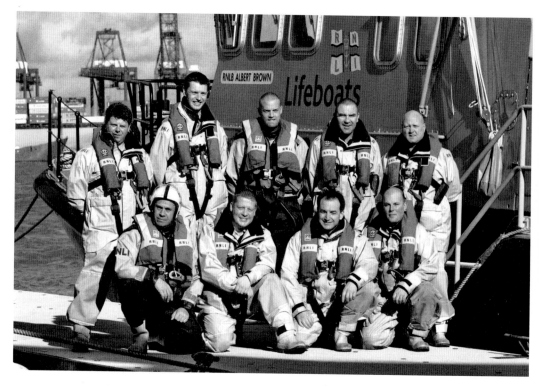

Lifeboat crew with RAF pilot John Nichol, author of the book Tornado Down. *He spent the day with the crew for a national newspaper which was writing an article about heroes. Asked to describe a hero, Nichol said the lifeboat volunteers, and so he went to Harwich to meet the local crew. (By courtesy of Harwich RNLI)*

24 August 2005 after Thames Coastguard requested both Harwich lifeboats stand by two small rigid-inflatable boats. The boats were seen to be in difficulty in force seven winds off Felixstowe. Lifeboat Operations Manager Rod Shaw discussed the situation with the watch manager, who was concerned about the sea conditions, and so the Atlantic 75 was launched at 6.30pm with a senior helmsman in charge and *Duke of Kent* was kept at immediate readiness.

The Atlantic located two rigid-inflatables, each with one person on board, travelling in company down the Felixstowe coast. As the craft still had to transit the turbulent waters off Landguard Point, the ILB helmsman considered it prudent to have *Duke of Kent* in attendance, so the all-weather boat put out to the three boats. The two lifeboats each escorted one boat as they rounded Landguard Point and reached the safety of Harwich harbour. Once both boats were in safe waters, the ILB escorted them to the local sailing club ramp for recovery and *Duke of Kent* returned to station. The two rigid-inflatables were acting as safety boats for a dragon boat race which had been cancelled due to the weather, but, manned by local fire brigade personnel, they decided to have a run in the heavy seas to test the boats capability. Their inexperience took them into severe sea conditions in excess of the boats' capabilities and safe operation, and so the lifeboats had to be called.

The last service by *Duke of Kent* at Harwich in 2005 took place on 10 October when she launched at 1.18am to the angling boat *Regardless*, which had five persons on board, one of whom had collapsed with chest pains. The casualty was two miles from the station and both Atlantic 75 B-789 and Rescue 125 helicopter from Wattisham were also tasked. The ILB was launched to get first aid to the casualty as quickly as possible, while the helicopter placed a winchman on board, who prepared the collapsed person, a fifty-year-old male, for a stretcher lift. *Duke of Kent* arrived as the helicopter commenced winching the casualty, so she stood by while winching was completed and then escorted the angling boat over the bar and back into the River Ore. With *Regardless* back in the river, both lifeboats returned to station.

During 2006 Harwich lifeboats performed a total of eighty-four services from standing by offshore towers on fire to medical emergencies and broken down boats. Although *Albert Brown* had returned to station in November 2005, after undertaking a further four services she was taken away again for repairs and *Duke of Kent* returned to the station on 3 May 2006 for a three-month stint and was involved in an unusual service on 23 June after the Roughs Towers caught alight due to a electrical fire. The tower, located about ten miles off Harwich, was the first of four naval forts designed by G. Maunsell to protect the Thames Estuary. *Duke of Kent* was tasked at 12.30pm to attend the scene as one person had been injured in the fire. An RAF rescue helicopter transferred

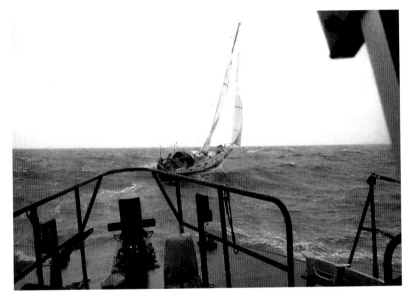

On 28 March 2008 Albert Brown launched to the 35ft yacht Permare with three persons on board. The yacht was located three miles off the North Shipwash, making slow progress towards Harwich in heavy seas and with limited fuel, so she was escorted into harbour by the lifeboat. (By courtesy of Harwich RNLI)

On 7 April 2008 the relief 17m Severn Fraser Flyer assisting the 20m sailing barge De Gebruder into harbour. The barge was found five miles south-east of Harwich near the Cork Sands with four persons on board and was in danger of grounding. (By courtesy of Harwich RNLI)

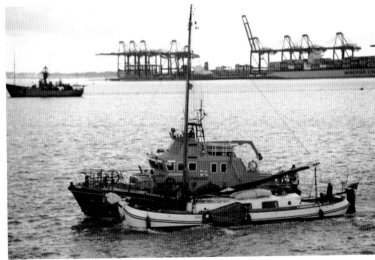

the person to Ipswich hospital, directly from the tower so the lifeboat stood by the tower until a local fire tug extinguished the fire.

Duke of Kent was busy during July and August, launching to a variety of craft, often assisting or assisted by B-789 *Sure and Steadfast*, which was even busier. On 15 July 2006 both Harwich lifeboats were tasked to help the 35ft motor boat *Deborah*, which encountered difficult sea conditions as it passed over the Deben Bar and proceeded to seaward. The skipper turned about to return to the river, but soon afterwards found water was coming on board and the boat was flooding fast. He put out a distress signal and the Atlantic 75 proceeded without delay with the salvage pump, followed by *Duke of Kent*. As the ILB was approaching the scene, a passing yacht reported *Deborah* had sunk and that the two persons who had been on board were being picked up. The ILB went alongside this yacht and found the two persons wet and tired but otherwise okay, so they were transferred to *Duke of Kent*, which had arrived on scene, and taken back to Harwich while the ILB searched the area to try and find signs of the wreckage.

The lifeboats, while mostly tasked to yachts and other pleasure craft, have also helped the local work boats around the harbour. During the evening of 23 July 2006 the local pilot boat *Haven Hawk* reported an engine room fire when eleven miles off the harbour, and required assistance, and so both lifeboats launched just after 7pm, with Rescue Helicopter 125 also responding as well as another pilot boat. *Haven Hawk's* crew had shut down the boat's engine compartment and were monitoring bulkhead temperature to ascertain the extent of the fire, and the temperatures appeared to be going down. Atlantic 75 B-789 *Sure and Steadfast* was first on scene, and found that the pilot boat crew had started the other engine and the boat was making headway towards Harwich. *Duke of Kent* arrived on scene and, with situation under control, the ILB was released while the lifeboat

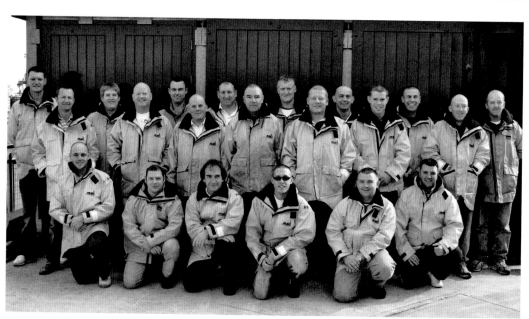

Harwich lifeboat crew in October 2008. Standing, left to right, Chris Glen Barber, Gavin Antiff, Paul Griffin, Simon Benham, Mark Darling, Lee James, John Reason, Paul Smith (Coxswain), Scott Wiltshire (Deputy Second Coxswain), Elliot Kemp, Stephen Amner (Third Mechanic), Michael Goddard, Jason Davis, Redford Moors, Andrew Moors (Assistant Mechanic). Front row, left to right, Robert Teatheredge, Stuart Vincent, John Teatheredge (Second Coxswain), Steve Emerson, Brendon Shaw and Stuart Henderson.

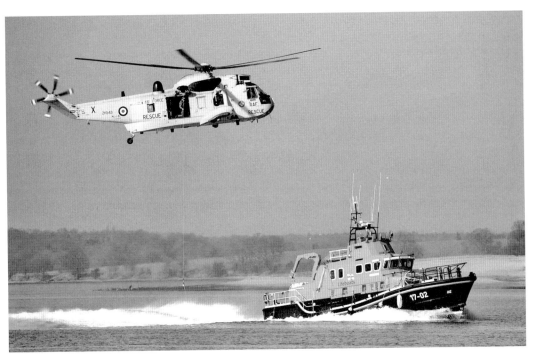

Relief 17m Severn The Will exercising with RAF Search and Rescue helicopter from Wattisham in the river Stour, February 2009. (Nicholas Leach)

escorted *Haven Hawk* back to Harwich. During the passage to Harwich the pilot boat's engine room was kept closed and she safely reached harbour, being berthed at the Harwich Pilot Station.

In 2007 the lifeboats performed ninety-nine services, with the Atlantic 75 completing sixty-nine of these. The most notable service came on 18 March 2007 when both lifeboats were launched at 12.26pm to five canoeists in trouble off the river Deben in gale force eight to nine north-westerly winds, accompanied by rough seas. The Atlantic 75 B-789 *Sure and Steadfast* launched at 12.32pm and within ten minutes was on scene, locating two of the missing five, a sixty-three-year-old man and twelve-year-old boy, in the water. The man was semi-conscious and hypothermic, and the boy told the lifeboat crew that his brother was still missing. Both were transferred onto *Albert Brown*, which arrived on scene soon after the Atlantic, and the Atlantic's crew then searched the area for further casualties, while *Albert Brown* rescued two more from the water. A rescue helicopter from RAF Wattisham arrived and was immediately requested to airlift two canoeists from the lifeboat that were in need of urgent medical attention. The last of the five persons, another child, was eventually located and rescued by the Atlantic. Subsequently all remaining persons were brought to the lifeboat station to a waiting ambulance to be medically examined. The three crew on the Atlantic 75, Scott Wiltshire, Matthew Preston and Stuart Henderson, were subsequently all recognised by the RNLI for the roles they played in this challenging rescue.

Less than a month later, both lifeboats effected rescues on the same day. On 15 April 2007 they were exercising in Harwich waters with four Duke of Edinburgh's award students when Thames Coastguard asked them to respond to two different incidents. The Atlantic 75 was called to the river Ore, together with Aldeburgh's inshore lifeboat, to help the 34ft yacht *Vagabond* which had two persons on board and had run aground on the banks. The vessel was pulled clear and escorted out of the river by the lifeboats. Meanwhile, *Albert Brown* was sent to the north of Harwich to

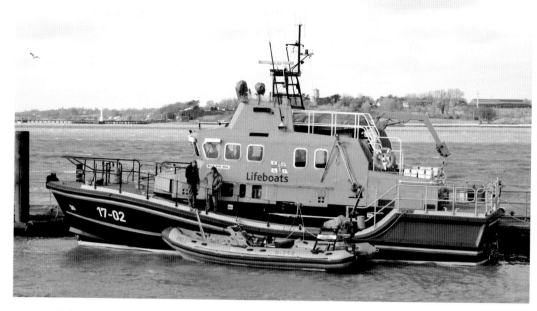

Relief 17m Severn The Will on duty in March 2009 while the mooring pontoon was under repairs. The lifeboat was moored temporarily at the Harbour Authority pontoons near Ha'penny Pier. The ILB launching davit was being repaired at the same time and so relief Atlantic 75 B-736 Toshiba Wave Warrior was on station and was kept afloat. (By courtesy of Harwich RNLI)

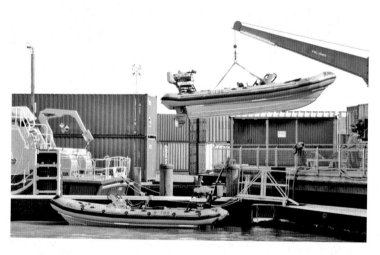

B-736 Toshiba Wave Warrior served on relief duty at Harwich while the launching davit was under repair; B-736 could be kept afloat as she had an anti-fouled hull. The boats are pictured swapping over after the completion of repairs in March 2009. (By courtesy of Harwich RNLI)

meet Aldeburgh lifeboat *Freddie Cooper*, which was towing the yacht *Templar* towards Harwich. The yacht had engine problems, and so the tow was transferred to the Harwich lifeboat which then proceeded to Shotley Marina with the casualty.

During the summer of 2007 Harwich lifeboats were particularly busy, responding to forty-six incidents compared to thirty-three the previous summer. The year was the hottest on record and this was undoubtedly a factor in attracting more people to the coast. On 19 May 2007 *Albert Brown* and her crew had a long service to the 56ft yacht *Louise* which was dismasted with eight persons on board twenty miles south-east of Harwich. Due to communication problems, the yacht's position was unclear and Walton lifeboat was also launched to assist, but *Albert Brown's* crew used the DF equipment to locate the yacht, which was towed to Harwich and berthed at the lifeboat station while the lifeboat crew helped to remove the mast and rigging from the water.

Another yacht was the cause of a major sea rescue operation less than a month later, on 14 June 2007. The 20ft yacht *Gentle Jane* had left Holland on 12 June bound for Harwich but had not arrived. The lifeboats put out at 3.42am with the Atlantic 75 B-789 *Sure and Steadfast* searching the harbour and Albert Brown searching an area from Harwich to thirty miles north-east of the harbour. Walton and Aldeburgh lifeboats were also tasked and searched to the north and south of Harwich, while an RAF helicopter and coastguard spotter plane also joined the search. The RAF helicopter eventually located the yacht forty-two miles north east of Harwich, so *Albert Brown* was sent to the yacht, which was located and towed to Harwich.

In early October 2007 the inshore lifeboat had three call-outs in twenty-four hours. The first came just after midday with the lifeboat launching to the yacht *Bellatrix*, which was disabled with fouled propellers at Felixstowe Dip. The yacht was freed and towed to Harwich harbour for further assistance. On leaving *Bellatrix*, at the request of Thames Coastguard the ILB was diverted to Walton Backwaters to the 27ft sloop *Lapalord*, which had run aground with one person on board. On proceeding to the scene, the ILB crew found that a local boat, which had also responded to the request for help, had now freed the vessel so the ILB returned to station. At 1.20am the ILB was again called out, this time to an unconscious male reported adrift on a boat at the Harwich Green area. The person was quickly found, recovered, and landed ashore to a waiting ambulance.

Of the eighty-four services undertaken in 2008, the Atlantic performed sixty-two and continued to be much in demand. *Albert Brown* went away for refit during March and April, with relief 17m

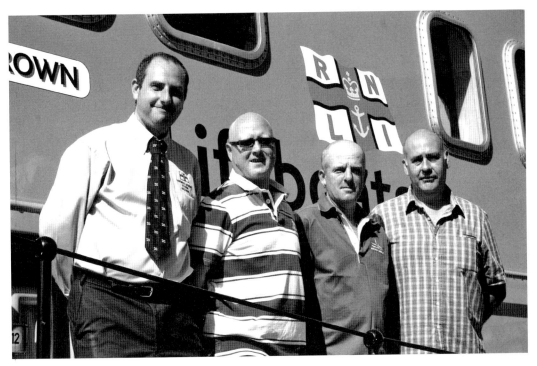

Harwich mechanics past and present: from left to right, David Thompson, Brian Hill, Andrew Moors and Jon Rudd. (By courtesy of Harwich RNLI)

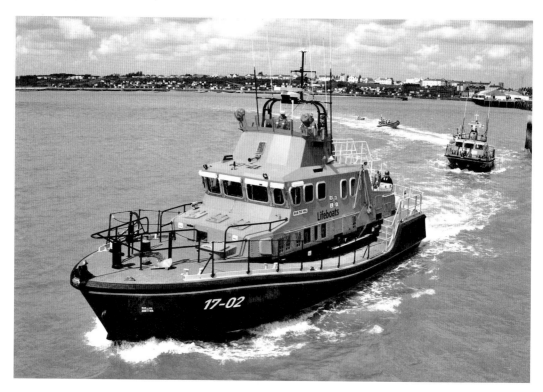

Essex lifeboats on exercise off Walton pier, June 2009. Relief 17m Severn The Will from Harwich leads Walton and Frinton lifeboat Kenneth Thelwall II, with (below) Atlantic 75s from Clacton-on-Sea (B-744) and Harwich also in attendance. (Nicholas Leach)

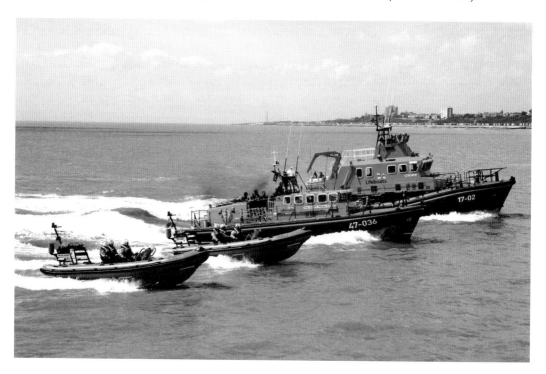

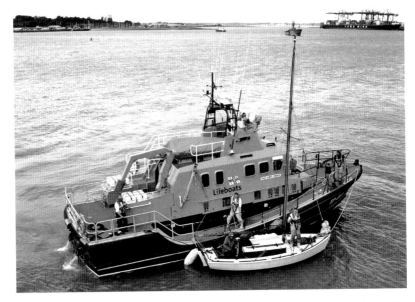

Severn *Fraser Flyer (Civil Service No.43)* coming in her place for a short stint during which she completed four services. On 28 March 2008 *Fraser Flyer* was launched to the 35ft yacht *Permare* with three persons on board requested assistance. The yacht was located three miles off the North Shipwash making slow progress towards Harwich in heavy seas with limited fuel. She was escorted into Harwich harbour. The all-weather lifeboat was launched after reports had been received that a crewman had been missing since 3am, presumed to have fallen overboard, from the ship *Baltic Sky 1* which was at anchor in the Sunk deep-water anchorage twelve miles east of Harwich. Lifeboats from Walton and Aldeburgh and air sea rescue helicopters from Wattisham and Dover joined in the search. A body was eventually recovered and flown to Ipswich Hospital. And on 20 April both Harwich lifeboats were launched to the 25ft sailing ketch *Sargasso*, which had run aground on the river Deben Sand bar, five miles east of Harwich, with one person onboard. She was towed clear of the sand bank by the inshore lifeboat and allowed to proceed into Harwich harbour unaided.

Albert Brown returned in early May 2008 ready for the summer season and had a long service on 31 May, launching at 9.14am to the 32ft yacht *Blubell*, which was in difficulty twenty-four miles east of Harwich. The yacht, with four persons on board, had fouled her propeller and was drifting in dense fog near the shipping lanes. She was located by the lifeboat crew using the directional equipment and towed to Shotley Marina. *Albert Brown* helped several other yachts during the summer, including one on 18 August 2008 when she launched in response to a Mayday call from the 28ft yacht *Auberge*, which was taking on water with engine and rigging failure in rough seas six miles east of Felixstowe. The yacht, with one elderly person on board, was having difficulties communicating with Thames Coastguard and unsure of his exact position. Once the lifeboat arrived on scene, the yacht was taken in tow and brought to the safety of Shotley Marina.

In 2009 Harwich lifeboats had a record year with 125 call outs. The previous highest total was in 2005, when 109 services were undertaken. During the year, twelve persons were saved and seventy-one people brought in, including kite surfers, yachtsmen, swimmers and fishermen, and two dogs were rescued as well. Captain Rod Shaw, Lifeboat Operations Manager, commented on the figures by saying, 'the increase in services gives cause for concern because it indicates the public are not taking adequate care and attention when using the sea for recreation. Poor maintenance of boats and failure to observe weather warnings are just two of the reasons for persons needing the services of the Harwich Lifeboats.' The lifeboat regularly operated well out in the North Sea and on 2 January 2009 assisted the Belgium trawler *Atlantis*, which was on fire thirty-five miles off Harwich with six persons onboard. The wheelhouse was blaze, and the RAF helicopter and Walton and Frinton lifeboat also attended the vessel. The crew on board the trawler had managed to extinguish the fire before the rescue craft arrived, so the lifeboats and helicopter stood by while a nearby trawler connected a tow and headed to Zeebrugge. The lifeboat, having launched at 10.45pm, returned to station at 2.30am on 3 January.

The station had a busy day on 28 July 2009 with, first, *Albert Brown* being called out at 12.10pm to assist the hundred-year-old 10m Gaffer sailing boat *Gwenili* twenty-one miles east of Harwich. The vessel, with four persons onboard, had sustained damage to her rigging and needed assistance into Harwich harbour. She was towed back to the lifeboat's pontoons where her rigging and sails were repaired. Later on the same day, Atlantic 75 B-789 *Sure and Steadfast* and a shore party from the station were called out after two members of the public reported a man in the water off Stone Pier. They had managed to throw a lifebelt ring to the stranded man, but been unable to pull him clear. On arrival, the ILB landed a crewman onto the pier and, with the assistance of the shore party, pulled the man to safety. He was transferred to the Coastguard mobile unit and driven along the pier to a waiting ambulance.

During 2010 the lifeboat crews responded to over 110 service calls. Both lifeboats were kept busy with the inshore boat responding to eighty incidents and the all-weather lifeboat thirty-one.

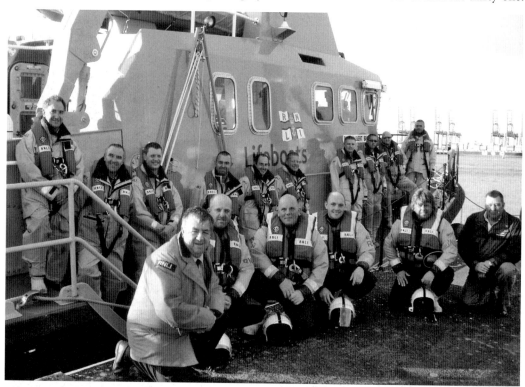

Harwich lifeboat crew, September 2009. On board Albert Brown are, left to right, Second Coxswain John Teatheredge, Coxswain Paul Smith, Chris Glen Barber, Mark Darling, Mechanic David Thompson, Elliot Kemp, Dan Sime, Steve Emerson, Brian Hill and Jason Davis. Kneeling in front are, left to right, Captain Rod Shaw, Andrew Moors, Lee James, Rob Teatheredge, Glen Merchant and Keith Churchman. (By courtesy of Andrew Moors)

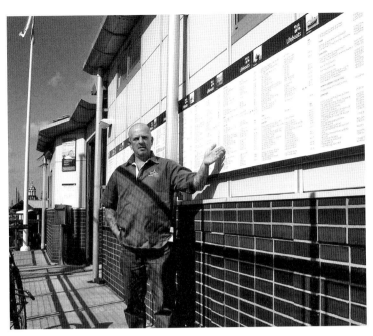

On 21 July 2010 a ten-year project to research the station's services was completed. Before this, the records were incomplete and when the new lifeboat station was built a project was started to research the history and display the information. Andrew Moors and Michelle Pierce obtained the information for the boards, which were mounted outside the boathouse on the Quay. A donor, who wished to remain anonymous, funded the display panels. The boards list the effective services by all station boats. (Keith Churchman)

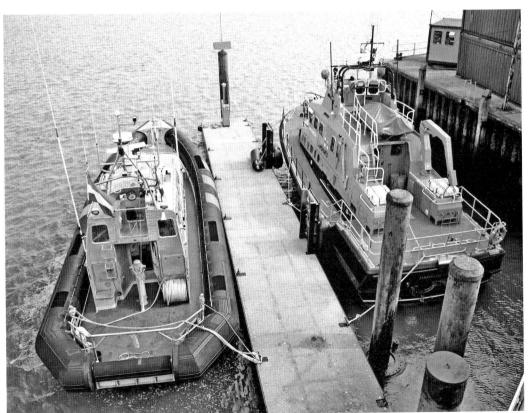

Hook of Holland lifeboat Jeanine Parqui berthed at Harwich with Albert Brown during the Dutch lifeboat's courtesy visit, July 2010. (Nicholas Leach)

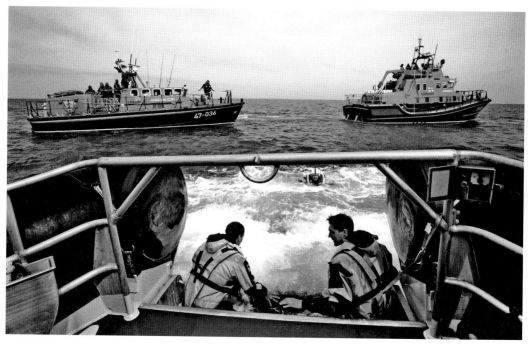

Walton lifeboat Kenneth Thelwall II and Harwich lifeboat Albert Brown stand by during a man overboard recovery exercise with Dutch lifeboat Jeanine Parqui. (Nicholas Leach)

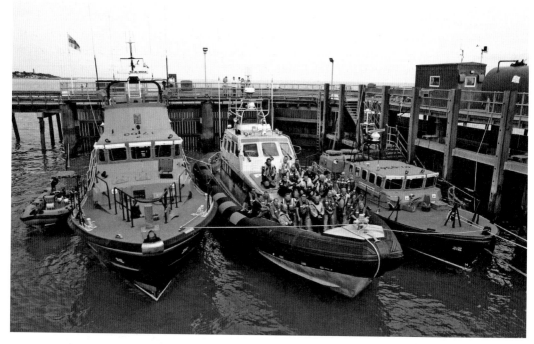

RNLI and Dutch lifeboat crews on board Dutch lifeboat Jeanine Parqui, flanked by Atlantic 75 B-789 Sure and Steadfast, Albert Brown and Kenneth Thelwall II (on right) in the boarding pen at Walton and Frinton, July 2010. (Nicholas Leach)

Ditched aircraft, grounded yachts, boats with engine failure, kite surfers, swimmers were just some of the incidents in which the lifeboats were involved. The first service by *Albert Brown* came on 20 February 2010 when she launched just after 2pm to recover a body reported about thirty-one miles east of Harwich by a passing survey vessel. The lifeboat was met by Essex Marina Police unit, who recovered the body from the water. The Atlantic 75 was busy throughout the year, and in July was called out more than twenty times. The boat was particularly busy on 10 and 11 July, with the first launch coming at 6.40am on 10 July to the ex-fishing vessel *Enterprise* with three persons on board at Stone Point, Walton Backwaters, which had run aground and was taking on water. At 2.25pm the ILB went to the aid of a swimmer in difficulties off Shingle Street and at 4.40pm took a salvage pump to the yacht *Estrella* on the river Stour, which had also run aground. The following day, B-789 assisted an upturned jet ski, attended an incident at the Orwell Bridge, assisted two yachts both of which had gone aground, and took out a salvage pump to the yacht *Thoma*, which was sinking at its mooring.

One of the longest services of the year came on 21 October 2010 after the skipper of the 30ft yacht *Aegis* requested assistance because he had been suffering severe seasickness for the previous twenty-four hours. When he called for urgent assistance, the yacht was north of the Galloper Banks, approximately thirty-five miles south-east of Harwich. *Albert Brown* launched at 3.15pm to proceed to the yacht, and assessed the condition of the captain and informed the coastguards of the situation. Because of the serious condition of the skipper he was transferred onto the lifeboat for immediate return to Harwich. A member of the crew was placed aboard the yacht to assist the remaining person still on board until the Aldeburgh lifeboat *Freddie Cooper*, which had also been launched, could make contact and take the yacht in tow. Paramedics met the lifeboat on her return to station at 6.40pm and immediately treated the casualty.

As well as the services, a number of other notable events happened during the year. In February 2010 the station was featured on the television series Deadly North Sea on Sky Bravo Channel. Tim Taggart, from the programme's production team, spent two weeks living and working alongside the lifeboat crews capturing rescues on film. And later in the year, during the first weekend in July, the KNRM lifeboat *Jeanine Parqui*, from the Hook of Holland station, visited Harwich for a weekend

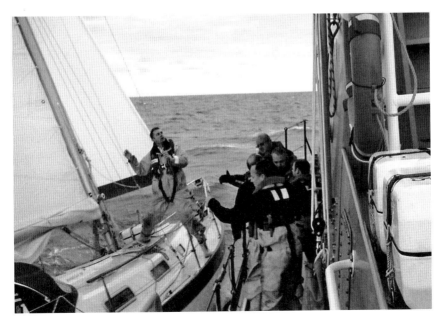

A crewman from Albert Brown is transferred on to the yacht Aegis on 21 October 2010. (By courtesy of Harwich RNLI)

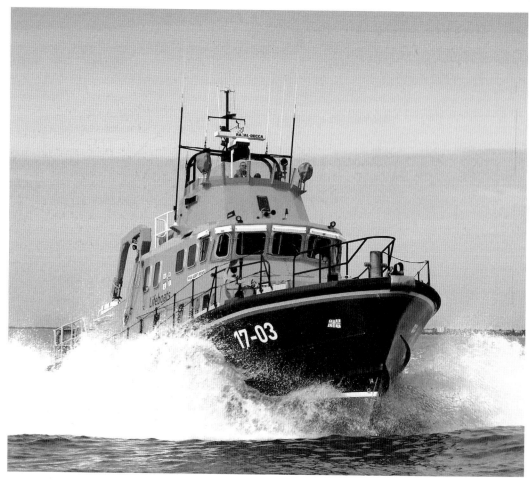

Harwich lifeboat 17m Severn Albert Brown at speed. (Nicholas Leach)

which started with an exercise off Essex. The Harwich and Hook boats were joined by the Walton and Frinton lifeboat *Kenneth Thelwall II* and the air-sea rescue helicopter from RAF Wattisham for winching exercises. Other rescue scenarios, including man overboard, lifeboat to lifeboat transfers and sea to lifeboat, were also undertaken by all boats. At the end of the exercise, the boats went to Walton pier to meet and greet their counterparts from across the North Sea, before the Harwich lifeboats returned to station, accompanied by *Jeanine Parqui*. The Dutch lifeboat returned to its home country the day after the exercise.

In describing the work of the lifeboat station in 2010, Lifeboat Operations Manager Captain Rod Shaw summed up not just the year, but the station's remarkable history, particularly since the station was re-established in the 1960s, when the number of rescues undertaken and lives saved has proved that Harwich is a key part of the RNLI's chain of lifeboat stations. He said: 'Call outs during the year placed great demand on the Harwich crews and tribute must be given to their total commitment and dedication to saving people's lives off Harwich and Felixstowe. Some services were long and arduous which required skill and expertise resulting in a successful rescue. Thanks must be recorded to our many local donors and loyal supporters whose fund raising efforts keep us operational and ensure we have the best boats for saving the lives of those in distress at sea.'

Appendices

A • LIFEBOAT SUMMARY

<hr>

███

Early lifeboats

c.1821			?	Melville
	Plenty	—		Essex Lifeboat Association
1821 – 1826			1821	Braybrooke
	N&S?	—		Essex Lifeboat Association

RNLI pulling lifeboats

1876 – 1881	35' x 9'	£432	1876	Springwell
(26/61)	Self-righter (10)	—	Woolfe, Shadwell	Miss E. Burmester, London
1881 – 1902	45'2" x 11'	£600	1881	Springwell
(94/82)	Self-righter (12)	317	Woolfe, Shadwell	Miss E. Burmester, London
1890 – 1891	38' x 9'	£452	1890	Reserve No.3
(1/39)	Self-righter (12)	206	Livie & Sons, Dundee	RNLI Funds
1904 – 1912	43' x 12'6"	£1,711	1904	Ann Fawcett
(16/15)	Watson (10)	517	Thames IW, Blackwall	Legacy of Miss Fawcett

Steam lifeboats

1890 – 1892	50' x 14'4"	£5,000	1889	Duke of Northumberland
(23/33)	Steam	231	R. & H. Green, Blackwall	RNLI Funds
1894 – 1897 &	52' x 16'	£2,639	1894	City of Glasgow
1898 – 1901 (23/32)	Steam	362	R. & H. Green, Blackwall	Glasgow Lifeboat Fund
1901 – 1917	56' x 14'8"	£4,190	1901	City of Glasgow
(99/87)	Steam	446	J. S. White, Cowes	Glasgow Lifeboat Fund

Motor lifeboats

1967 – 1980	44' x 12'8"	£26,500	1967	Margaret Graham
(173/77)	Waveney	1004	Brooke Marine, Lowestoft	Anonymous gift
1980 – 1996	44' x 12'8"	£260,000	1980	John Fison
(244/99)	Waveney	1061	Fairey Marine, Cowes	Gift of Mrs D. E. Fison and others
1996 –	17m x 5.5m	£1,580,000	1995/6	Albert Brown
	Severn	1202	Hull by Green Marine/ fit out Berthon Bt Yd	Bequest of Victoria Maisie Brown

Inshore lifeboats

1965 – 1970	15'3" x 6' 3" RFD PB16	£750 D-71	1965	— —	
1.1971 – 12.1973	15'3" x 6' 3" RFD PB16	D-201	1971	— —	
1.1974 – 1975	15'3" x 6' 3" RFD PB16	D-206	1971	— —	
11.3.1976 – 13.11.1977	15'3" x 6' 3" Zodiac II	D-240	1975	— —	
2.1978 – 10.1987	22'9" x 7'6" Atlantic 21	B-526	1978	— Lady D. E. G. Hunt.	
31.10.1987 – 10.2002	22'9" x 7'6" Atlantic 21	B-571	1987 ILB Centre, Cowes	British Diver II The British Sub-Aqua Club	
15.10.2002 –	24' x 8'8" Atlantic 75	B-789	2002 ILB Centre, Cowes	Sure and Steadfast The Boys' Brigade Appeal	

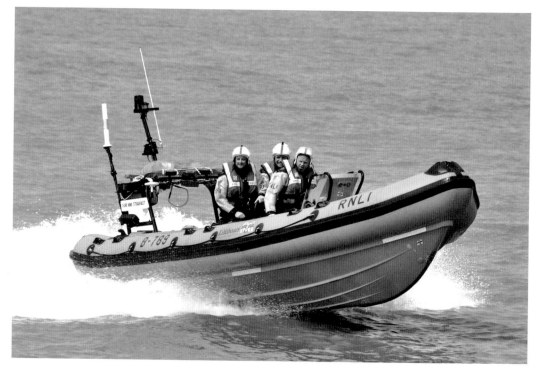

Atlantic 75 B-789 Sure and Steadfast has been on station since October 2002 and is the third Atlantic to serve Harwich. (Nicholas Leach)

Springwell

On *station*	January 1876 – 1881
Record	26 launches, 61 lives saved
Dimensions	35ft x 9ft
Type	Self-righter, 10 oars double-banked
Built	1876, Woolfe, Shadwell
Donor	Gift of Miss Ellen Burmester, London
Cost	£433
Disposal	Capsized on service 1881, returned to London 1881.

Springwell

Official Number	317
On station	1881 – 1902
Record	94 launches, 82 lives saved
Dimensions	45ft x 11ft x 5ft 5in
Type	Self-righter, 12 oars double-banked
Built	1881, Woolfe, Shadwell
Donor	Gift of Miss Ellen Burmester, London
Cost	£800
Disposal	Broken up in June 1902.

Ann Fawcett

Official Number	517
On station	No.1, March 1904 – 1912
Record	16 launches, 15 lives saved
Dimensions	43ft x 12ft 6in
Type	Watson, 10 oars
Weight	11 tons 4 cwt
Built	1904, Thames Iron Works, Blackwall, yard no.TK47
Donor	Legacy of Mrs A. Fawcett, London
Cost	£1,711
Disposal	Served at Kingston (Dun Laoghaire) from 1913 to 1919. Sold out of service 1920.

Duke of Northumberland

Official Number	231
On station	19 September 1890 – 26 July 1892
Record	15 launches, 33 lives saved
Dimensions	50ft x 14ft 3in x 5ft 9in
Type	Steam
Engines	Horizontal, direct-acting compound and surface condensing with two cylinders and a 12-inch stroke, developing 170hp
Weight	24 tons
Built	1889, R. and H. Green, Blackwall, yard no.G227
Donor	RNLI funds.
Cost	£5,000
Disposal	The first steam lifeboat built for the RNLI. After Harwich, she served at Holyhead 1892-93 and 1897-1922, and New Brighton 1893-97, before being sold out of service in 1923.

City of Glasgow

Official Number	362
On station	No.2, 7 November 1894 – 24 November 1897; and February 1898 – October 1901
Record	9 launches, 4 lives saved
Dimensions	53ft x 16ft x 5ft 6in, 48ft waterline
Type	Steam
Engines	Penn patent water-tube boiler driving two vertical turbines through a compound engine of 200hp
Weight	28 tons
Built	R. and H. Green, Blackwall
Donor	City of Glasgow Lifeboat Fund.
Cost	£2,639 10s 0d
Disposal	Served at Gorleston November 1897 to February 1898. Sold out of service in October 1901 for £105 to Mr M. Lemon, Harwich.

City of Glasgow

Official Number	446
On station	May 1901 – May 1917
Record	99 launches, 87 lives saved
Dimensions	56ft 6in x 15ft 9in x 5ft 8in
Type	Steam
Engines	180hp engine, single propeller, 1 mast, also carried forelug and jib; top speed 9.66 knots
Weight	31 tons 15 cwt, displacement 32.6 tons
Built	J. Samuel White & Co Ltd, Cowes
Donor	City of Glasgow Lifeboat Fund, in connection with the Lifeboat Saturday demonstrations of 1893 and 1894.
Cost	£4,191 0s 0d
Disposal	The last steam lifeboat built by the RNLI. Sold out of service in December 1917 to the Admiralty for use as a patrol vessel, renamed **Patrick**, and sent to the Nile.

Margaret Graham

Official Number	1004 (operational number 44-005)
On station	September 1967 – March 1980
Record	173 launches, 77 lives saved
Dimensions	44ft x 12ft 8in
Type	Waveney
Engines	Twin 215hp Cummins V6 Cummins six-cylinder diesels; re-engined in 1982 with twin 203hp Caterpillar D3208 eight-cylinder diesels
Weight	17 tons 16 cwt
Built	1967, Brooke Marine, Lowestoft; yard number B351
Donor	Anonymous gift
Cost	£43,020
Disposal	Served in the Relief Fleet from 1980 to 1986 and then at Amble from June 1986 to July 1999; she was the last 44ft Waveney lifeboat to be in RNLI service. Sold out of service in August 1999 to Scarborough Borough Council for use as a pilot boat operated by Whitby Harbour Board, renamed *St Hilda* of Whitby.

John Fison

Official Number	1060 (operational number 44-021)
On station	11 March 1980 – October 1996
Record	244 launches, 99 lives saved
Dimensions	44ft x 12ft 8in
Type	Waveney, steel-hulled
Engines	Twin 250hp Caterpillar 3208T diesels
Weight	18 tons 16 cwt
Built	1980, Fairey Marine, Cowes; yard number 687
Donor	Gift Mrs D. E. Fison, in memory of her husband; Mrs Knowles; legacy of Mrs Sutcliffe; and a gift from Fisons Ltd
Cost	£243,487
Disposal	Served in the Relief Fleet from 1996 to 1999, and sold out of service in August 1999 to the Raglan Volunteer Coastguard of New Zealand; she was shipped to New Zealand and renamed Hamilton Rotary Rescue. In 2007 she was sold by the Coastguard and became a harbour cruiser at Fremantle, Australia.

Albert Brown

Official Number	1202 (operational number 17-03)
On station	2 October 1996–
Dimensions	17m x 5.5m x 3.3m
Type	Severn, fibre reinfocred composite hull
Engines	Twin 1,050hp Caterpillar 3412TA diesels
Weight	41 tonnes
Built	1995, hull by Green Marine,Lymington; fitted out by Berthon Boat Co., Lymington
Donor	Bequest of Victoria Maisie Brown, London, in memory of her husband
Cost	£1,563,238

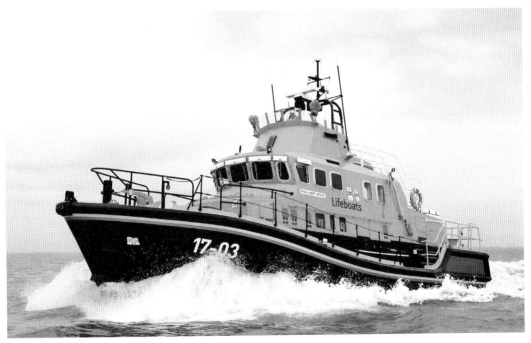

17m Severn Albert Brown, Harwich lifeboat since 1996. (Nicholas Leach)

Braybrooke Lifeboat [Essex Association lifeboat, record probably incomplete]

1822	May	Assisted to refloat vessel
1823	Jan 15	HM cutter *Surly*, assisted vessel
1824	Nov 3	Brig *Northumberland*, of Sunderland, landed crew from *Caledonia*, of Sunderland

Springwell Lifeboat [first RNLI lifeboat]

1876	Dec 12	Schooner *Exhibition*, of Colchester, rendered assistance
	29	Brigantine *Willie*, of Llanelly, assisted to save vessel
1877	Dec 2	Barque *Jacob Langstrum*, of Gothenburg, saved 8
1879	Feb 16	Barque *Pasithea*, of Liverpool, saved (including 10 smacksmen) 23
	17	Barque *Pasithea*, of Liverpool (second service), stood by and saved 1
1881	Jan 6	Spanish schooner *Rosita*, saved 8
		Spanish schooner *Rosita* (second service), saved 3
	20-1	Steamship *Ingrid*, of Rotterdam, saved 7
	Oct 23	Barque Iris, of *Gefle*, saved (and afterwards assisted to save vessel) 12

Springwell (second) Lifeboat

1882	Apr 25	Schooner *Henrietta*, of London, saved 4
1883	Feb 7	Barque *Lorely*, of Memel, saved 11
1884	Jan 24	Barge *Jessie*, of Rochester, saved abandoned barge
	Oct 11	Three-masted schooner *Moreford and Trubey*, of Aberdeen, saved 2
1886	Dec 4	Ship *Constanze*, of Hamburg, assisted to save vessel
1888	Mar 14	Brig *William and Anthony*, of Folkestone, saved vessel and 8
	Nov 9	Brig *Carl Gustaf*, of Christiania, saved 9
1890	Mar 2	Schooner *Mary and Maria*, of Hull, assisted to save vessel and 3

Reserve No.3 Lifeboat

| | | See details of five services in the steam lifeboat listing |

Springwell (second) Lifeboat

1892	June 5	Barque *Ephrussi*, of Brevik, stood by vessel
1893	Jan 17	Steamship *Helsingfor*, of Elsinore, landed 18 from Long Sand LV
	Nov 4	Steamship *Rockliff*, of West Hartlepool, rendered assistance
	10	Barque *St Olof*, of Mariehamn, saved 12
1894	Feb 19	Barque *Ebor*, of Liverpool, assisted to save vessel and 13
1897	Jan 23	Schooner *Sancho Panza*, of Faversham, saved 6
		Boat of Smack, saved 5
1898	Oct 17	Barque *Inga*, of Laurvig, stood by
1899	Nov 2	Barquentine *Pactolus*, of London, saved 5

Ann Fawcett Lifeboat

1911	April 5	Brigantine *Lenore*, of Faversham, saved vessel and 6
	June 25	Schooner *L'Espoir de l'Avenir*, of Rotterdam, assisted to save vessel and 6
1912	Jan 6	Barge *Monarch*, of London, assisted to save vessel and 3

Duke of Northumberland Lifeboat

1890	Oct 8	Brigantine *Ada*, of Faversham, stood by
	20	Steamship *Achilles*, of Sunderland, assisted to save vessel and 21
	Nov 13	Three-masted schooner *Christine Elizabeth*, of Haugesund, assisted to save vessel and 21
1891	Jan 6	Ketch *Day's*, of Barrow, saved 2
		Ketch *Day's*, of Barrow, (second launch), landed a body
	Mar 3	Three-masted schooner *Mercury*, of Aberdeen, saved 12

City of Glasgow Lifeboat

1895	June 6	Schooner *Hans*, of Rendsburg, saved vessel and 4
1897	Oct 25	Barque *Triton*, of Rostock, assisted to save vessel
1898	Mar 26	Steamship *Pampa*, of Hamburg, assisted to save vessel
1899	Jan 30	Long Sand lightvessel, landed 2 mechanics
	Dec 7	Steamship *Lambeth*, of London, landed 8, also a dog, and boat, from Sunk Light-vessel
1901	Mar 30	Schooner *Rose*, of Ipswich, saved 4

City of Glasgow (second) Lifeboat

1901	May 17	Schooner *Harriet*, of Goole, stood by
1904	Nov 23	Steamship *Tyne*, of Newcastle, assisted to save vessel
1905	Jan 21	Schooner *Dashing Wave*, of Fowey, assisted to save vessel
	Nov 23	Brigantine *Thirza*, of Faversham, assisted to save vessel and 7
		Steam tug *Spray*, of Harwich, gave help
1906	Dec 25	Barque *Earlshall*, of Dundee, stood by
1908	April 7	Schooner *Notre Dame de Toutes Aides*, of Nantes, saved 9
	Sep 9	Schooner barge *San Pedro*, of Rio de Janeiro, saved barge and 5
1909	May 14	Smack *Tripper*, of Harwich, stood by
1910	Aug 19	Barque *Fox*, of Arundel, stood by
	Oct 27-8	Steamship *Baltzar von Platen*, of Hamburg, gave help
	Dec 16	Barge *Baltic*, of London, stood by
1911	April 5	Brigantine *Volant*, of Hull, assisted to save vessel and 6
	Oct 30	Barge *Antje*, of London, saved (also a dog) 3
1912	Dec 30	Barge *Agnes and Constance*, of Rochester, saved barge and 3
1913	Aug 21	Schooner *Christabel*, of Whitstable, assisted to save vessel
	Oct 25	Pilot cutter *Will o' the Wisp*, of London, saved cutter and 9
1914	Mar 18	Ketch *Malvoisin*, of London, assisted to save vessel and 2
1915	Jan 1-2	Steamship *Obidense*, of Bergen, landed 25 and saved 2
	Sep 22	Steamship *Koningin Emma*, of Amsterdam, saved 20
1916	Jan 7-8	Steamship *Zeeland*, of Rotterdam, stood by and assisted to save vessel

Margaret Graham Lifeboat

1967	Oct 17	Motor tanker *Astrid Elizabeth*, of Bergen, stood by
	Dec 16	Kentish Knock lightvessel, landed a sick man
1968	Feb 20	Motor gas tanker *Arguimedes*, of Panama, took doctor to injured man
	June 4	Motor vessel *Hermar*, of Haven Ems, gave help
	Aug 10	Yacht *Platapus*, escorted yacht
	22	Yacht *Sandora*, of London, landed 6 and saved yacht
	Sep 15	Yacht *Skipjack*, saved yacht
	28	Barge *Spithead*, of London, landed an injured man
	Oct 24	Motor vessel *Flity*, of London, took doctor to injured man
	Dec 5	Motor vessel *Viking III*, of Oslo, took out doctor and landed 3
1969	Jan 17	Motor vessel *Doni*, of Groningen, in tow of tug *Sauria*, of London, stood by and escorted vessels
	Feb 3	Catamaran, saved catamaran and 2
	May 19	Motor tanker *Siluna*, of Oslo, stood by

44-001 Relief Lifeboat

	July 1	Trimaran *Three Wishes*, gave help and landed 3 (including a sick child)

Margaret Graham Lifeboat

	Sep 28	Yacht *Jacranda*, saved yacht and 2
1970	May 3	Motor boat *Dangerous*, gave help
	June 25	Motor vessel *Nereide*, of Monrovia, landed a sick man
	27	Yacht *Viola*, saved yacht and 3
		Yacht, saved yacht and 2
		Harwich Inshore Rescue Boat, gave help
	July 14	Yacht *Patsy Ann*, in tow of motor vessel *Pass of Melfort*, of London, gave help
	19	Motor yacht *Sea Spray*, gave help
	31	Trawler *Evald Tammlaan*, of Tallinn, landed a sick man
	Aug 4	Yacht *Bombardier*, landed a woman and a sick child
	26	Motor vessel *City of Winchester*, of London, landed an injured man

44-001 Relief Lifeboat

	Nov 15	Cabin cruiser *Qualo*, gave help
	18	Man on drilling pontoon, gave help

Margaret Graham Lifeboat

1971	Jan 1	Motor vessel *Thuroklint*, of Thurso, recovered a life raft
	10	Dinghies *Red Elf*, *Three Nuns*, *Jacqueline* and HH.88, gave help
	Apr 7	Motor vessel *Barford*, of London, landed an injured man, saving 1
	21	Drilling rig, saved 4

	June 2	Rowing boat, saved boat
	7	Sailing dinghy, escorted dinghy
	17	Catamaran, gave help
	Aug 27	Motor cruiser *Lady N*, gave help
	28	Yacht *Fanfare*, saved yacht and 4
	Sep 14	Fishing boat *Joan L*, gave help
	26	Tanker *Thuntank 6*, of Newcastle, took out doctor
	29	Tanker *Viva*, of Arendal, landed a sick man, saving 1
	Oct 29	Cabin cruiser *Tiger* of Chichester, gave help
	Nov 12	Cabin cruiser, gave help
	21	Cabin cruiser *Andy Ross*, saved boat & 5
		Two motor cruisers, gave help

44-001 Relief Lifeboat

	Dec 11	Motor boat *Leo*, in tow of fishing vessel *Midas*, gave help
1972	Feb 17	Two crashed aircraft, landed a pilot

Margaret Graham Lifeboat

	Mar 11	Motor vessel *Taiping*, of London, gave help regarding injured man
		Motor vessel *Tod Head*, took out doctor and landed injured man
	July 15	Yacht *Jenny Lyn*, gave help
	21	Motor vessel *Kathe-Marie*, of Hamburg, took out doctor and landed injured man
	Sep 14	Motor vessel *Inga*, of Helsingborg, landed 4
	22	Motor vessel *Rhon*, of Rostock, landed a sick man
	Oct 6	Cabin cruiser *Chadorlee*, saved cruiser and 2
	Nov 9	Fishing boat *Lodestar*, saved boat and 2
	19	Motor tug *Kinghow*, of Preston, stood by
	Dec 16	Galloper lightvessel, landed a sick man
		Fishing boat, saved boat and 2
1973	Jan 23	Motor boat, gave help and landed 6
	Apr 27	Tanker *British Fulmar*, of London, landed a sick man
	June 3	Fishing boat *Kingfisher* (IH 94), of Ipswich, saved boat and 4
	9	Dredger *Pen Stour*, of Southampton, landed an injured man, saving 1
	11	Sick man aboard Russian tanker *Lyubertsuszr*, landed sick man, saving 1
	July 18	Oil tender *Nordic Service*, landed 10
	19	Dredger *Norstone*, landed an injured man
	Aug 14	Motor vessel *Finn Seal*, of Krotka, landed a sick man, saving 1
	Sep 12	Fishery research vessel *Clione*, of Lowestoft, landed a sick man, saving 1
	28	Fishing boat *Wavecrest* (HH 88), saved boat and 1
		Yacht *Boxer*, of Burnham, saved yacht and 2
	Nov 5	Yacht *Avena*, gave help
	16	Outboard dinghy, gave help
1974	June 8	Motor vessel *Olympic Alliance*, of Monrovia, landed an injured man

44-001 Relief Lifeboat

July 28	Yacht *Janetta*, saved yacht and landed 3
Aug 4	Yacht *Gillian*, saved yacht and 3
10	Yacht *Irene*, landed 9
	Yacht *Irene*, landed 4 and saved boat
24	Yacht *Estella*, saved boat and 3
Sep 1	Yacht *Banjo*, saved boat and 5
	Motor launch *Teal*, gave help
4	Customs launch *Orwell Hunter*, saved boat and 3
15	Motor vessel *Geestrom* in collision with sloop *Naseby*, recovered wreckage
Dec 12	Angling boat, saved boat and 2

Margaret Graham Lifeboat

1975	Feb 24	Sick man on board Liberian motor vessel *Cape Sea*, landed a sick man
	June 22	Injured man on board Swedish cargo vessel *Victoria*, landed an injured man
	28	Sunk lightvessel, landed an injured man
	July 8	Spanish cargo vessel *Rio Limay*, landed a sick man
	Aug 1	Two canoes, saved canoes and 5
		Yacht *Evening Star*, saved yacht and 2
	15	Yacht *Ortu*, gave help
	Sep 8	Yacht *Eipararon*, gave help
		Cabin cruiser *Gloriette*, saved boat and 5
		Yacht *Bella Pais*, gave help
	9	Yacht *Tuskar*, saved yacht and 2
	14	Yacht *Tiamo*, gave help
	18	Yacht *Eriskay*, saved yacht and 2
	Oct 24	Dinghy *Torus*, landed 2
	Nov 15	Tender to motor vessel *Coral*, of Cyprus, saved 4

44-001 Relief Lifeboat

Nov 30	Dinghy, landed 2
	Fishing boat *Roker*, gave help
Dec 1	Small boat, recovered wreckage
	Tanker *Astroman*, landed a body

Margaret Graham Lifeboat

1976	Apr 23	Motor vessel *Manta*, of Liverpool, escorted
	May 4	Motor vessel *Lagarfoss*, of Rekjavik, landed a sick woman
	Aug 18	Dredger, landed a body
	Oct 24	Trawler *Le Boulonnais*, of France, landed an injured man
	Nov 9	Survivors of cargo vessel *Judert II*, on board Russian trawler *Omulew*, of Czezin, stood by
	16	Fishing boat *Kingfisher Too*, stood by
1977	Feb 13	Motor vessel *Tatrina*, took out doctor for a sick man
	May 4	Motor vessel *El Gezira*, of Port Sudan, landed a sick man, saving 1
	June 25	Yacht *Miura*, gave help
	July 9	Cutter *L'Atlanta*, saved yacht and 6
	Sep 17	Yacht *Wet Dream*, of The Netherlands, saved 2

44-001 Relief Lifeboat

Nov 2	Motor vessel *Frederick Hughes*, of London, escorted
30	Motor fishing vessel *Lindfar*, escorted

1978	Jan 8	Motor boats, gave help

Margaret Graham Lifeboat

	Feb 1	Motor vessel *El Barat*, of Liberia, landed a sick man
	17	Gas tanker *Methane Princess*, of London, took out doctor and landed sick man
	Mar 11	Boys cut off by tide, saved 2
	29	Motor cable layer *Iris*, took out doctor and landed an injured man
	May 3	Motor vessel *Tania*, of Havana, took out doctor and landed an injured man
	June 8	Tanker *Al Badiah*, landed a body
	July 23	Norwegian motor vessel *Viking III*, of Oslo, took out doctor and landed an injured man
	Aug 5	Yacht *Wistikal*, gave help
	21	Dredger *Bowknight*, of London, took doctor to 3 injured men
	Sep 9	Tanker *Matco Thames*, took out doctor and landed a sick man
	24	Motor vessel *Nadina*, of Seattle, took out doctor and to an injured man
	Nov 22	Sunk lightvessel, took out doctor and landed a sick man
	25	Motor vessel *Bravo Aries*, of London, landed a sick man
	Dec 6	Vehicle carrier *Cobres*, took out doctor and landed a sick man
	18	Tanker *Helmsman*, of London, took out doctor and landed a sick man
	29	Cabin cruiser *Swinge*, gave help
1979	Jan 19	Radio ship *Mi Amigo* of Panama, landed 5
	29	Fishing boat Angelina, saved 2
	Feb 22	Sick man on board cargo vessel *Baltic Enterprise*, of London, took out doctor and landed a sick man thereby saving 1
		Injured man on board cargo vessel *Dettifoss*, of Iceland, landed injured man
	Mar 10	Injured man on board pilot boat *Pathfinder*, of London, took out doctor
	May 5	Cargo vessel *Isle del Atlantico*, of Spain, stood by vessel
	26	Cargo vessel *Queenford*, of Rye, landed 1
	July 21	Injured man on board cargo vessel *Neugraben*, took out doctor
	Aug 9	Yacht *Vitacha*, gave help
	13	Yacht *Quiet Moment*, gave help
	Sep 14	Cabin cruiser *Butembu*, gave help
	Nov 3	Fishing boat, gave help
1980	Jan 25	Cargo vessel *Arlington*, stood by vessel

John Fison Lifeboat

	June 28	Sick man on board tanker *British Poplar*, of London, took out doctor, landed a sick man
	July 12	Yacht *Lady of Longcombe*, gave help
	18	Yacht *Snow Goose*, saved boat and 3
	Aug 29	Yacht *Champion*, of The Netherlands, saved boat and 5
	Nov 28	Cargo vessel *Moon Trader*, of West Germany, escorted vessel
1981	May 25	Catamaran *Artac*, saved boat and 6
	June 18	Sick man on board minesweeper HMS *Stubbington*, took out doctor
	24	Motor cruiser *Comet IV*, gave help

	Dec 2	Cargo vessel *Rolsion*, escorted vessel
1982	Mar 25	Injured man on board tanker *Matco Avon*, landed an injured man
	May 31	Yacht *Chimp*, gave help
	Sep 27	Yacht *Etiquette*, stood by boat
	Dec 7	Yacht *Monsun*, saved boat and 3
	19	Passenger/cargo ferry *European Gateway*, of London, landed 3 bodies, gave help
1983	June 30	Yacht *Tudor Rose*, gave help
	July 5	Yacht, gave help
	Nov 18	Injured man on board passenger/cargo vessel *Prinz Hamlet*, of West Germany, landed an injured man
	Dec 13	United States Air Force safety boat, stood by
1984	Jan 3	Cargo vessel *Gladonia*, of Goole, stood by
	Mar 22	Sick man on board motor vessel *Orion III*, landed a body
	May 9	Yacht *Yassou*, landed 4, recovered life raft
	23	Injured man on board trawler *Tom Grant*, of Kuwait, landed an injured man
	31	Yacht, of Belgium, landed 1
	June 1	Sick man on board tanker *Swan Lake*, of Piraeus, landed a sick man
	3	Yacht, of Belgium, saved boat and 6
	8	Schooner *Stina*, gave help
	July 11	Injured man on board motor vessel *Finn Merchant*, landed an injured man
	Nov 15	Dinghy, gave help
	Dec 28	Motor boat, saved boat
1985	Jan 6	Sealink ro-ro cargo vessel *Speedlink Vanguard*, of London, escorted vessel

44-001 Relief Lifeboat

	July 19	Yacht *Anne Chien*, of Holland, saved boat and 4
	28	Yacht *Marna Jane*, gave help
	Aug 7	Yacht *Sabre*, gave help
	Sep 18	Cabin cruiser ex-lifeboat *Moby Dick*, gave help

John Fison Lifeboat

	Nov 19	Motor vessel *Amina*, of Casablanca, escorted
1986	Apr 5	Sick man on board passenger ferry *Dana Anglia*, of Denmark, landed a sick man
	May 21	Cabin cruiser *Lenten Rose*, of Portsmouth, saved boat and 4
	July 5	Cabin cruiser *Old Bunbury*, escorted boat
		Yacht Nomad, stood by boat
	July 22	Injured child on board passenger/cargo ferry *Tor Brittania*, of Denmark, landed injured child
	Aug 30	Cabin cruiser *Frepau*, of York, escorted
	Sep 3	Yacht *Glen Mist II*, saved boat and 4
	9	Sick man on board dredger/sand carrier *Arco Tyne*, of Southampton took out doctor and landed a sick man thereby saving a life
	Oct 13	Two injured men on board container ship *Dorothee*, of West Germany, took out doctor and landed 2 injured man
	18	Yacht *Cavalier of Kent*, gave help
	28	Fishing vessel *La Vestale*, of Lowestoft, saved boat
1987	Jan 21	Injured man on board container vessel *Adabelle Lykes*, of USA, gave help

Khami Relief Lifeboat

	May 21	Cabin cruiser *Retreat*, saved boat and 2
	June 8	Yacht *Gandeo*, craft brought in– gave help
	14	Trawler *Mary La*, gave help
	July 18	Yacht *Horizon*, craft brought in– gave help

John Fison Lifeboat

	July 31	Yacht *Jusim VIII*, saved yacht and gave help
	Sep 6	Yacht *Magic Dragon*, saved yacht and 2
	12	Catamaran *Elizabeth*, saved craft and 4 (and a dog)
	Oct 16	Chemical tanker *Silver Falcon*, stood by
	Nov 2	Israeli container vessel *Vered*, landed 1
1988	Jan 27	Belgian minesweeper *Van Haverbeke*, took out doctor
	Mar 24	Passenger ship *Nordic Ferry*, of London, stood by
	Apr 6	Yacht *Lotus*, of Netherlands, craft brought in– gave help
		Yacht *Homespun*, saved boat and 3
	May 29	Yacht *B Natural*, craft brought in
	Aug 7	Fishing boat *Nellie*, brought in– gave help
	12	Yacht *Tuesday Girl*, saved yacht and 3
	19	Yacht *Copine*, of Netherlands, escorted
	Sep 18	Injured man on Roughs Tower Lighthouse, took out doctor
	Oct 17	Barge *Real*, saved craft and 2
	20	Cabin cruiser *Maikos 2*, craft brought in– gave help
	Nov 14	Sick man on board cargo vessel *Shamrock Endeavour*, landed a sick man
1989	Jan 26	Passenger ferry *Hamburg*, of Bahamas, landed a sick person
	30	Cargo vessel *Inci V*, landed a sick person

Khami Relief Lifeboat

	Apr 28	Yacht *Charisma C*, gave help

John Fison Lifeboat

	May 10	Gas tanker *Lissy Shulte*, gave help
	June 17	Motor vessel *Nordvik*, landed a sick girl
	27	Passenger ferry *Tor Britannia*, of Denmark, landed a sick person
	July 1	Catamaran *Pavona*, craft brought in– gave help
	16	Fishing vessel *Boy Tom*, landed a sick person
	17	Yacht *Westwind of Stour*, stood by and landed 11
	Aug 28	Injured man on board yacht *Tookie*, took out doctor
		Yacht *Tookie*, gave help
	Oct 8	Yacht *Shwaiy-Shwaiy*, gave help
	10	Passenger ferry *St Nicholas*, of Bahamas, landed a sick person
	20	Yacht *Jack Galloper*, saved boat and 3
	Nov 8	Injured man on board cargo vessel *Niels*, took out doctor
1990	Feb 22	Fishing boat *Amy M*, landed body and recovered wreckage
	Mar 18	Speedboat *Sum Speed*, gave help
	27	Dredger/sand carrier *Arco Axe*, landed a sick person

Khami Relief Lifeboat

	May 1	Fishing boat *Seeker*, brought in– gave help

John Fison Lifeboat

July	12	Ketch *Marana F*, gave help
	14	Yacht *Smooth Torquer*, gave help & landed 4
	20	Dredger *Redcliffe Sand*, landed injured person
Aug	17	Dredger *Cambrae*, gave help
Sep	1	Yacht *Ajaia*, craft brought in– gave help
	7	Yacht *Sujuva II*, gave help
Oct	6	Yacht *Morning Glory*, craft brought in– gave help
Nov	22	Yacht *Kahamsin*, gave help and escorted
Dec	14	Naval tanker *Sealift Pacific*, of United States, landed a sick person
	28	Cargo vessel *Mill Supplier*, gave help
1991	Jan 7	Ship *Foka Gas I*, stood by
	June 12	Cabin cruiser *Sanchia*, craft brought in– gave help
	15	Yacht *Patpocius*, of Walton, saved boat and 2

Khami Relief Lifeboat

July	1	Ship *Cherry Valley*, landed a sick person
Aug	15	Government research vessel *Seaspring*, landed a sick person
	17-8	Trawler *Rival II*, craft brought in– gave help

John Fison Lifeboat

Sep	22	Yacht *Jenever*, craft brought in– gave help
Oct	24	Trawler *Sivia*, craft brought in– gave help
Dec	14	Motor vessel *Eliza Heeren*, took out doctor and landed a sick person
1992	May 16	Motor vessel *DSR Baltic*, stood by
		Motor vessel *Montlhery*, landed an injured person
	28	Survey vessel *Bermuda*, landed injured person
	June 24	Motor ship *Stena Seatrader*, of Netherlands, gave help, assisted by prototype lifeboat ON.1179
	July 15	Tanker *Echoman*, landed a sick person
	Aug 16	Yacht *Bluster*, gave help
	22	Yacht *Eskimo Knell*, craft brought in– gave help
	30	Yacht *Brazillian Legacy*, towed to Gorleston, gave help
	Sep 1	Yacht *Fantasea*, saved 4
	9	Cabin cruiser *Seacat*, gave help
	Dec 18	Pilot boat *Prospect* taking on water, escorted
1993	Feb 7	Dredger *Formalhaut*, landed injured person
	Mar 18	Catamaran *Tikkitak II*, gave help
	Apr 4	Motor fishing vessel *Tom Pepper*, craft brought in– gave help
	15	Cabin cruiser *Katrina*, brought in– gave help
	May 1	Yacht, escorted boat
	24	Dutch yacht *Vaarwel*, brought in– gave help
	31	Yacht *Blush*, saved boat and 8
	June 14	Cabin cruiser *Rising Star of Sunbury*, landed an injured person
	15	Tanker *Northia*, of London, took out doctor and landed a sick person
	22	Yacht *Louern*, craft brought in– gave help
	July 6	Yacht *Capricornus*, brought in– gave help
	14	Yacht *Mary Josephine*, gave help
	Aug 2	Yacht *Pulsate*, saved 2
	5	Cabin cruiser *Lady Linda*, craft brought in– gave help
	12	Ketch *Anju*, craft brought in– gave help
	15	Yacht *Bluster*, landed an injured person

Sep	3	Tanker *Star Bergen*, took out doctor and landed a sick person
	4	Passenger/roro cargo ship *Hamburg*, took out a doctor
	12	Yacht *Moonpenny*, stood by
	17	Yacht *Zuiderkruis*, craft brought in– gave help
	18	Catamaran *Soggy Moggy*, landed 2
Oct	15	Bulk carrier *Sir Charles Parsons*, took out doctor and landed an injured man
	22	Yacht *Petra*, saved boat and 2
Nov	14	Cargo vessel *Teano*, in tow of rig support vessel *Granite*, escorted vessels
Dec	18	Cabin cruiser *Sealand 2*, saved boat and 2

Khami Relief Lifeboat

1994	Feb 12	Yacht *Camarada*, saved boat

John Fison Lifeboat

May	28	Sick man onboard Russian bulk carrier *Kapionos Stulpinas*, landed a sick man
	29	Sick woman onboard passenger\roro cargo ferry *Stena Europe*, took out doctor
June	13	Yacht *Get Kracking*, two persons and craft brought in
July	2	Two injured men onboard sailing barge *Gladys*, landed one injured man
	3	Cabin cruiser *Mary Rose*, saved boat & 4
		Yacht *Ale Dancer*, four persons and craft brought in
	11	Fishing vessel *Boy Andrew*, assisted to save vessel and 1
	17	Yacht *Kantele*, saved boat and 3
Aug	10	Yacht *Maruna*, eight persons brought in
Sep	15	Yacht *Narnia*, landed 4 & craft brought in
	24	Yacht *Skean Dhu*, two persons and craft brought in
	30	Sick woman on board ferry *Princess of Scandinavia*, landed a sick woman
1995	Jan 6	Motor boat *Leviathan*, one person and craft brought in, saved by another lifeboat

Khami Relief Lifeboat

Mar	23	Yacht *Pamela Ann*, three persons and craft brought in

John Fison Lifeboat

May	30	Yacht *Iris*, gave help
July	10	Yacht *Red Wing*, saved boat and 2
Aug	20	Yacht *Whipper Snapper*, three persons and craft brought in
	27	Yacht *Evita*, landed 4 and craft brought in
Sep	1	Harwich ILB B-571, gave help
Oct	8	Yacht *Bosun*, landed 2 and craft brought in
	30	Yacht *Lulotte*, two persons and craft brought in

Albert Brown Lifeboat [on trials]

Dec	29	Barge *Sirius*, escorted boat

John Fison Lifeboat

1996	Feb 7	Ro-ro cargo vessel *Roseanne*, stood by
	Mar 6	Fishing vessel *Thomasam*, four persons and craft brought in
	May 4	Yacht *Ruskina*, two persons and craft brought in

	22	Yacht *Challenge*, six persons and craft brought in
June 8		Yacht *Shamu*, landed 4 & craft brought in
	15	Cabin cruiser *Aegir*, landed 3 and craft brought in
	29	Yacht *Off Licence*, six persons and craft brought in
July 28		Motor cruiser *Malachite*, two persons and craft brought in
Aug 5		Passenger/ro-ro/cargo ferry *Koningin Beatrix*, stood by craft
	7	Yacht *Mad Carew*, five persons and craft brought in
	23	Yacht *Gwen II*, saved craft and 2
	26	Yacht *Eye of the Wave*, escorted craft
		Yacht *Polly Anna*, five persons brought in – saved by another lifeboat
		Helicopter winchman, one person brought in – saved by another lifeboat
	29	Injured man onboard cargo vessel *Panama Senator*, took out doctor
Sep 14		Yacht *Peer den Schuymer*, three persons and craft brought in

Albert Brown Lifeboat

	Nov 6	Yacht *E. F. Language*, escorted craft
	12	Cargo vessel *Union Venus*, stood by
1997	Jan 19	Cabin cruiser *Deben Cork*, landed 3 and craft brought in
	Apr 2	Injured man on board tanker *Celtic Terrier*, injured man brought in
	21	Injured man on board tanker *Windsor*, injured man brought in
	28	Yacht *Verge*, gave help
	30	Fishing vessel *Tide Cheater*, one person and craft brought in
	May 10	Yacht *Sasparilla*, two people and craft brought in – saved by another lifeboat
	June 29	Cabin cruiser *Lady Floss*, gave help
	July 14	Injured woman on board passenger vessel *Aegean I*, injured woman brought in
	27	Yacht *Queen Mini*, landed 5 and saved craft
	Aug 2	Yacht *Blue Sapphire*, three people and craft brought in
	18	Fishing vessel *Yvonne Anne*, four people and craft brought in
	23	Yacht *Explorer*, saved craft and 5
	24	Injured man on board barge carrier *Condock V*, injured man brought in
	30	Cabin cruiser *Bagheera*, landed 2 and craft brought in
1998	May 12	Injured woman on board passenger/ro-ro cargo ferry *Dana Anglia*, injured woman brought in
	13	Sick man on board fishing vessel *Marleen*, escorted craft
	28	Injured man on board fishing vessel *Wilmar*, injured man brought in

Duke of Atholl Relief Lifeboat

| | June 9 | Yacht *Ficato*, landed 2 and craft brought in |

Albert Brown Lifeboat

| | July 13 | Cabin cruiser *Bertie*, two people and craft brought in |

	17	Yacht *Scott* in tow of pilot vessel Progress, escorted craft
	18	Yacht *Francipam*, escorted craft
Aug 1		Cabin cruiser *Bounty*, five people and craft brought in
	20	Yacht *Louise*, escorted craft
	23	Yacht *Victoria*, saved craft and 2
	26	Yacht *Pilgrim*, saved 2
	27	Yacht *Zeehond*, three people and craft brought in
	Oct 3	Yacht *Sea Shanty*, saved craft and 1
1999	Apr 12	Yacht *Proud Maeve*, craft brought in
	June 6	Sick man on board tanker *Dali*, landed a sick man
	12	Yacht *Indigo*, stood by
	17	Sick man on board floating trawler museum *Hatherleigh*, took out doctor
	28	Yacht *Silver Lining*, landed 4 and craft brought in
	July 17	Man overboard from cabin cruiser *Purdy*, saved craft and 1
	Aug 13	Yacht *Widgeon*, three and craft brought in
	29	Sick woman on board passenger ship *Maasdam*, one person brought in
	Sep 5	Yacht *The Bear*, landed 2 & craft brought in
	Oct 17	Yacht *Black Rose*, stood by
	26	Sick man on board merchant vessel *Rodona*, landed 1

Fraser Flyer Relief Lifeboat

2000	Jan 9	Powerboat *Boy Darren*, landed craft and 3
	Mar 19	Yacht *Take Two*, landed craft and 4
	21	Angling craft *Melanchory*, escorted craft
	22	Angling craft *Short Straw*, landed craft and 2
		Yacht *Polytropos*, escorted craft
	May 28	Yacht *Rose Bank*, stood by

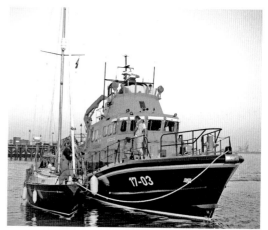

Albert Brown bringing in the 30ft yacht Chevin Star on 2 July 2009. The yacht, with three persons onboard, was adrift eight miles east of Harwich and had become entangled with fishing gear around her propeller and rudder. She was taken in tow back to the lifeboat pontoons. (By courtesy of Harwich RNLI)

Albert Brown Lifeboat

	July 20	Trawler *Goede Hoop*, assisted to save craft
	Sep 6	Yacht *I Like It*, saved craft and 2
	Nov 5	Missing person, landed 1
	Dec 1	Sick man on board merchant vessel *Lykes Liberator*, landed a sick person
2001	May 27	Yacht *Brown Eyes*, landed craft and 4

Volunteer Spirit Relief Lifeboat

	Jun 30	Sail catamaran, gave help
	July 2	Yacht *Siga-Siga*, landed craft and 4
	10	Cabin cruiser *Snodgrass*, saved craft and 2
	15	Yacht *Denaria*, escorted craft
	24	Cabin cruiser *Mitzatori*, landed craft & 1
	31	Yacht *Venturer*, landed craft and 4
	31	Yacht *Ada Rose*, gave help
	Aug 1	Yacht *Chardenae*, landed craft and 2
	12	Yacht *Baleen*, landed craft and 4
	14	Cabin cruiser *Moonstone*, landed craft & 1
	Sep 23	Yacht *Nancy Blackett*, landed craft and 3

A. J. R. and L. G. Uridge Relief Lifeboat

2002	Feb 21	Dredger *Arco Bourne*, escorted craft

Albert Brown Lifeboat

	May 8	Fire on Felixstowe pier, gave help
	June 7	Human body to be brought ashore from fishing vessel *Cirolana*, landed a body
	23	Sick man on board yacht *Seawind II*, four people brought in
	30	Yacht *Seawolf*, landed craft and 6
	30	Yacht *Miracle*, landed craft and 3
	July 8	Fishing vessel *Flamingo*, landed two bodies
	17	Three yachts, craft brought in
	31	Yacht *Emma*, gave help
	Aug 10	Angling vessel *Ocean Obsession*, three people and craft brought in – handed over tow to another vessel
	16	Sick man on board cruise liner *Minerva*, landed sick man
	26	Yacht *Seawork*, landed craft and 2
	Sep 10	Yacht *Little World*, gave help
	Oct 20	Yacht *Smebre*, landed craft and 2
	31	Yacht *Gold Dust*, escorted craft
2003	Jan 30	Pilot launch *Haven Heron*, landed craft and 3

The Will Relief Lifeboat

	Mar 20	Rowing boat, gave help
	21	Yacht *Happy Wanderer*, landed craft and 3

Albert Brown Lifeboat

	Apr 14	Fishing vessel *Yvonne Anne*, landed 1 and craft brought in
	May 8	Motor boat *Arcadia*, landed craft and 3
	June 3	Sailing dinghy, craft brought in
	5	Yacht *Helena*, landed craft and 3
	July 12	Injured man on board merchant vessel *Strilbas*, landed injured man

The Will Relief Lifeboat

	Aug 7	Yacht, landed craft and 4
	9	Fishing vessel *Hiva OA*, landed craft and 1
	14	Yacht *Wench*, landed 3 people
	24	Yacht *Carpe Diem*, escorted craft
	Dec 20	Yacht *Kalidos*, landed craft and 3

2004	Mar 24	Tanker *Apollo*, landed 1 person
	29	Yacht *Stern*, landed craft and 5

Albert Brown Lifeboat

	Apr 25	Power boat *Aqua Juliet*, gave help – transferred first aider
	June 4	Power boat *Antares*, landed craft and 4
	7	Merchant vessel *Nedlloyd Damieta*, landed 1
	18	Yacht *Rhynhor*, landed craft and 2
	July 25	Fishing vessel *Boy Andrew*, saved 3
	26	Yacht *Entropy*, landed craft and 2
		Yacht *Brulo*, landed craft and 6
	Aug 30	Yacht *Coquine*, landed craft and 1
	Sep 9	Sail training vessel *Lord Nelson*, landed 1

Osier Relief Lifeboat

	Sep 17	Yacht *Vita Breves*, of the Netherlands, landed craft and 3

Albert Brown Lifeboat

2005	Apr 30	Power boat, escorted craft
	30	Yacht *Luskentyre*, landed craft and 4
	May 4	Yacht *Cross Over*, landed craft and 4
	4	Yacht *Mar Ia Lecerne*, landed craft and 2
	June 21	Yacht *Siesta*, landed 2

Duke of Kent Relief Lifeboat

	July 18	Yacht *Sweet Promise*, landed craft and 1
	28	Yacht *Paradox*, landed craft and 3
		Yacht *Catchwind*, landed craft and 2
	29	Yacht *Orton Lady*, landed craft and 4
	Aug 1	Yacht *White Horses*, landed craft and 4
		Conveyed injured man from merchant vessel *Contship Tamarind*, landed 1
	6	Conveyed injured person from cruise liner *Thomson Celebration*, landed 1
	13	Yacht *Adrian Dream*, landed craft and 2
		Yacht *Eclipse*, landed craft and 2
	24	Power boat, escorted craft
	29	Yacht *Boogie*, landed craft and 4

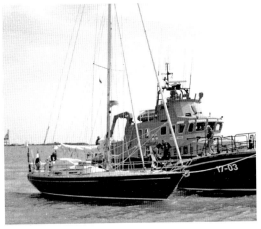

Albert Brown assisting the Dutch yacht Kobbe on 9 August 2009 which, with two persons on board, suffered engine failure forty-six miles east of Harwich. (Andrew Moors)

	Sep 11	House boat, gave help – assisted to contain fire
	11	Power boat *Lydia B*, landed craft and 3
	Oct 1	Yacht *Kangei*, landed craft and 1
	10	Sick person on board power boat *Regardless*, stood by

Albert Brown Lifeboat

	Dec 16	Dinghy, recovered craft
2006	Apr 2	Yacht *Panther*, landed craft and 7

Duke of Kent Relief Lifeboat

	May 6	Angling vessel *Dunflyin*, landed craft & 7
	18	Yacht *Kent*, landed craft and 2
	28	Yacht *Simba*, landed craft and 4
	29	Yacht *Al Cardondas*, landed craft and 4
	Jun 2	Yacht *Redfes*, landed craft and 2
	23	Injured person on Rough Tower, stood by Yacht *Wiggen 5*, landed craft and 1
	28	Sick man on passenger vessel *Balmoral*, landed 1
	July 13	Yacht *Gisborg*, landed craft and 4
	15	Powered boat *Deborah*, landed 2
	17	Yacht *Exuo*, landed craft and 4
	23	Pilot launch *Haven Hawk*, escorted craft
	Aug 5	Powered boat *Sahara*, landed craft and 4

Albert Brown Lifeboat

	Sep 20	Yacht *Jackolope*, landed craft and 2
	Oct 15	Yacht *Varic*, landed craft and 3
	Oct 15	Yacht *Kingfisher*, landed craft and 6
	Dec 3	Yacht *Gentoo of Antartica*, escorted craft
	Dec 9	Powered boat *Shirley June*, landed craft and 2

Duke of Kent Relief Lifeboat

2007	Mar 9	Tanker *Alfa Britannia*, landed 1

Albert Brown Lifeboat

	Mar 18	Canoes, saved two canoes and 2
	Apr 15	Yacht *Templar*, gave help
	May 7	Powered boat *Toomix*, stood by
	May 10	Yacht *Oh Susanhah*, two people and craft brought in
	16	Dutch Yacht *Daikin*, landed craft and 8
	18	Yacht *Nightwind*, landed craft and 2
	19	Yacht *Louise*, landed craft and 8
	June 3	Yacht *Bare Necessity*, landed craft and 2
	9	Orwell Bridge, landed a body
	14	Yacht *Gentle Jane*, landed craft and 2
	19	Lifeboat from tanker *British Cygnet*, gave help
	20	Pilot boat *Haven Hawk*, saved craft
	26	Yacht *Aegle* landed craft and 2
	July 1	Yacht *Joshua* landed craft and 2
	9	Fishing vessel *Yvonne Anne*, landed craft and 3
	13	Yacht *Gavia*, landed 2
	14	Yacht *Mid Life Crisis*, landed craft and 4

Duke of Kent Relief Lifeboat

	31	Sick man on tanker *Sten Baltic*, landed sick man
	Aug 3	Dutch Yacht *Speer*, saved craft and 4

Albert Brown Lifeboat

	Aug 12	Dive boat, landed craft and 3
	30	Barge *Martina*, landed craft and 3
	Sep 16	Yacht *Morning Star*, landed craft and 3
2008	Feb 5	Container vessel *Cap Rojo*, stood by
	20	Powered boat *Basset*, landed craft and 2
	Mar 04	Injured man on merchant vessel *Dirhami*, landed 1

Fraser Flyer Relief Lifeboat

	May 28	Yacht *Permare*, escorted craft
	Apr 7	Yacht *De Gebruder*, landed craft and 5
	20	Yacht *Sargasso*, stood by

Albert Brown Lifeboat

	May 31	Yacht *Bluebell*, landed craft and 4
	June 20	Powered boat *Wild Goose*, landed craft and 2
	29	Yacht *Lynx*, landed craft and 2
	July 19	Yacht *Cyano*, gave help
	Aug 18	Yacht *Auberge*, landed craft and 1
	31	Powered boat *Hooker*, landed craft and 3
	Oct 15	Yacht *Charisma*, of Germany, gave help- refloated craft
	18	Fishing vessel *Catherine Lucy*, landed craft and 2
	Nov 28	Pilot launch *Prospect*, landed craft and 4
	Dec 21	Yachts *Try Star* and *Robinetta*, stood by

The Will Relief Lifeboat

2009	Jan 3	Belgian trawler *Atlantis*, stood by
	Apr 5	Fishing vessel *Patricia Rose*, landed craft & 2
	May 10	Powered boat *Sallmine*, landed craft and 2
	19	Powered boat *Eminence*, landed craft & 3
	29	Yacht *Miss Behaving*, landed craft and 5
	30	Yacht *Onia*, escorted craft
	31	Yacht *Fennig 3*, landed craft and 5

Albert Brown Lifeboat

	June 27	Yacht *Guapa*, landed craft and 2
	July 2	Yacht *Chevin Star*, landed craft and 3
	11	Polish yacht *Merkury*, landed craft and 9
	17	Yacht *Louise*, landed craft and 1
	23	Dutch yacht *Stroom*, landed craft and 4
	28	Yacht *Gwenili*, landed craft and 4
	Aug 3	Yacht *Kathleen II*, landed 1
	9	Dutch yacht *Kobbe*, landed craft and 2
	25	Yacht *Fiddler*, one person brought in
	28	Yacht *Saorsamhairi*, landed craft and 2
	Sep 1	Yacht *Amazon Countess*, landed craft & 1
	Nov 10	Human body landed a body
	15	Kite surfer, assisted to save a life
	30	Yacht *Beatrice Bee*, landed craft and 2
2010	Feb 20	Human body, gave help – assisted to recover
	Mar 6	Powered boat *Suka*, landed 2 and craft brought in
	7	Powered boat *Horatio*, landed 2 and craft brought in
	11	Yacht *Strata 6*, two people & craft brought in
	Apr 24	Powered boat *Venture*, three people and craft brought in
	May 4	Yacht, two people and craft brought in
	23	Diver support craft *Pacific*, four people and craft brought in

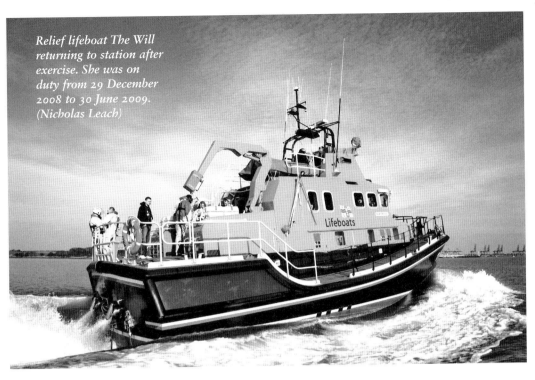

30	Yacht *Black Magic*, four people and craft brought in	2011 Feb 22	Person on Orwell Bridge, landed 1
June 4	Powered boat *Ard Graft*, landed 2 and craft brought in	Mar 19	Fishing vessel *Blue Angel*, two persons and craft brought in
5	Yacht *Baleeka*, landed 2 & craft brought in	May 13	Yacht *Sagarmata*, two persons and craft brought in
July 4	Human body, gave help	20	Yacht *Lodestar*, four persons and craft brought in
26	Yacht *Wizard*, four people & craft brought in	21	Yacht *Halcyon*, stood by
Aug 3	Sick man on catamaran *Pelican*, landed 1 and craft brought in	28	Yacht *Avocet*, two persons and craft brought in
8	Yacht *Wind Harp*, landed 4 and craft saved	June 2	Yacht *Sealord* with injured man on board, one person and yacht brought in
16	Powered boat *Stella Blue*, landed 2 and craft brought in	19	Yacht, gave help
Sep 1	Aircraft, gave help	July 5	Injured man on board Belgian warship, landed an injured man
11	Yacht *Albatross*, landed 2 & craft brought in	10	Trawler *Rasmine*, craft brought in
18	Powered boat *Julies Pride*, four people and craft brought in	12	Sick man on board yacht, landed 1
Oct 4	Yacht *Maggie B*, two people and craft brought in	13	Yacht *Bakaruda 2*, eight persons and craft brought in
9	Yacht *Margovillat*, landed 2 and craft brought in	17	Motor vessel *Scooby Doo 2*, craft brought in
21	Yacht *Teleost*, escorted craft	18	Yacht *Sea Otter*, two persons and craft brought in
22	Sick man on yacht *Aegis*, landed 1	24	Diving boat, three persons and craft brought in
	Yacht *Aegis*, gave help - took over tow from Aldeburgh lifeboat	Aug 2	Angling boat, seven persons and craft brought in
Nov 2	Yacht *Passo Da Onca*, gave help - refloated casualty		
5	Yacht *Anny B*, three people and craft brought in		
28	Men overboard from ferry *Stena Britannica*, landed 2		

No.71 (later D-71) inshore lifeboat

1965	June 18	Dinghy, gave help
	July 29	Yacht, gave help
	Sep 2	Cabin cruiser *Taifung*, gave help & landed 1
	Oct 10	Motor boat *Scimitar*, saved boat
	31	Yacht *Pandora*, gave help
1966	Apr 23	Yacht *Tintana II*, escorted
	May 8	Four small boats, escorted two boats
	28	Motor boat, gave help
	30	Yacht, saved 2
1967	Mar 29	Yacht, landed 2
	31	Body in the water, landed a body
	May 13	Dinghy, gave help
	14	Motor launch *Princess Royal*, landed 2
	21	Sailing dinghy, saved 4
	28	Yacht *Aquiulla*, gave help
	June 14	Dinghy, saved dinghy and 2
	July 12	Pram dinghy, gave help and landed 2
	22	Dinghy *Emma Peel*, saved 2
	Oct 4	Dinghy, saved dinghy
1968	Apr 6	Speedboat, gave help
	June 12	Children cut off by tide, saved 2
	July 2	Rowing dinghy, saved dinghy and 1
		Rubber dinghy, saved dinghy and 1
	11	Yacht *Yeomac*, stood by
	21	Speedboat, gave help
	29	Canoe, saved canoe and 2
	Aug 22	Yacht *Sandora*, gave help
1969	Feb 13	Landed the body of a diver
	Sep 25	Sailing yacht *Mewtra De Sintra*, gave help
	Nov 9	Tender to yacht *Solent Sprite*, saved tender and 2
1970	Apr 13	Rowing boat, saved boat and 1
	Sep 5	Sailing dinghy *Soectrum*, saved dinghy & 2
	Oct 11	Yacht *Star Stream*, stood by
	18	Yacht *Deben Gipsy*, stood by
	Nov 15	Cabin cruiser *Qualo*, gave help
		Motor boat, saved boat and 3
	18	Pontoon drifting, saved 1

D-201 inshore lifeboat

1971	Mar 28	Landed two boys cut off by the tide
	Apr 17	Landed six persons cut off by the tide
	June 29	Three persons cut off by tide, saved 3
	Aug 27	Motor cruiser *Lady IV*, gave help
	28	Yacht *Fanfare*, gave help
	Sep 5	Canoe, saved canoe and 1
	Nov 21	Dinghy, saved dinghy and 2
		Pram dinghy, gave help
1972	Jan 20	Motor boat, saved boat and 2
	May 28	Sailing dinghy, gave help and landed 2
		Sailing dinghy, saved dinghy and ld 1
	29	Sailing dinghy, saved boat and 2
	30	Sailing dinghy, saved 3
		Canoe and dinghy, saved boats and 1
	Aug 15	Bather, saved 1
	24	Yacht *Hyskier III*, landed 2 including an injured girl
	28	Motor cruiser *Marracheen*, stood by
1973	June 23	Persons cut off by tide, saved 2

	Aug 13	Sailing cruiser *Lohara*, gave help
	Nov 12	Fibreglass dinghy, saved 1
	24	Dinghy, gave help

D-206 inshore lifeboat

1974	Jan 10	Persons stranded by the tide, saved 1
	Apr 9	Yacht, saved 1
	25	Customs launch, gave help
	June 21	Yacht, saved yacht and 3
	23	Cabin cruiser *Sea Jane*, landed 2
	Aug 10	Ketch, stood by and saved 9
	12	Sailing dinghy *Bone Dry*, landed 2 and saved dinghy
1975	Aug 23	Dinghy, landed 1
	25	Dinghy, gave help
	Sep 14	Yacht *Sara*, landed 2

D-240 inshore lifeboat

1976	Apr 2	Dinghy, saved dinghy and 2
	18	Dinghy, saved dinghy and 2
	May 16	Cabin cruiser, gave help
	July 1	Helicopter, stood by
	18	Yacht *Tenacity* of Mayland, escorted
	Aug 18	Dredger, took a doctor to an injured man
	Sep 10	Sailing dinghy, saved dinghy and 2
	Oct 22	Person cut off by tide, saved 1
	Nov 24	Dinghy, saved 2
1977	Feb 27	Motor boat *Distant Star* in tow, stood by
	Apr 11	Speedboat, gave help
	June 12	Yacht *Anros*, gave help
	July 17	Sailing dinghy, gave help
	24	Persons cut off by tide, saved 4
	26	Persons stranded in old lighthouse, landed 4
	Aug 23	Yacht *See Gee III*, gave help
	Nov 14	Dinghy, saved 3

D-225 inshore lifeboat

1978	Feb 4	Fishing boat *Gale Haytor*, gave help
	14	Boys cut off by tide, landed 6

B-526 Atlantic 21

	Apr 16	Motor cruiser, gave help
	May 1	Injured man stuck in mud, saved 1
	Aug 8	Sailing dinghy, gave help
	Oct 1	Fishing boat *Puffin*, gave help
	Nov 2	Motor boat, gave help
1979	Apr 23	Cabin cruiser *Rolyat*, gave help
	May 6	Yacht, gave help
	31	Two injured swimmers on lighthouse, landed 2
	Aug 12	Dinghy *Squire*, gave help
	Sep 20	Yacht *Zura*, saved boat and 1
	Nov 7	Dinghy, stood by boat
1980	Mar 8	Catamaran *Sail Craze*, saved boat and 2
	10	Rescue boat, gave help
	May 18	Dinghy, landed 1
	June 12	Woman overboard from ferry *Princes Beatrix*, gave help
	17	Yacht, landed 2
	22	Sailing dinghy, gave help
	Aug 18	Three persons cut off by tide, saved 3

	Aug 26	Man overboard from ferry *Princess Beatrix*, gave help
	29	Yacht *Lara*, saved boat and 4
	30	Two boys cut off by tide, saved 2
	Sep 5	Yacht *Beehive III*, escorted boat
	29	Cabin cruiser *Zelia*, gave help
	Oct 15	Rescue boat, saved boat and 5
	Nov 1	Dinghy, saved 1
1981	Jan 10	Sailboard, saved board and 1
	Apr 17	Yacht *Dunkit*, gave help
	May 3	Sailing dinghy, saved board and 2
	June 5	Yacht *Evening Star*, saved 3
	7	Fishing boat *Lady Owen*, gave help
		Dinghy, gave help
	28	Sailboard, escorted
	July 4	Yacht *Rifardo*, gave help
	Aug 4	Airbed, landed 2
1982	Apr 9	Persons cut off by tide, gave help
	26	Sailing dinghy, saved board and 1
	June 11	Yacht, saved boat and 3
	25	Yacht *Wings*, saved boat and 2
	Aug 13	Rubber dinghy, saved boat and 3
	24	Yacht *Karisma*, landed 2
	29	Yacht, saved boat and 2
		Yacht *Mahopak*, stood by
	Sep 5	Two sailboards, gave help
		Lifeguard's rescue boat, gave help
	8	Sailboard, saved board and 1
	20	Sailboard, gave help
	29	Sailing school safety boat, gave help
	Oct 19	Speedboat, saved boat and 3
1983	Apr 18	Dinghy, saved 1
	May 10	Surfboard, saved board and 1

B-542 *William Yeo*

	29	Speedboat, gave help
	June 5	Cabin cruiser *Calypso*, saved boat and 1
	18	Motor boat *Marjo*, gave help
	20	Cabin cruiser *Amazing Grace*, landed 2

B-526 Atlantic 21

	July 5	Ferry *Brightlingsea*, landed 99
	17	Sailing dinghy, saved boat and 2
	24	Sailboard, gave help
	Aug 1	Yacht *Pecotty*, gave help
	Sep 4	Speedboat, saved boat and 6
	Oct 1	Yacht *Cariad*, gave help
	19	Sailboard, saved board and 1
1984	Mar 2	Motor cruiser *The Carol*, saved 1
	18	Canoe, gave help
	July 24	Sick man on board motor cruiser *Lucky Dip*, landed a sick man
	Aug 31	Sailing dinghy, saved boat and 2
1985	Jan 20	Man overboard from liberty boat, landed a body
	Apr 7	Sailboard, landed 1
	May 26	Sailboard, gave help
		Canoe, gave help
	29	Catamaran *Dogboat*, gave help
	Aug 4	Cabin cruiser *Penang Girl*, gave help
	14	Sloop *Hengor*, gave help
	30	Motor boat, saved 1
	Sep 1	Sailboard, saved board and 1
	Oct 4	Yacht *Manhana*, saved boat and 2
	24	Yacht *Sea Mist*, saved boat and 3

B-513 *William McCunn & Broom Church Youth Fellowship*

	Nov 19	Motor boat *Scorpion*, gave help
	24	Sailboard, saved board and 1
		Motor boat, gave help
1986	Jan 16	Radio station *Communicator*, stood by and saved 2
	Apr 30	Dinghy, gave help
	May 4	Yacht *Harriet*, gave help
	11	Sailing dinghy *Saucy Nancy*, saved boat and 2
	24	Sailing dinghy, saved boat and landed 2

B-526 Atlantic 21

	July 17	Yacht *Miura*, gave help
	20	Cabin cruiser *Medlar*, escorted boat
	23	Sailing dinghy, saved boat and 2
	29	Sailing dinghy, escorted boat
	Aug 2	Yacht *Camarada*, gave help
	3	Yacht *First of June*, gave help
		Yacht's safety boat, gave help
		Catamarans, gave help
	13	Diver's boat on service to sunken fishing vessel *Pescado*, stood by boat
	25	Catamaran, recovered wreckage
	28	Fishing boat *Hunter*, gave help
1987	Jan 10	Motor boat, gave help
	Apr 11	Man fallen from breakwater, gave help
	17	Sailboard, saved board and 1
	May 4	Sailboard, saved board and 1
	June 27	Man fallen from lighthouse, landed 1
	Aug 3	Sailboard, saved board and 1
		Two sailboards, gave help
	23	Sailboard, gave help
	25	Injured man on board yacht *Libra*, landed an injured man
	30	Yacht, gave help
	Sep 6	Sailing dinghy, saved 3

B-571 *British Diver II*

	Dec 24	Cabin cruiser, saved boat and 2
1988	Jan 20	Sailboard, gave help
	24	Sailboard, gave help
	30	Rubber dinghy, saved boat and 2
		Motor boat, saved boat and 2
	Feb 16	Dinghy, landed 1 and a body
		Yacht, gave help
	Mar 23	Cabin cruiser, saved boat and 2
	24	Passenger/roro cargo/ferry *Nordic Ferry*, stood by vessel
	Apr 6	Yacht *Home Spun*, gave help
	May 7	Yacht *Prelude*, gave help
	21	Yacht *Brigand*, gave help
	June 5	Sick man on board yacht *Katie*, gave help
	19	Yacht *Malo*, gave help
	July 3	Yacht, saved boat and 3
	9	Yacht *Helen*, gave help
	22	Yacht *Jerkana*, gave help
	24	Dinghy, saved boat
		Yacht club safety boat, escorted boat
		Sailboard, saved board and 1
	25	Sailboard, saved board and 1
	31	Yacht *General C*, gave help

Aug 9	Yacht *Aghia 2*, gave help
11	Sick man on board yacht *Navicula*, took out doctor and landed a body
14	Catamaran, saved boat and landed 2
16	Two sailboards, landed 2 and recovered 2 boards
Sep 8	Yacht *Helle*, gave help
23	Felixstowe Sailboard Club rescue boat, saved boat and 2
24	Motor boat *Gregory Girl*, saved boat
27	Yacht *Thirdygree*, gave help
Oct 1	Fishing vessel *Niblick*, gave help
15	Yacht *Copperas*, gave help
29	Cabin cruiser *Tudor Rose*, gave help

1989	Apr 6	Sailboard, saved board and 1
	7	Fishing vessel *Christe Lee*, escorted
	May 12	Yacht *Harnser*, saved boat and 2
	20	Injured man on board yacht *John Bull*, landed an injured man
	27	Yacht *Becky Too*, gave help
	June 4	Yacht Club Safety boat, saved 1
		Sailboard, gave help
		Cabin cruiser *Cubra II*, gave help
	8	Yacht *Hunraken*, gave help
	July 3	Speedboat, gave help
	8	Fishing vessel *Emma Jane*, gave help

B-514 *Guide Friendship I*

16	Sick man on board fishing vessel *Boy Tom*, took out doctor and stood by
17	Yacht *Westwind of Stour*, saved 11
22	Power boat *Draco*, gave help
26	Sailboard, gave help
	Sailing dinghy, gave help
Aug 13	Yacht *Gannet*, escorted boat
	Sailing dinghy, gave help
22	Yacht *Misty*, saved boat and 2
28	Cabin cruiser, gave help
	Injured man on board yacht *Tookie*, landed an injured man

B-571 *British Diver II*

	Sep 2	Sick man on yacht *Pleindievre*, gave help
	8	Yacht *Quoir II*, landed 3
	10	Cabin cruiser *Barbie*, landed 5
	Oct 8	Sailboard, saved 1
	14	Motor boat, landed 2
	29	Sailboard, saved board and 1
		Sailing dinghy, saved boat and 1
	Nov 2	Yacht *Folklore*, saved boat, tender and 1
	Dec 14	Rowing boat, gave help
1990	Jan 14	Ill crewman on motor vessel, landed an ill person
	Feb 14	Sailboard, saved board and 1
	Mar 26	Yacht, landed 1
	31	Safety boat capsized, landed 2
	Apr 7	Sail multihull with sail failure, landed craft
	May 20	Yacht, gave help
	26	Yacht, gave help
	June 2	Catamaran, saved craft and 4
	30	Sailing dinghy, gave help
	July 1	Sailing dinghy, landed craft
	12	Yacht, gave help
	14	Sailing dinghy, gave help

	22	Yacht, stood by
	26	Yacht, landed 2
	Aug 3	Motor boat, landed craft
	9	Bather drowning, saved 1
	24	Power boat out of fuel, craft brought in
	26	Ill crewman on board yacht, landed 1
	29	Rowing boat, landed craft
	Sep 2	Yacht, gave help
	19	Yacht, saved casualty and 1
	Oct 21	Yacht, gave help
	Nov 1	Person cut off by tide, saved 1
1991	Jan 6	Yacht *Blue Dolphin*, gave help
		Yacht *Arwen Pallister*, landed 2
	Mar 6	Yacht *Oriel-S*, escorted boat
	Apr 17	Sailboard, saved board and 1
	22	Yacht *Buckler*, gave help
	June 1	Sail training yacht *Salex*, gave help
	23	Sailing dinghy, saved 2
	26	Yacht *Vlieter*, stood by boat
	July 13	Catamaran *Pikinini Truganini*, gave help
		Catamaran *Pikinini Truganini*, saved boat and 1
	Aug 8	Sailing dinghy, gave help
	12	Injured man on board yacht *Charlotte*, landed an injured man

B-586 *Clothworker*

Aug 18	Yacht *Rival II*, saved boat and assisted to save 2
22	Cabin cruiser *Gristina*, landed 1
Oct 2	Speedboat *Ti-Cal*, gave help
	Man in sea, gave help
Nov 24	Sailboard, saved board and 1
Dec 20	Sailboard, landed 1

B-571 *British Diver II*

1992	Mar 9	Dinghy, landed a body
	21	Cabin cruiser *Inigma*, in tow of Police launch, escorted boats
	Apr 22	Man cut off by tide, landed 1
	23	Canoe, saved boat and 1
	May 9	Sailboard, saved board and 1
	16	Power boat, gave help
	26	Two sailing dinghies, gave help
	June 13	Yacht *Arwen* of Burnham, g help
	14	Sailing dinghy, saved boat and 1
	17	Catamaran, saved boat and 2
	21	Sailing dinghy, saved boat and 2
	30	Man overboard from passenger ferry *Stena Britannica*, gave help
	July 1	Fishing boat *Saturn*, gave help
	18	Yacht *Mouymang*, gave help
	27	Sailboard, saved board and 1
		Yacht, gave help
	31	Three persons cut off by tide, gave help
	Aug 24	Yacht *Haura*, gave help
		Yacht *Haura*, gave help
	28	Yacht *Trineke of Denem*, saved boat and 2
	29	Yacht *Crinan Lass*, gave help
	30	Yacht *St Peter*, stood by boat
		Yacht, stood by boat
		Yacht *Silver Meridian*, escorted
	Sep 13	Yacht *Our Tern*, gave help
	15	Yacht *Saljahan*, gave help

	Oct 3	Yacht *Spider II*, gave help
	11	Tender to yacht *Stardust*, recovered boat
	31	Injured man on board cargo vessel *Ardent*, landed an injured man
	Nov 1	Sailing dinghy, stood by boat
		Yacht *Blazer*, gave help
	8	Passenger ro-ro ferry *Dana Anglia*, stood by
	14	Yacht *Fluglia*, escorted boat
	Apr 4	Motor cruiser *Tom Pepper*, gave help
	May 17	Yacht *Dissem*, saved boat and 2
	20	Yacht *No Problem*, gave help
	June 1	Yacht *Mistique*, gave help
	9	Speedboat, gave help
	14	Injured man on board cabin cruiser *Rising Star of Sunbury*, gave help
	26	Catamaran, landed 2
	July 3	Sailboard, saved board and landed 1
		Sailing dinghy, gave help
		Swimmer, stood by
		Catamaran, gave help
	July 11	Sailing dinghy, saved boat and 2
	14	Yacht *Mary Josephine*, escorted
	19	Cabin cruiser *Enterprise Ranger*, gave help
	22	Sailing dinghy, saved boat
	25	Sailing dinghy *Hamburger*, saved boat and 2
	Aug 2	Yacht *Allegro*, stood by boat
		Yacht *Pulsate*, gave help
	5	Sailboard, saved board and 1
		Cabin cruiser *Lady Linda*, stood by
	11	Sailing dinghy, saved boat and 2
	12	Two canoes, saved boats
		Rubber dinghy, saved boat
	15	Yacht *Bluster*, gave help
	18	Harbour launch, gave help
	21	Catamaran, gave help
	Sep 5	Yacht *Sweet Return*, gave help
	12	Yacht *Moonpenny*, saved boat and 1
	18	Catamaran *Soggy Moggy*, saved boat
	21	Sailboard, saved board and 1
	Oct 10	Cabin cruiser *Elizabeth*, landed 5, gave help
	14	Sailboard, saved board and 1
	18	Woman swept off promenade into sea, recovered a body
	24	Cabin cruiser *Westall*, in tow of harbour patrol boat *Valentine*, escorted
1994	Jan 30	Dinghy, saved boat and 2
	Feb 12	Yacht *Camarada*, saved 2
	Apr 4	Motor boat, landed 2
	8	Yacht, escorted boat
		Yacht *Satsuma*, saved boat and 2
	May 11	Yacht *Taeke Hadewych*, escorted
	12	Yacht *Seneca*, gave help
	31	Speedboat, two persons and craft brought in
	31	Yacht *Patti-Sing*, two persons and craft brought in
	June 11	Yacht *Bird of Paradise*, landed 1
	12	Yacht *Dawn Voyager*, two persons and craft brought in
	29	Three child bathers, landed 3
	July 3	Cabin cruiser *Mary Rose*, stood by
	10	Man over board fm jet ski, sd jet ski and 1
	11	Fishing vessel *Boy Andrew*, assisted to save vessel and 1
	17	Yacht, gave help
	17	Yacht *Kantele*, gave help

	22	Dinghy, two persons and craft brought in
	28	Sailboard, landed 1 and craft brought in
	Aug 2	Sailing dinghy One person landed
	7	Yacht *Pollette*, landed 5
	9	Yacht *Troll*, gave help
	10	Yacht *Maruna*, gave help
	10	Yacht *Lara of Albany*, saved boat and 2
	27	Yacht *Tanti*, escorted and gave help
	29	Yacht *Splinter Group*, saved boat and 6
	Oct 9	Sick woman onboard yacht *Getaway*, escorted boat
	17	Yacht *Balchis*, three and craft brought in
	25	Motor boat, escorted boat
	Dec 4	Motor boat, saved boat and 2
1995	Jan 2	Dinghy, saved 2
	Apr 7	Sailing dinghy, saved boat and 2
	25	Sailing dinghy, saved boat
	May 4	Tug *Gray Vixen*, gave help
	16	Yacht *Menina*, three persons and craft brought in
	22	Yacht *Water Buffaloe*, two persons and craft brought in
	30	Yacht *Iris*, gave help
	June 5	Two sailboards, landed 2 and two craft brought in
	16	Sick man on yacht *Cynara*, landed a body
	26	Motor boat *Wittiwake*, two persons and craft brought in
	30	Rubber dinghy, escorted boat
	July 22	Two girls cut off by tide, saved 2
	25	Yacht *Walrus*, gave help
		Yacht *Walrus*, landed 4 and craft brought in
	Aug 1	Rubber dinghy, saved dinghy and 2
	4	Yacht in tow of fishing boat, escorted
	10	Yacht *Libertijn*, gave help
	20	Yacht *Whippper Snapper*, gave help
		Sailing dinghy, saved 3
	27	Yacht *Roseidon*, one person brought in
		Rubber dinghy, saved boat and 1
		Yacht *Sigtta of Culne*, two persons and craft brought in
		Sailing dinghy, gave help
	28	Yacht, two persons and craft brought in
	Sep 1	Yacht *Prudence*, saved boat and 2
	9	Yacht *Whistfull*, two persons brought in
	16	Yacht *Green Ginger*, four persons and craft brought in
	Oct 1	Yacht *Lorien*, gave help
	5	Yacht *Samsar*, two persons & craft brought in
	8	Yacht *Bosun*, gave help
	Nov 12	Two persons over board from roro/cargo ferry *Hamburg*, saved 2
	Dec 29	Barge *Sirius*, gave help
1996	Jan 1	Motor boat *Cormorant*, escorted
	8	Sailboard, saved board
	22	Boy washed into sea, recovered a body

B-536 Relief Atlantic 21

	Mar 6	Fishing vessel *Thomasam*, stood by
	Apr 11	Motor cruiser *Noreen Anne*, escorted
	May 18	Woman fallen from sea wall, gave help
	22	Yacht *Sunnyside 2*, gave help
		Yacht *Challenge*, gave help
		Yacht *Sunnyside 2*, gave help
	26	Yacht *Isles of the Seas*, saved craft & 6

May 31   Yacht *Dhowmoa*, two persons and craft brought in

June 15   Sailing dinghy, two persons & craft brought in

25   Yacht *Bonella*, gave help

29   Sailboard, saved 1
Yacht, gave help

30   Yacht *Hoppinn*, gave help

July 15   Two sailboards, landed 1 and saved board

18   Swimmer, saved 1
Two youths cut off by tide, one person brought in

23   Four persons stranded on Low Lighthouse, landed 2

Aug 3   Yacht *Pirrha B*, gave help

5   Sailboard, saved 1
Catamaran, saved 1
Passenger/roro cargo ferry *Koningin Beatrix* Stood by craft

9   Yacht *Piccanin*, gave help
Yacht *Templer*, gave help

18   Yacht, stood by craft

23   Jet ski, landed 1 and saved 1
Fishing vessel *Alex Maria*, one person and craft brought in

24   Sailboard, saved board and 1
Sailing dinghy, saved craft and 2

26   Yacht *Suzy K*, gave help
Yacht *Lady Grace*, gave help
Yacht *Polly Anna*, saved 5
Helicopter winchman, saved 1

31   Injured woman onboard yacht *Peter Witch*, injured woman brought in

Sep 1   Yacht *Legal Eye*, two persons brought in and gave help

4   Yacht *Paliamma*, gave help

B-571 *British Diver II*

Sep 18   Sailing dinghy, saved craft and 1

29   Sailboard, saved 1

Oct 3   Yacht *Wild Mouse*, saved craft and 2

6   Rowing boat, escorted craft

26   Motor boat, three persons & craft brought in

Dec 8   Injured man on board motor boat *Fontainne of Worth*, landed an injured man
Motor boat, escorted craft

1997   Apr 2   Yacht *Mistress Quickly*, gave help

3   Harbour ferry *S-Express*, landed 3 and craft brought in

28   Sailing dinghy, one person & craft brought in

May 10   Yacht *Sasparilla*, saved craft and 2
Yacht *Kantara*, three people and craft brought in

21   Yacht *Kanga of Maldon*, two people and craft brought in

28   Yacht *Linda*, five people brought in

June 15   Diver support craft *Tornado I*, four people and craft brought in

21   Catamaran, landed 2 and saved craft

24   Sailing dinghy, gave help

July 21   Yacht *Serlio*, escorted craft

25   Yacht *Pzazz*, gave help

26   Sailboard, landed 1 and board brought in

27   Yacht *Nancy Blacket*, gave help

Aug 4   Two sailing dinghies, escorted craft

7   Yacht *Albora*, stood by craft

9   Yacht *Ayesha*, two and craft brought in
Yacht *Mellonita*, landed a sick man
Yacht, three people, two dogs and craft brought in

10   Motor boat, gave help

11   Yacht *Kiki II*, took out doctor and injured woman brought in

18   Four swimmers, four people brought in

27   Sailing dinghy *Venture*, landed 2 and craft brought in

28   Rubber dinghy *Rhapsody*, escorted

Sep 26   Yacht *Balchis*, escorted craft

Oct 1   Speedboat, two persons & craft brought in

14   Survey boat *Shamrock*, gave help

19   Yacht *Sea Victor*, one person and craft brought in

Nov 21   Body in river, landed a body

Dec 23   Motor boat *Winkle III*, saved boat and 2

29   Cabin cruiser *Freddie Fly*, five people and craft brought in

1997   Apr 2   Yacht *Mistress Quickly*, gave help

3   Harbour ferry *S-Express*, landed 3 and craft brought in

28   Sailing dinghy, one person & craft brought in

May 10   Yacht *Sasparilla*, saved craft and 2
Yacht *Kantara*, three people and craft brought in

21   Yacht *Kanga of Maldon*, two people and craft brought in

28   Yacht *Linda*, five people brought in

June 15   Diver support craft *Tornado I*, four people and craft brought in

21   Catamaran, landed 2 and saved craft

24   Sailing dinghy, gave help

July 21   Yacht *Serlio*, escorted craft

25   Yacht *Pzazz*, gave help

26   Sailboard, landed 1 and board brought in

27   Yacht *Nancy Blacket*, gave help

Aug 4   Two sailing dinghies, escorted craft

7   Yacht *Albora*, stood by craft

9   Yacht *Ayesha*, two and craft brought in
Yacht *Mellonita*, landed a sick man
Yacht, three people, two dogs and craft brought in

10   Motor boat, gave help

11   Yacht *Kiki II*, took out doctor and injured woman brought in

18   Four swimmers, four people brought in

27   Sailing dinghy *Venture*, landed 2 and craft brought in

28   Rubber dinghy *Rhapsody*, escorted

Sep 26   Yacht *Balchis*, escorted craft

Oct 1   Speedboat, two persons and craft brought in

14   Survey boat *Shamrock*, gave help

19   Yacht *Sea Victor*, one person and craft brought in

Nov 21   Body in river, landed a body

Dec 23   Motor boat *Winkle III*, saved boat and 2

29   Cabin cruiser *Freddie Fly*, five people and craft brought in

1998   Mar 8   Fishing vessel *Klystron*, gave help

13   Cabin cruiser, two and craft brought in

16   Person fallen from Orwell Bridge, landed body

Apr 6 Motor boat *Kezmea*, two people and craft brought in
29 Woman stranded on breakwater, stood by
May 9 Yacht *Morning Mist*, stood by craft
29 Yacht *Eater Hacker*, stood by craft
June 8 Yacht *Eyrlk*, gave help
Yacht *Antaries*, one person & craft brought in
20 Cabin cruiser *Aquarian Dawn*, landed 2 and craft brought in
July 4 Motor boat, three and craft brought in
Boy stuck in mud, stood by
10 Yacht *Sjonest*, gave help
11 Yacht *Kajanus*, landed 2 and craft brought in
Man fallen from Orwell Bridge, landed body
18 Cabin cruiser, landed 1 and craft brought in
Yacht *Francipam*, gave help
Speedboat *Double 00*, three people and craft brought in
Aug 1 Tender to yacht *Ampersand*, stood by
4 Two bathers, saved 2
12 Air bed, saved air bed and 3
20 Yacht *Baripama*, landed 2 and craft brought in
Yacht *Chrisdan*, two people & craft brought in
21 Woman in sea, saved 1
Yacht *Zest*, gave help
23 Motor boat, two people & craft brought in
Sep 5 Sailing dinghy *Sirius*, escorted
Sailing dinghy *Rainbow*, saved dinghy and 2
Sailing dinghy *Osprey*, landed 3 and craft brought in
23 Yacht *Snowfire*, saved yacht and 1
Oct 10 Youth in sea, saved 1
20 Yacht *Wuir*, gave help
24 Yacht *Rumpty III*, gave help
Nov 7 Yacht *Determination*, one person brought in
21 Cabin cruiser Teal, two & craft brought in
Dec 6 Motor boat *Bananna Boy*, two people and craft brought in
27 Sailing dinghy, saved craft
1999 Feb 6 Motor boat *Kirsty Lee*, two people and craft brought in
Mar 12 Cabin cruiser *Lyn Vick Gem*, two people brought in
17 Yacht Sun *Downer*, escorted craft
21 Speedboat *Mandy Jayne*, three people and craft brought in
Apr 5 Yacht *Sun Mist*, gave help
12 Yacht *Proud Maeve*, gave help
18 Yacht *Sandpiper*, gave help
19 Motor boat, two people & craft brought in
20 Rowing boat, saved craft
May 11 Yacht *Matina*, two people & craft brought in
31 Diver support craft B SAC 54, four people and craft brought in
June 8 Yacht *Sabre*, landed 4 and craft brought in
11 Yacht *Vashti*, gave help
12 Yacht *Indigo*, escorted craft
20 Yacht *Whim-A-Wag*, gave help
21 Yacht *Pee Jay III*, four people and craft brought in
Sailboard, saved board
Yacht *Chalice*, saved craft
27 Sailing dinghy, saved craft and 2
Yacht *Deva*, two people & craft brought in
July 3 Speedboat, craft brought in
5 Yacht *Disting*, two and craft brought in
9 Yacht *Silver Bugle*, gave help
10 Yachts *Beestie* and *Miss Siagon*, gave help
12 Motor boat, saved craft and 3
21 Yacht Mooie Meid, gave help
31 Bather, saved 1
Aug 2 Yacht Arriuist, gave help
11 Yacht She, gave help
22 Yacht Frances Josephine, gv help
25 Yacht Anna Cray, escorted craft
26 Yacht *Barbarie Dream*, four people and craft brought in
27 Yacht *Joliebrise*, craft brought in
30 Yacht, one person and craft brought in
Sep 5 Yacht *The Bear*, gave help
8 Yacht *Orca*, gave help
9 Speedboat, gave help
10 Speedboat, one person and craft brought in
18 Man overboard from ferry *Stena Discovery*, stood by
25 Yacht *Mistress*, stood by
29 Swimmer, landed 1
Oct 12 Yacht *Folksong*, one and craft brought in
17 Sailing dinghy, gave help
Yacht *Black Rose*, landed 6
18 Sick man on board tug *Beaver*, one person brought in
23 Yacht *Sarah*, landed 4 and craft brought in
Nov 26 Powerboat *Chardway*, two people and craft brought in
Dec 11 Powerboat *Jean Ann*, three people and craft brought in
29 Two people cut off by tide, two people brought in
2000 Jan 9 Power boat *Boy Darren*, gave help
31 Man stranded on town pier, stood by
Feb 27 Yacht, gave help
Mar 19 Yacht *Take Two*, gave help
Power boat *Freedom*, escorted craft
25 Angling craft *Nemo II*, landed craft and 2
Apr 3 Yacht *Alona*, landed craft and 3
4 Yacht *Wild Gull*, landed craft and 3
10 Yacht *Nostromo*, gave help
23 Cabin cruiser *Coreen*, landed two people
May 3 Yacht *Minky*, landed craft and 1
4 Yacht *Pamela Jane*, landed craft and 1
15 Yacht, landed craft and 2
22 Yacht *Polytropos*, landed craft and 2
25 Yacht *Catehrines Mist*, landed craft and 1
June 6 Yacht *Regal Warrior*, gave help
July 13 Yacht *Antares*, gave help
31 Powerboat, landed craft and 2
Aug 7 Powerboat, landed craft and 2

B-590 *Wolverson X-Ray*

13 People stranded, landed 2
18 Yacht *Infinity*, landed craft and 2
26 Yacht *Syn Fye*, gave help
28 Yacht *Brierly*, saved craft and 1
29 Powerboat, escorted craft
30 Sailing dinghy *Taz*, gave help
Sep 20 Sailing dinghy, craft brought in
24 Sailing dinghy, recovered dinghy and 2
Yacht with steering problems, towed craft

Oct 7 Yacht, gave help and escorted
     9 Yacht, craft brought in
    10 Yacht, landed craft and persons
    16 Yacht, escorted craft
    18 Suicide Orwell Bridge, recovered body
    21 Fishing vessel, craft brought in
Nov 22 Sailing dinghy, craft brought in
Dec 14 Person cut off by tide, landed 1
2001 Jan 7 Two people stranded, stood by
Feb 18 Person stranded on Orwell Bridge, stood by
    21 Cabin cruiser, escorted craft
Mar 10 Fishing vessel *Pedro*, landed craft and 1
    11 Cabin cruiser *Gorn Queen*, landed craft & 6
Apr 12 Two people cut off by tide, brought in 2
         people
    13 Body in water, recovered body

B-571 *British Diver II*

May 5 Yacht *Minstrel*, landed craft and 4
        Yacht *Sapphire*, gave help
     6 Yacht *Odessa*, landed craft and 9
        Yacht *Catherine*, landed craft and2
    19 Tender to yacht, gave help
        Powerboat, landed craft and 2
    22 Yacht *Whim-Away*, gave help
    26 Yacht *Maid Marrion*, landed craft and 4
    27 Yacht *Orion*, gave help
        Three people cut off by tide, stood by
    28 Cabin cruiser *Sammy B*, two people brght in
June 2 Yacht *Blade Fisher*, gave help
    20 Cabin cruiser *Emma*, landed craft and 1
    25 Speedboat, landed craft and 2
    30 Sail catamaran, landed craft and 2
        Yacht *Schnuky*, landed craft and 4
July 4 Yacht *Pee Jay III*, landed craft and 2
    17 Yacht *Chow Chou San*, gave help
        Yacht *Griffon*, gave help
    18 Speedboat, landed craft and 1
    30 Sailing dinghy, landed craft and 2
Aug 1 Speedboat, landed craft and 2
     5 Rowing boat, landed craft and 3
    10 Yacht *Bells Down*, gave help
    16 Yacht *Fliss*, stood by
    19 Inflatable dinghy, craft brought in
    22 Injured woman on board
        Yacht *Selana*, stood by
Sep 6 Canoe, one life and craft saved
     7 Yacht *Critical Care*, landed craft and 3
        Yacht *Possum*, landed craft and 2
Oct 7 Sailing dinghy, saved craft
    14 Powerboat, gave help
        Yacht *Pretender*, landed craft and 1
    18 Yacht *Jeni Be Good III*, landed craft and 8
    20 Powerboat, landed craft and 2
2002 Jan 13 Three children stuck in mud, landed 1
Feb 2 Rowing dinghy, landed craft and 1
    10 Yacht *Illusion*, landed craft and 1
    17 Powerboat *Adventurer*, landed craft and 3
Mar 9 Yacht *Roussillon*, landed craft and 2
    26 Person in water, landed a body
    30 Yacht *Sarbande*, gave help
        Yacht *Christena*, escorted craft
    31 Powerboat, landed craft and 3

Apr 5 Sail dinghy, gave help
     7 Yacht *Bumble Bee*, gave help
    13 Jet ski, landed craft and 1
        Two people overboard from sailboards, two
         people landed 2
    26 Yacht *Mimsy*, escorted craft
May 6 Powerboat *Pugwash*, landed craft and 2
    18 Injured crewman on board yacht *Thames
         Shipwight*, one person brought in
    26 Man overboard from sailboat, saved craft
         and 1
    27 Yacht *Ragged Robin III*, gave help
    27 Yacht *Ragged Robin III*, landed craft and 2
June 7 Yacht *Marionette*, landed craft and 3
        Yacht *Mandarin*, gave help
     8 Person on Orwell Bridge, stood by
    11 Yacht *Witbow*, gave help
    20 Yacht, one person brought in
    23 Sick man on board yacht *Seawind II*, gave
         help
        Sailing dinghy, landed craft and 1
    30 Yacht *Eleanor of Porvan*, gave help
July 4 Two people cut off by tide on Orwell Bridge,
         landed 2
     8 Sail training vessel *Black Magic*, gave help
        Yacht, landed craft and 8
    17 Three yachts, gave help
    22 Sick crewman on board yacht *Twyde Sop*,
         one person brought in
        Yacht *Twyde Sop*, gave help
    24 Yacht *Mouse*, gave help
    26 Horse in river, stood by
Aug 11 Yacht *Meltemi*, landed craft and 2
    21 Yacht *Blue Cascade*, gave help
    26 Powerboat, landed craft and 2
    30 Person fallen from man made structure,
         landed a body
Sep 1 Yacht *Vita Nova*, gave help
     5 Rowing boat, gave help
    10 Yacht *Trinovante*, gave help
        Yacht *Little World*, one person brought in
    13 Person on Orwell Bridge, stood by
    15 Yacht *Spirit of Sukford*, gave help
    15 Speedboat, gave help
    22 Yacht, gave help
    28 Motor boat, landed craft and 2
Oct 4 Person in water, saved 1
     6 Motor boat, landed craft and 5
    14 Yacht *Diana*, landed craft and 3

B-789 *Sure and Steadfast*

Dec 1 Yacht *Lady October*, landed craft and 3
     6 Motor boat *About Time*, landed craft & 1
     8 Cabin cruiser *Frantic*, landed craft and 3
    14 Motor boat *Joint Venture*, landed craft and 2
    25 Person on bridge, stood by
    27 Person in distress on breakwater, stood by
2003 Jan 11 Angling boat *Joint Venture*, landed craft & 2
    18 Cabin cruiser, landed craft and 1
    25 Angling boat *Kaipee*, escorted craft
    26 Person in water, landed body
Mar 1 Motor boat, two people brought in
     1 Motor boat, gave help
     2 Cabin cruiser, landed craft and 3
     4 Human body, landed a body

Mar 20	Rowing boat, saved 1
28	Motor boat, landed craft and 3
Apr 9	Motor boat, landed a body
18	Tender to yacht *Mambury*, landed craft & 2
19	Motor boat *Nalor*, landed craft and 2
20	Motor boat *Lydia*, landed craft and 2
May 1	Yacht, escorted craft
2	Yacht *Adventurer*, landed craft and 3
9	Yacht *Butterfly*, landed craft and 2
29	Motor boat, gave help
June 3	Sailing dinghy, gave help
8	Diver support craft, saved craft and 6
	Cabin cruiser Katrine, landed craft and 10
18	Yacht Katie Lou, landed craft and 1
22	Yacht, stood by
July 4	Three people cut off by tide, three people brought in
10	Powerboat, landed craft and 3
15	Yacht *Aspara*, gave help
	Yacht *Aspara*, landed craft and 2
	Motor boat, landed craft and 2
21	Four people stranded, four people brought in
21	Eight people in the sea, stood by
27	Yacht *Ivy*, craft brought in
Aug 8	Yacht, craft brought in
14	Yacht *Wench*, landed craft and 1
24	Yacht *Carpe Diem*, landed craft and 4
24	Powerboat, landed craft and 4
27	Yacht *Polski Len*, gave help
27	Yacht *Polski Len*, landed craft and 8
Sep 4	Jet ski, landed craft and 2
18	Sail craft, landed people and craft
24	Man overboard, escorted craft
26	Powerboat *Ria*, landed craft and 3
29	Yacht *Crescent Moon*, landed craft and 1
Oct 8	People in danger of drowning, saved craft and 2
	Yacht *Maldon Maid*, landed craft and 2
11	Yacht *Amista*, landed craft and 2
12	Yacht *Amulet*, landed craft and 2
14	Yach *Sea Walker*, landed craft and 1
23	Powerboat, saved craft
Nov 22	Yacht, landed craft and 1
Dec 18	Sick youth on board yacht, landed 1
20	Yacht *Trinwamelle*, landed 3
	Yacht *Tantina*, landed craft and 3
	Yacht *Kalidos*, gave help
21	Lifebuoy, gave help
22	Yacht *Runaway*, gave help

2004	Jan 11	Man overboard from powerboat *Lydia*, landed 1
	Feb 1	Human bodies, landed two bodies
	7	Human bodies, gave help – transferred crew member to yacht
	17	Tug *Otter*, landed craft and 2
	29	Canoe, gave help – search
	Mar 28	Human body, landed a body
	29	Weather balloon, gave help – located and brought in weather balloon
	Apr 12	Rowing boat, saved craft
	21	Powered boat, landed craft and 3
	25	Powered boat *Aqua Juliet*, gave help - transferred first aider

May 8	Yacht *Baruna*, landed craft and 5
17	Powered boat, landed craft and 3
21	Powered boat, landed craft and 2
June 3	Yacht *Curlew*, escorted craft
4	Powered boat *Antares*, gave help
6	Yacht *Passepart Out*, gave help
	Yacht *Passepart Out*, landed craft and 3
14	Powered boat, landed craft and 4
23	Tender to yacht, stood by
25	Yacht *Anneaa 2*, landed craft and 3
28	Sailing dinghy, landed craft and 1
30	Yacht *Manana*, landed craft and 4
July 3	Power boat *Shore Thing*, landed craft and 2
6	Powered boat, escorted craft
6	Yacht *Dulcinea*, landed craft and 3
22	Powered boat, landed craft and 2
25	Yacht *Duo*, landed 1
28	Yacht *Meltemi*, gave help
Aug 8	Swimmer, stood by
	Swimmers, stood by
9	Person in sea, stood by
11	Yacht *Bonnie Lee*, landed craft and 2
16	Yacht *Bonnie Lee*, landed craft and 2
20	Sailboat, landed sailboard and 1
20	Sailboat, landed sailboard and 1
30	Yacht *On Site*, landed craft and 2
Sep 1	Yacht *Sea Horse*, landed 2
3	Human body, landed body
4	Sailing dinghy, landed 2
4	Sailing dinghies, stood by
6	Child in danger of drowning, landed a child
7	Fire under jetty, gave help
Oct 1	Sick man on board tug *Gray Vixen*, stood by
Nov 2	Powered boat, landed craft and 2
5	Powered boat Shelly, gave help

2005	Jan 23	Yacht, gave help
	Apr 11	Person at risk on the Orwell Bridge, stood by
	22	Yacht, landed craft and 1
	30	Yacht, gave help
	May 2	Power boat, landed craft and 6
	4	Yacht *Ejay*, escorted craft
	6	Yacht *First Avenue*, landed craft and 3
	8	Yacht *Arkola*, landed craft and 1
	8	Yacht *Te Arawa*, landed craft and 3
	14	Catamaran *Nina of Daresbury*, landed craft and 2
	20	Injured person on rocks, landed body
	28	Yacht *Eastermay*, gave help
	June 3	Yacht *Ellen Dora*, landed 10 people
	3	Powered boat *Sharon J*, landed craft and 1
	4	Injured crewman on board Yacht *Signus*, one person landed
	16	Powered boat *Layla J*, gave help
	July 8	People over tender to yacht *Dun Leanin*, saved 2
	8	Yacht *Cantana*, landed craft and 4
	9	Yacht *Southern Comfort*, gave help
	13	Sick man on board yacht Butterfly, one person brought in
	17	Yacht *Hiawather*, stood by
	17	Yacht *Witch of Hoo*, escorted craft
	18	Yacht *Witch of Hoo*, escorted craft
	21	Sailing dinghy, one person & craft brought in
	24	Sailing dinghy, saved 1

25	Powered boat *Bassa*, two people and craft brought in	
28	Yacht *Paradox*, gave help – pumped out	
28	Yacht *Catchwind*, gave help – assisted ALB to connect tow to casualty	
29	Yacht *Orton Lady*, gave help – towed casualty to deeper water	
30	Yacht *Scallion*, four people & craft brought in	

Aug 1 Yacht *White Horses*, gave help – completed tow
12 Sailing dinghy, landed 1 & craft brought in
13 Person in danger of drowning, landed 1
18 Yacht, stood by
24 Powered boats, escorted craft
Sep 3 Yacht *Pentoma*, escorted craft
Powered boat, two people & craft brought in
4 Yacht *Fargo II*, escorted craft
11 Houseboats, gave help – searched area
15 Yacht *British Beagle*, gave help – assisted to clear obstruction
16 Yacht *So What*, one person & craft brought in
28 Powered boat *Sand Piper*, one person and craft brought in
Oct 10 Sick person on board powered boat *Regardless*, stood by
16 Yacht *Prime Time*, stood by
Injured person on board yacht *Roca*, gave help – assisted with transfer 1 to helicopter
Nov 19 Dog, gave help
20 Powered boat *Casa*, three people and craft brought in
Dec 4 Tug *Norsund* and powered boat *Glave*, gave help
29 Powered boat, two people brought in
2006 Feb 12 Human body, landed a body
Mar 27 Yacht *Rival of Sharlee*, gave help
27 Yacht *Rival of Sharlee*, gave help
Apr 2 Yacht *Panther*, gave help
16 People cut off by the tide, two people brought in
17 Yacht *Selena Rose*, landed craft and 2
27 Catamaran, craft brought in
May 19 Sailing dinghy, stood by
27 Powered boat *Fairwinds*, gave help
28 Yacht *Simba*, gave help
28 Powered boat *Caritas*, gave help
29 Sailing dinghies, saved 2
June 7 Powered boat, landed craft and 2
7 Person in sea, landed a body
19 Jet ski, landed craft and 1
23 Yacht *Wiggen 5*, gave help
July 1 Powered boat *Kingfisher*, landed craft and 2
15 Powered boat *Deborah*, gave help
15 Yacht *Athenia*, gave help
15 Kiteboard, gave help
22 Inflatable dinghies, stood by
23 Powered boat, landed craft and 5
30 Powered boat *Jacabe One*, escorted
Aug 13 Yacht *Charissa*, gave help
15 Kiteboard, landed kiteboard and 1
20 Yacht *Audere*, gave help
20 Powered boat, landed craft and 3
28 People cut off by tide, two brought in
Sep 2 Powered boat, landed craft and 3
15 Tender to yacht *Atlantis*, landed craft and 1
19 Person at risk on stone pier, stood by

Sep 26 Person in river, landed 1
30 Powered boat, landed craft and 2
Oct 9 Kiteboard, landed board and 1
15 Yacht *Busy Bee*, landed craft and 2

B-755 *London's Anniversary 175*

30 Catamaran *Tu Tu Tango*, one person brought in
Dec 3 Yacht *Gentoo of Antartica*, gave help
2007 Jan 17 Yacht *Tango*, gave help
28 Angling vessel *Pecan*, landed 1, one person and craft brought in

B-789 *Sure and Steadfast*

Mar 18 Canoes, saved three canoes and 3
Apr 2 Yacht, two people and craft brought in
3 Yacht *Rival of Sharlee*, gave help
9 Powered boat *Toni's Lady Swan*, two people and craft brought in
12 Powered boat, gave help
15 Yacht *Vagabond*, gave help
16 Yacht *Zee Zeiler*, gave help
29 Yacht *Tellia*, landed 1 & craft brought in
May 7 Powered boat *Toomix*, gave help
8 Sailboard, sailboard brought in and saved 1
June 3 Yacht *Spindrift*, three people and craft brought in
6 Yacht *Indeweer*, one person and craft brought in
9 Injured man, gave help
26 Yacht *Aegle*, gave help
July 8 Powered boat, two people & craft brought in
13 Yacht *gavia*, gave help
14 Yacht *Mid Life Crisis*, stood by
16 Yacht *Notredame*, gave help
28 Kiteboard, saved 1
Aug 1 Yacht *Suli Suli*, two people & craft brought in
3 Yacht *Speer*, gave help
6 Yacht *Winafre*, gave help
8 Person in the sea, saved 1

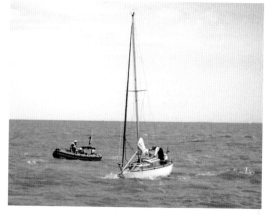

Working with Albert Brown, B-789 Sure and Steadfast pulls the 31ft yacht Lynx off the Cork Sands, six miles south-east of Harwich. The yacht, with 2 persons onboard, had run aground early and needed assistance to refloat. (By courtesy of Harwich RNLI)

Aug 18	Sailing dinghy, landed 1, craft brought in
26	Sick man on beach, gave help
Oct 1	Yacht *Bellatrix*, two and craft brought in
2	Powered boat, landed 1
11	Powered boat *Pegasus*, two people brought in
17	Yacht *Seduction*, gave help
27	Kiteboards, two people and kiteboards brought in
28	Powered boat *Nichola Anne*, two people and craft brought in
Nov 11	Missing persons, landed a body
Dec 20	Powered boat *Sax Angler*, one person and craft brought in
2008 Jan 8	Person on Orwell Bridge, others coped
13	Man overboard from jet ski, resolved unaided
Mar 15	Human body, unsuccessful search
25	Missing person unsuccessful search
Apr 20	Yacht *Sargasso*, gave help - refloated casualty
27	Missing person, unsuccessful search
May 1	Tender to *Silver Queen*, two people and craft brought in
4	Person stranded on sandbank, false alarm
16	Yacht *Dingle*, gave help – refloated casualty
20	Yacht *Tromba*, gave help – refloated casualty
24	Injured man, landed 1
26	Yacht *Boru*, craft brought in
31	Yacht *Rodia*, gave help – freed propeller
June 2	Yacht *Chiron of Hoyle*, false alarm
7	Powered boat *Ondora*, others coped
11	Person on Orwell Bridge, others coped
29	Yacht *Lynx*, gave help
29	Inflatable dinghy, resolved unaided
July 6	Inflatable dinghy, others coped
17	Sailing dinghy, gave help
19	Yacht *Cyano*, two and craft brought in
22	Jet ski, one person and jet ski brought in
22	Yacht *Qudam*, two people & craft brought in
27	Yacht *Ardtalla*, two people & craft brought in
28	Yacht *Samingo II*, gave help – refloated
29	Yacht *Blue Streak*, gave help – refloated
Aug 2	Swimmer, resolved unaided
7	Missing person, unsuccessful search
8	Powered boat, four people & craft brought in
14	Yacht *Nimrod*, two people brought in
16	Yacht *Blue Sprit*, two people and craft brought in
16	Yacht *Andrea*, gave help – laid anchor
24	Tender to yacht, one person and craft brought in
30	Yacht, gave help
Sep 1	Sailing dinghy, resolved unaided
6	Yacht, craft brought in
12	Yacht *Misbehave*, two people and craft brought in
22	Injured man on Stoke Bridge, landed 1
26	Yacht *Genevive*, gave help – refloated
Oct 6	Person in river Deben, unsuccessful search
8	Person on Orwell Bridge, others coped
28	Yacht *The Pearl*, gave help - refloated
Nov 23	Tender, landed 2
28	Pilot launch *Prospect*, stood by
28	Catamaran, gave help
2009 Feb 27	Yacht *Annabel*, escorted craft
28	Powered boat, two person & craft brought in

Mar 3	Tender, two person and craft brought in

B-736 *Toshiba Wave Warrior*

Mar 22	Yacht *Pirouette*, stood by
Apr 11	Powered boat *Charlotte Michael*, gave help – laid anchor
11	Powered boat *Charlotte Michael*, landed 5 and craft brought in
12	Yacht *Nazca 2*, gave help – towed to deeper water
12	Yacht *Corina of Hamble*, gave help – laid anchor
18	Yacht *Swedish Lass*, two person and craft brought in
27	Kiteboard, resolved unaided

B-789 *Sure and Steadfast*

Apr 29	Dog, gave help – rescued dog
May 7	Yacht *Snowbird*, two person and craft brought in
16	Powered boat *Abanna*, others coped
17	Person at risk, false alarm
25	Yacht *Minx*, gave help - laid anchor
26	Yacht *Fulmar*, two and craft brought in
26	Inflatable toy, landed 3 children and inflatable toy brought in
28	Yacht Puffin, gave help – laid anchor
30	Man overboard from ro-ro cargo ship *Maersk Importer*, false alarm
31	Powered boat, five and craft brought in Powered boat *Baja 26*, four person and craft brought in
June 6	Yacht *Hope Floats*, two person and craft brought in
10	Person in river, recovered body
15	Yacht *Hobo*, one person and craft brought in
30	Commercial vessel *Triton*, two person and craft brought in
July 3	Missing person, false alarm
19	Sailboard, landed 1 and saved sailboard

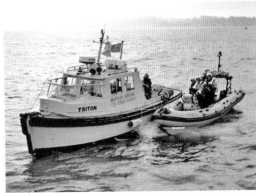

On 30 June 2009 B-789 Sure and Steadfast diverted from exercise to assist the workboat Triton, which was adrift at the Ganges Buoy with gearbox failure. Triton, with two persons on board, was towed to the pontoons at the lifeboat station. (By courtesy of Harwich RNLI)

	19	Yacht *Sundowner*, craft brought in
	19	Yacht *Jackie B*, others coped
	19	Powered boat *Tatum*, two person and craft brought in
	20	Person in the river, assisted to save 1
	25	Yacht *Dr No*, landed 1
	26	Tender, craft brought in
	28	Person fallen from pier, landed 1
Aug 2		Yacht *Bellanova*, saved 1
	3	Yacht *Kathleen Two*, gave help
	4	Dog in the sea, gave help
	9	Swimmer, resolved unaided
	10	Yacht *Xanthos*, gave help – towed to deeper water
	13	Yacht *Summer Wind*, landed 1 and craft brought in
	16	Powered boat, four and craft brought in
	17	Yacht *Jemini*, three and craft brought in
	18	Yacht *Samica*, three and craft brought in
	18	Yacht *Highland Dance*, gave help – refloated casualty
	19	Yacht *Zuzeppi*, gave help – laid anchor
	20	Inflatable toy dinghy, landed 2 and inflatable toy dinghy brought in
		Tender *Hope II*, craft brought in
	21	Yacht, two person and craft brought in
	22	Kiteboard, landed 1, kiteboard brought in
	22	Person in the river, resolved unaided
	24	Kiteboard, landed 1, kiteboard brought in
	25	Yacht *Fiddler*, escorted craft
	27	Yacht *Saorsa Mhairi*, gave help – attached tow to ALB
	30	Yacht *Myth*, escorted craft
Sep 1		Yacht *Amazon Countess*, stood by
	18	Powered boat, one person & craft brought in
	28	Powered boat *Dee S*, false alarm
Oct 3		Yacht *Ceilidh*, gave help – recovered anchor
	6	Canoes, escorted craft
	10	Yacht *Muskoka Mons*, landed 4, craft saved
	11	Tender to yacht *Dorkas*, gave help
	28	Person on Orwell Bridge, others coped
Nov 15		Powered boat, resolved unaided
		Kiteboard, assisted to save 1
	24	Fishing vessel *Sunrise*, gave help – pumped out craft
Dec 12		Yacht *Solo*, one person & craft brought in
	12	Ferry *Stena Britannica*, landed 1
	13	Yacht *Solo*, one person & craft brought in
2010	Feb 8	Human body, landed a body
	20	Yacht *Serin*, gave help – refloated craft
Mar 21		Ferry *Dana Sirena*, landed 1
Apr 2		Yacht *Renegade Runner*, two people and craft brought in
	6	Powered boat *Kingfisher*, one person and craft brought in

B-736 *Toshiba Wave Warrior*

May 3		People overboard from tender, gave help
	22	Powered boat *Melvin 3*, five people and craft brought in
		Yacht *Little Rascal*, three people and craft brought in
	24	Yacht *Tinkertess*, gave help – refloated casualty
June 9		Tender, landed 4 and craft brought in
	17	Yacht, gave help – assisted to craft

B-789 *Sure and Steadfast*

June 26		Powered boat, four and craft brought in
July 4		Human body, landed a body
	5	Tender, craft brought in
	9	Powered boat, craft brought in
	10	Powered boat *Enterprise*, gave help – pumped out casualty
		Yacht *Estrella*, gave help – pumped out
		Yacht *Erica*, two people and craft brought in
	11	Jet ski, one person and jet ski brought in
		Yacht *One Bamboo*, gave help – pumped out craft
		Yacht *Thomas*, landed 1 and craft brought in
	19	Canoes, landed 1, craft brought in, saved 1
	24	Powered boat, two people & craft brought in
	30	People cut off by tide, landed 2
	30	Kiteboard, one person and board brought in
Aug 8		Yacht, gave help – refloated casualty
	11	Powered boat *Lady Lane*, one three people and craft brought in
	15	Yacht *Karabela of Wight*, four people and craft brought in
	20	Person in the sea, landed 1
	24	Powered boat, six people brought in and dog rescued
	28	Sailing dinghy, gave help – righted craft
	30	Yacht *Hannah*, four and craft brought in
Sep 1		Aircraft, gave help
	4	Yacht *Powder Monkey*, two people and craft brought in
	6	Yacht *Slipper*, gave help – laid anchor
	7	Swimmer, stood by
	12	Person on Orwell Bridge, stood by
	22	Yacht *Sunshine*, gave help – laid anchor
	28	Missing person, gave help – assisted to ambulance
Oct 9		Yacht *Sirus of Avon*, gave help – laid anchor
	26	Yacht *Rustler*, escorted craft
Nov 2		Yacht *Passo Da Onca*, gave help
	21	Powered boat *Alf*, two people and craft brought in
	28	Men overboard from ferry *Stena Britannica*, gave help – transferred casualty to ALB
2011	Feb 22	Person on Orwell Bridge, landed 1
	Apr 11	Yacht *Hallelujah*, three persons and craft brought in
	17	inflatable dinghy, landed 2
		Yacht *Rival of Shalee*, gave help
	25	Fishing vessel *Mermaid*, three persons and craft brought in
	May 10	Capsized dinghy, assisted to land 2
	14	Yacht *Indabia*, gave help
		Yacht *Parana*, gave help
	21	Yacht *Halcyon*, gave help
	22	Tender to yacht, landed 1
	30	Yacht *Wyvern*, two persons and craft brought in
	June 2	Four persons cut off by tide, gave help
	5	Yacht, gave help and landed 1
	July 7	Yacht, landed 2
	10	Injured man on board yacht *Pickle*, landed 1
		Yacht *Bliss*, one person and craft brought in
	17	Sailing dinghy, gave help
	25	Dinghy, two persons and craft brought in
	30	Yacht *Three Fortunes*, gave help
	31	Yacht *Dusk*, craft brought in

G • THE LIFEBOAT MUSEUM

The Harwich lifeboat museum operates out of the old lifeboat house with the former Clacton-on-Sea offshore lifeboat *Valentine Wyndham-Quin* as the centrepiece. This 37ft Oakley class lifeboat was stationed at Clacton between 1968 and 1984, launching 179 times and saving 61 lives, before going to Clogher Head in Ireland for a further four years. When she finished as an operational lifeboat in 1989 she was moved to Cromer where she was placed on display on the seafront, close to the Henry Blogg Museum. She was moved from Cromer to Harwich in 1993 at which point the old lifeboat house was reopened and refurnished to accommodate her. The lifeboat museum now contains a large collection of general and local lifeboat artefacts. The museum is run by the Harwich Society and is open to the public during the summer period. For more information see the Society's website at www.harwich-society.co.uk.

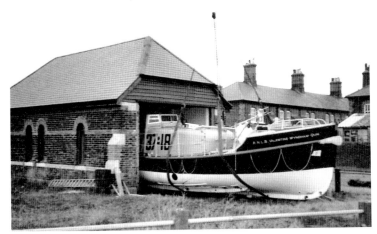

The old lifeboat house has been refurbished and fitted out as a Lifeboat Museum housing Valentine Wyndham-Quin. The former Clacton 37ft Oakley was brought to Harwich (left) in 1993 and craned into the boathouse to become the museum's centrepiece. (Left: Harwich RNLI; below left: Nicholas Leach; below: Graeme Ewens)

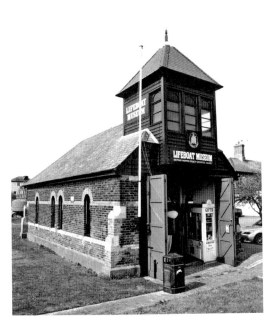

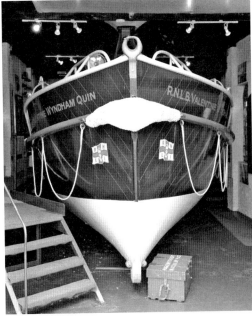

Honorary Secretaries

William S. Richmond	1876 – 5.1879
Arthur P. Bray	5.1879 – 5.1881
Lucas T. Cobbold	5.1881 – 2.1882
Dr Samuel Evans	2.1882 – 4.1889
William Mullinson	4.1889 – 8.1889
James N. Justice	11.1889 – 2.1896
John Paterson	2.1896 – 7.1920
Capt Derek Gibson	1965 – 6.1973
Capt Richard Coolen	29.6.1973 – 5.1985
Capt Rod Willis Shaw	1.6.1985 –

Coxswains

Pulling Lifeboat

John Tye	1876 – 1880
William Britton	1880 – 8.1883
William Tyrrel	1883 – 1890
Ben Dale	1890 – 12.1904
Benjamin Dale	1.1905 – 17.8.1912

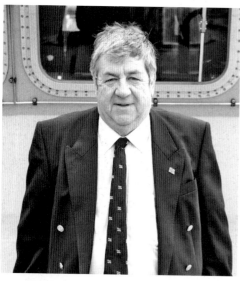

Rod Shaw

Captain Rod Shaw, then assistant harbour master (operations), was appointed as Honorary Secretary in June 1985, having been involved with the station in some capacity since 1975. The title of the post subsequently changed to Lifeboat Operations Manager.

Steam Lifeboat

William Tyrrel	1890 – 4.1904
Matthew Scarlett	4.1904 – 12.4.1916
Adam Garnett	7.1916 – 1.1917

Motor Lifeboat

Peter Burwood*	1967 – 1991
David Gilders	1991 – 9.1992
Peter Ronald Dawson	1.9.1992 – 1.2003
Paul Smith	6.2.2003 –

Chief Engineers (steam lifeboats)

Arthur Simmons	1890 – 1892
George Armstrong	1894 – 1917

Mechanics (motor lifeboats)

Peter Burwood*	1967 – 1991
Brian Jon Rudd	8.4.1991 – 2002
Brian Hill	6.2002 – 10.2008
David Thompson	12.2008 –

*Coxswain Mechanic joint position

Assistant Mechanics

Doug Jennings	1967 – 1970
Jeff Sallows	1970 – 1977
Charlies Moll	1977 – 1986
Robert Ramplin	1986 – 1991
Ken Brand	1991 – 2001
Andrew Moors	2001 –

Second Coxswains

Pulling Lifeboat

Ben Dale	1881 – 1890
James Dale	1890 – 17.8.1912

Steam Lifeboat

John Lambeth	1889 – 3.1898
Matthew Scarlett	3.1898 – 1904
Adam Garnett	7.1904 – 1916
Benjamin Dale	7.1916 – 1917

Motor Lifeboat

Les Smith	1967 – 1989
David Gilders	1989 – 1991
Paul Smith	1991 – 2.2003
John Teatheredge	2.2003 –

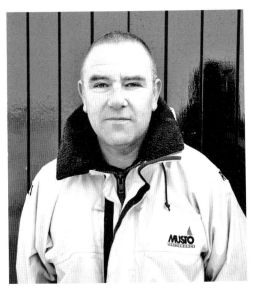

Paul Smith

Paul Smith joined the crew in November 1982 and was Second Coxswain for twelve years before becoming full-time Coxswain. He was stand-in Coxswain for three months after David Gilders retired and before Peter Dawson took over. (Harwich RNLI)

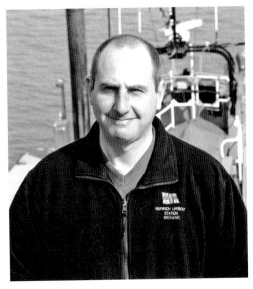

David Thompson

David Thompson was appointed full-time mechanic on 1 December 2008 having served as relief mechanic at the station previously. Originally from Newcastle, he was a volunteer crewmen at Tynemouth station for ten years. (Nicholas Leach)

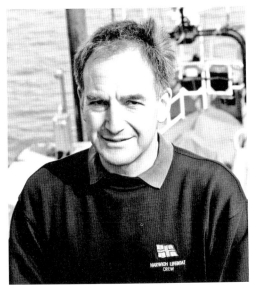

John Teatheredge

John Teatheredge has been on the crew since 1977 and became third coxswain before becoming second coxswain on 9 March 2003. He works as a pilot launch coxswain for Harwich Haven Authority. (Nicholas Leach)

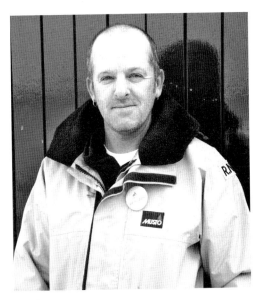

Andrew Moors

Andrew Moors is the second mechanic and works as a coxswain for Harwich Haven Authority. He has been on the crew since January 1991, and has been second mechanic since January 2002. (Harwich RNLI)

1 • LIFEBOATS ON PASSAGE

Harwich is regularly visited by lifeboats on passage, whether they are on trials out of the local boatyard at Levington or travelling between another yard and their own station. Harwich, with its good facilities and sheltered berth, is a natural stop-off point for lifeboats being moved along the east coast heading to or coming from the RNLI's Depot at Poole in Dorset, and numerous lifeboats have called at the port. New lifeboats, especially those destined for east coast stations and Scotland, visit during crew training passages, while many of the former Arun lifeboats destined for China came to Harwich prior to being loaded onto container ships to be taken to their new homes.

Merchant Navy
The 33ft Brede Merchant Navy served in the Relief Fleet from 1983 to 1987 and called at Harwich on 25 June 1983 on passage to Gothenburg for the International Lifeboat Conference. (Ken Brand)

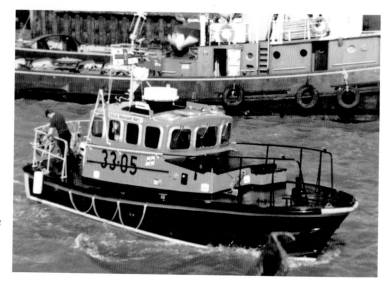

Sam and Joan Woods
The relief 47ft Tyne Sam and Joan Woods, built in 1982, called at Harwich on 16 September 1985 while on passage from Poole to Fraserburgh. (Ken Brand)

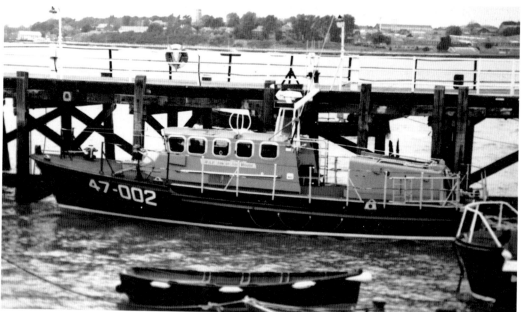

Margaret Frances Love

The 52ft Arun Margaret Frances Love being lifted aboard a container ship at Felixstowe for transportation to China. A number of old Aruns sold by the RNLI came to Harwich prior to being taken across the harbour to Felixstowe to be loaded onto container ships. (Andrew Moors)

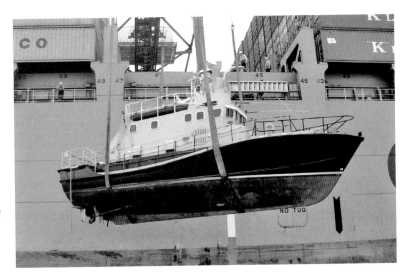

Dora Foster McDougall

The relief 14m Trent Dora Foster McDougall at Harwich in 2006 while on passage. Built in 1997, she has served in the Relief Fleet. (Andrew Moors)

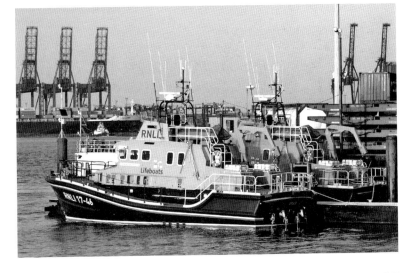

Margaret Joan and Fred Nye

The 17m Severn Margaret Joan and Fred Nye alongside the lifeboat pontoon on 5 April 2009. The lifeboat, built in 2004 for service in the Relief Fleet, had been re-engined with MTU marine diesels and was visiting stations so the crews could assess the boat with the new powerplants. (Graeme Ewens)

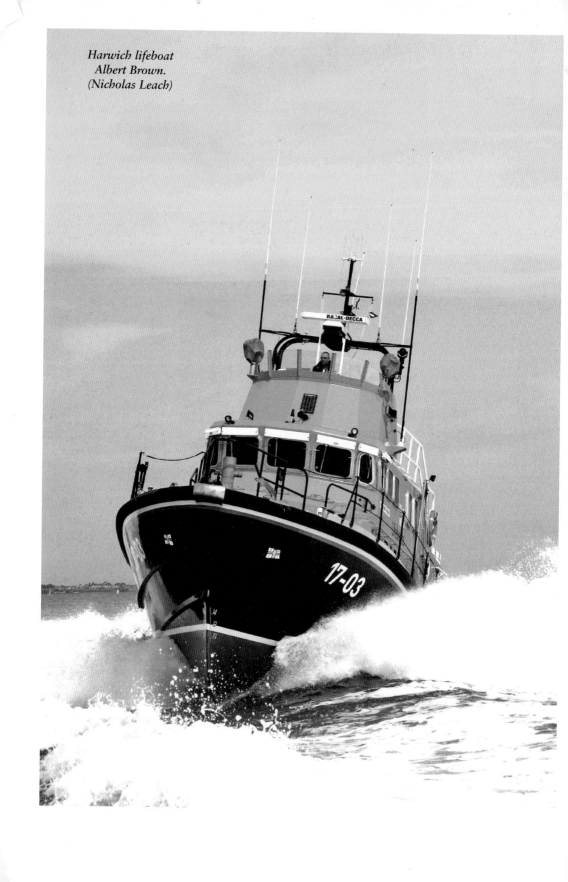

*Harwich lifeboat
Albert Brown.
(Nicholas Leach)*